Traumatic Brain Injury

Second Edition

Traumatic Brain Injury

A Multidisciplinary Approach

Second Edition

Edited by

Peter C. Whitfield
University Hospitals Plymouth NHS Trust and Peninsula Medical School, Plymouth, UK

Jessie Welbourne
University Hospitals Plymouth NHS Trust, Plymouth, UK

Elfyn Thomas
University Hospitals Plymouth NHS Trust, Plymouth, UK

Fiona Summers
NHS Grampian and Honorary Lecturer, University of Aberdeen, UK

Maggie Whyte
NHS Grampian and Honorary Lecturer, University of Aberdeen, UK

Peter J. Hutchinson
Addenbrooke's Hospital, University of Cambridge, UK

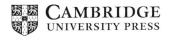

CAMBRIDGE
UNIVERSITY PRESS

CAMBRIDGE
UNIVERSITY PRESS

University Printing House, Cambridge CB2 8BS, United Kingdom

One Liberty Plaza, 20th Floor, New York, NY 10006, USA

477 Williamstown Road, Port Melbourne, VIC 3207, Australia

314–321, 3rd Floor, Plot 3, Splendor Forum, Jasola District Centre,
New Delhi – 110025, India

79 Anson Road, #06–04/06, Singapore 079906

Cambridge University Press is part of the University of Cambridge.

It furthers the University's mission by disseminating knowledge in the pursuit of
education, learning, and research at the highest international levels of excellence.

www.cambridge.org
Information on this title: www.cambridge.org/9781108430869
DOI: 10.1017/9781108355247

© Cambridge University Press 2009, 2020

First published 2009
Second edition 2020

Printed in the United Kingdom by TJ International Ltd, Padstow Cornwall

A catalogue record for this publication is available from the British Library.

ISBN 978-1-108-43086-9 Paperback

Contents

Contributors

Gareth Allen, MBBCh, BaO, FFARCSI, DIBICM
Consultant in Anaesthesia and Critical Care Medicine, Belfast City Hospital, Belfast, UK

Lindsey Beedie, MA, DClinPsychol
Clinical Psychologist, Beedie Psychology Services, Aberdeen, UK

Catherine Best, BSc, PhD
Faculty of Health Sciences and Sport, University of Stirling, Stirling, UK

Rowan Burnstein, MBBS, FRCA, PhD, FFICM
Consultant in Anaesthesia and Intensive Care, Addenbrooke's Hospital, Cambridge University NHS Trust, Cambridge, UK

Jonathan Coles, MB, ChB, DA, FRCA, PhD
Honorary Consultant and Academy of Medical Sciences/Health Foundation Clinician Scientist, Cambridge University Department of Anaesthesia, Cambridge University Hospitals NHS Foundation Trust, Cambridge, UK

Giles Critchley, MA, MD, FRCS (SN)
Consultant Neurosurgeon, South East Neurosurgery, Brighton and Sussex University Hospitals NHS Trust, Haywards Heath, West Sussex, UK

Bruce Downey, MA (Hons), DClinPsychol
Consultant Paediatric Neuropsychologist, NHS Grampian, Aberdeen, UK

Ellie Edlmann, BMBS, MRCS, PhD
Speciality Registrar and Clinical Lecturer in Neurosurgery, Plymouth University Peninsula School of Medicine, University Hospitals Plymouth NHS Trust, Plymouth, UK

Antoinette Edwards
Institute of Population Health, University of Manchester, Manchester, UK

Jonathan J. Evans, BSc (Hons), DClinPsychol, PhD, FBPsS
Institute of Health and Wellbeing, College of Medical, Veterinary and Life Sciences, University of Glasgow, UK

Judith Fewings, BSc (Physiotherapy), PG Cert Neurological Physiotherapy and Critical care
Consultant Therapist in Neurosurgery and Honorary University Fellow, South West Neurosurgery Centre, University Hospitals Plymouth NHS Trust, Plymouth, UK

Clare N. Gallagher, MD, PhD, FRCS (C)
Division of Neurosurgery, Department of Clinical Neurosciences, University of Calgary, Calgary, Alberta, Canada

Helen M. K. Gooday, MBChB, MRCPsych
Consultant in Rehabilitation Medicine, Department of Rehabilitation Medicine, NHS Grampian, Aberdeen, UK

Andrew Gvozdanovic, MBBS
Division of Neurosurgery, Department of Clinical Neurosciences, University of Cambridge, Cambridge, UK

Jane Halliday, FRCS (SN)
Neurosurgery Consultant, Oxford University Hospitals NHS Foundation Trust, Oxford, UK

Jackie Hamilton, MA (Hons), DClinPsychol, PGDip
Clinical Neuropsychologist, Department of Clinical Neuropsychology, NHS Grampian, Honorary Lecturer, University of Aberdeen, Aberdeen, UK

Emma Hepburn, MA (Hons), DClinPsychol, PGDip
Clinical Psychologist, Department of Clinical Neuropsychology, NHS Grampian, Honorary Lecturer, University of Aberdeen, Aberdeen, UK

Camilla Herbert, MA, MSc, DClinPsychol, FBPsS
Consultant Clinical Neuropsychologist, East Sussex UK

Ciaran S. Hill, MBBS, BSc (Hons), MSc, MCSP, MRCS, MRCP, DMCC, DOHNS, FHEA
Neurosurgery Registrar and Honorary Senior Lecturer, Cambridge University Hospitals NHS Trust, Cambridge, UK

David Hilton, MD, FRCPath
Consultant Neuropathologist and Honorary Reader, University Hospitals Plymouth NHS Trust, Plymouth, UK

Stephen Honeybul, FRACS, FRCS (SN)
State-wide Director of Neurosurgery, Department of Neurosurgery, Sir Charles Gairdner Hospital, Royal Perth Hospital and Fiona Stanley Hospital, Perth, Western Australia, Australia

Peter J. Hutchinson, PhD, FRCS (SN)
Professor of Neurosurgery, Division of Neurosurgery, Department of Clinical Neurosciences, Addenbrooke's Hospital, University of Cambridge, Cambridge, UK

Greg James, PhD, FRCS
Consultant, Department of Neurosurgery, Great Ormond Street Hospital for Children and

Senior Lecturer, Great Ormond Street Institute of Child Health, University College London, London, UK

Matt Jamieson, MA, MSc, PhD
Research Associate, University of Glasgow, Glasgow, UK

Deva S. Jeyaretna, MD, FRCS (SN)
Consultant Neurosurgeon, Oxford University Hospitals NHS Foundation Trust and Nuffield Department of Clinical Neurosciences, University of Oxford, Oxford, UK

Anthony Kehoe, MB ChB, MSc, MRCSEd, FRCEM
Consultant in Emergency Medicine, University Hospitals Plymouth NHS Trust, Plymouth, UK

W. Hiu Lam, BMedSci (Hons), BM BS, FRCA, FRCP, MSc (ML)
Consultant in Neuroanaesthesia, University Hospitals Plymouth NHS Trust, Plymouth, UK

Thérèse Lebedis
Consultant Occupational Therapist in Stroke, NHS Grampian, Aberdeen, UK

Fiona Lecky, MB, ChB, FRCS, DA, MSc, PhD, FCEM
Clinical Professor of Emergency Medicine, University of Sheffield, School of Health and Related Research, Sheffield, UK

Paul McArdle, BDS, FDSRCS, MBChB, FRCS, FRCS (OMFS), MSc
Consultant Oral and Maxillofacial Surgeon, Department of Oral and Maxillofacial Surgery, Derriford Hospital, Plymouth, UK

Anjum Memon, MBBS, DPhil (Oxon), FFPH
Professor of Epidemiology and Public Health Medicine, Brighton and Sussex Medical School, Falmer, Brighton, UK

Amr H. Mohamed, FRCS (SN)
Locum Consultant Neurosurgeon,
Neurosurgery Department, Cardiff and
Vale University Hospital Trust, Heath Park
Way, Cardiff

Brian O'Neill, BA, MSc, DClinPsychol, MBPS
Consultant in Neuropsychology and
Rehabilitation, Brain Injury Rehabilitation
Trust and University of Glasgow,
Glasgow, UK

Hiren C. Patel, PhD, FRCS (Neurosurgery)
Consultant Neurosurgeon, Salford Royal
NHS Trust, Salford, UK

Nicola Pilkington, BMBS, FRCA, PGCE, FHEA
Consultant in Paediatric Anaesthesia,
Royal Manchester Children's Hospital,
Manchester, UK

Puneet Plaha, MBBS, MS, MD, FRCS (SN)
Consultant Neurosurgeon, Oxford
University Hospitals NHS Foundation
Trust, Oxford, UK

Thomas M Price, BMBS, BMedSci, FRCA, FFICM
Specialist Registrar in Anaesthesia and
Intensive Care, Royal Victoria
Hospital, UK

Ann-Marie Pringle, MA (Hons), Dip, PhD
Consultant Speech and Language
Therapist, Astley Ainslie Hospital,
Edinburgh, UK

Richard Protheroe, MBBS, MRCS, FRCP, FRCA, FFICM
Consultant Neuroanaesthesia and Critical
Care, Salford Royal NHS Foundation Trust,
Salford, UK

Chiara Robba, MD
Department of Clinical Neurosciences,
Addenbrooke's Hospital, University of
Cambridge, Cambridge, UK

Imogen Rogers, PhD
Research Fellow in Epidemiology, Brighton
and Sussex Medical School, Falmer,
Brighton, UK

Won Hyung A. Ryu, MSc, MTM, MD
Department of Clinical Neurosciences,
University of Calgary, Calgary, Alberta,
Canada, UK

Mark Sair, PhD, FRCP, FFICM
Consultant in Intensive Care and
Anaesthetics, Intensive Care Unit,
Derriford Hospital, Plymouth, UK

Aggie Skorko, MBBS, BSc, MRCP, FFICM
ST6 Intensive Care Medicine
Bristol Royal Infirmary, Bristol, UK

Peter Smielewski, PhD
Brain Physics Group, Department of
Clinical Neurosciences, Addenbrooke's
Hospital, University of Cambridge,
Cambridge, UK

Martin Smith, MBBS, FRCA, FFICM
Department of Neuroanaesthesia and
Neurocritical Care, The National Hospital
for Neurology and Neurosurgery,
University College London Hospitals NHS
Foundation Trust, London, UK

Fiona Summers, BSc, MA (Hons), DClinPsychol
Consultant Clinical Neuropsychologist,
Department of Clinical Neuropsychology,
NHS Grampian and Honorary Lecturer,
University of Aberdeen, Aberdeen, UK

Tamara Tajsic, PhD, MRCS
Division of Neurosurgery, Department of
Clinical Neurosciences, University of
Cambridge, Cambridge, UK

Elfyn Thomas, BSc MBBS, FRCA, FFICM
Consultant in Intensive Care Medicine and
Anaesthesia, University Hospitals,
Plymouth NHS Trust, Plymouth, UK

Matthew J. C. Thomas, FRCA, MRCP
Consultant in Anaesthesia and Intensive Care Medicine, Bristol Royal Infirmary, Bristol, UK

Robbie Thorpe, FRCA, FFSEM (RCSI), PGCMEAnaes (Dund)
Consultant Anaesthetist, Consultant NI Helicopter Emergency Services, Royal Victoria Hospital, Belfast, Northern Ireland

Ivan Timofeev, PhD, FRCS
Division of Neurosurgery, Department of Clinical Neurosciences, University of Cambridge, Cambridge, UK

Ceri Trevethan, PhD, DClinPsychol, PGDip CPsychol
Lecturer and Honorary Principal Clinical Psychologist, University of Aberdeen, NHS Grampian, Aberdeen, UK

Rikin A. Trivedi, MRCP(UK), MRCS, PhD
Division of Neurosurgery, Department of Clinical Neurosciences, Addenbrooke's Hospital, University of Cambridge, Cambridge, UK

Martin B. Walker, MB, BS, FRCA
Consultant in Intensive Care Medicine and Anaesthesia (Retired), Derriford Hospital, Plymouth Hospitals NHS Trust, Plymouth, UK

Adam J. Wells, MBBS, BMedSc, PhD, FRACS (Neurosurgery)
Division of Neurosurgery, Department of Clinical Neurosciences, Addenbrooke's

Hospital, University of Cambridge, Cambridge, UK and

Clinical Academic Consultant Neurosurgeon, The Royal Adelaide Hospital and Senior Clinical Lecturer, The University of Adelaide, Adelaide, South Australia

Laura White
National Training and Support Officer, The Trauma Audit and Research Network, Salford Royal NHS Foundation Trust, Salford, UK

Kathrin J. Whitehouse, BSc, MBBCh, MClinEd, FRCS (SN), FHEA
Locum Consultant Neurosurgeon, Caridd and Vale University Health Board, Cardiff, UK

Peter C. Whitfield, BM (Distinction), PhD, FRCS England, FRCS (SN), FHEA, FAcadMEd
University Hospitals Plymouth NHS Trust and Peninsula Medical School, Plymouth, UK

Maggie Whyte, BSc (Hons), DClinPsychol
Consultant Clinical Neuropsychologist, Department of Clinical Neuropsychology, NHS Grampian and Honorary Lecturer, University of Aberdeen, Aberdeen, UK

Mark Wilson, BSc, MBBChir, PhD, FRCS (SN), MRCS, FIMC, FRGS
Professor of Neurosurgery and Prehospital Care, Imperial College NHS Trust, London, UK

Foreword to First Edition

There are many types of head injury, they affect many people and their care demands input from many disciplines. No one person can know everything needed to provide effective comprehensive management, yet this is the key to improving outcome – in acute and late phases. This book provides a much-needed, coherent but concise account that sets out the principles and practice of management within a discipline and also what each discipline needs to know about each other. This reflects the wide spread of expertise in its multi disciplinary authorship – encompassing pathology, neurosurgery, maxillofacial surgery, anaesthesia, intensive care, emergency medicine, neuropsychology, neurology, rehabilitation specialists, public health physicians and basic science. Most come from the UK, in particular from the Cambridge 'school', but the perspective is international and integrated. It will benefit all kinds of personnel involved in caring for head-injured people -from the site of the injury, through acute assessment, investigation and intervention to recovery, rehabilitation and dealing with long-lasting sequelae. These are disturbingly frequent after either an apparently mild or a severe initial injury, so the expectation that their impact will be reduced through the clinical application of the knowledge and wisdom set out here is greatly valued.

Sir Graham M Teasdale

Emeritus Professor of Neurosurgery, University of Glasgow,
Chairman NHS Quality Improvement Scotland
Editor in Chief of *Acta Neurochirurgica,* the European Journal of Neurosurgery

Past President of the Royal College of Physicians and Surgeons of Glasgow,
Chairman of the European Brain Injury Consortium and of the
International Neurotrawna Sodety
MB, BS Dunelm, FRCS Edinburgh,
FRCPS Glasgow, FRCP London, FRCP Edinburgh

Honorary FRCS England, Ireland
MD Hon Causae, Athens,
Honorary International Fellow, American College of Surgeons
Fellow of the Academy of Medical Sciences
Fellow of the Royal Society of Edinburgh

Foreword to Second Edition

At long last, the global healthcare burden created by traumatic brain injury (TBI) is becoming recognised by governmental policy makers worldwide. TBI is the leading cause of mortality and disability in young people in high-income countries. There are over one million attendances per annum at Emergency Departments in the UK for head injury. The majority of these are minor, as defined by the degree of loss of consciousness, but even many of these may have long-term cognitive consequences with stress on family relationships, employability and mental health. Head injuries in young people may lead to subsequent criminality. Sport-induced concussion and blast injuries may predispose to subsequent dementia.

There have been remarkable advances in prevention, early detection of avoidable secondary insults, and intensive care of patients after TBI that have resulted in improved outcomes. Neurorehabilitation is advancing. TBI has attracted high quality randomised controlled trials. Recently, Class 1 evidence has been secured for the value of decompressive craniectomy and ultra-early use of tranexamic acid. In contrast, RCTs for novel neuroprotective agents have been negative. In part, this stems from failure to take adequate account of the truism that no two human head injuries are the same. Heterogeneity has been the bane of TBI research. We are only now developing the tools to define the various pathophysiological processes and their interactions that may contribute to an individual patient's outcome after TBI in order to personalise and advance their care using the approaches of the new neurobiology such as genetics, neuroplasticity, stem cells and implant devices.

Crucially, all stages of the care pathway for TBI patients from initial ictus through to reintegration into the community require a multidisciplinary approach. All players in this pathway must understand each other's roles and the realistic goals of management. Newcomers to the world of TBI from all the neuroscience disciplines need an authoritative, concise and lucid account that sets out the principles and practice of head injury management. The second edition of this book, first published in 2009, provides just such an internationally relevant and up to date account. It is a fitting successor to such classics as John Potter's *Practical Management of Head Injuries* from the pre-CT era.

Professor John Pickard CBE, FMedSci, MChir, FRCS, FRCSEd,
Docteur Honoris Causa (Liege, Belgium).

Emeritus Professor of Neurosurgery, University of Cambridge
Emeritus Professorial Fellow, St Catharine's College, Cambridge
Honorary Director, National Institute for Health Research
Brain Injury MedTech Cooperative
Honorary Civilian Consultant in Neurosurgery to the Army.

Chapter 1

Epidemiology of Head Injury

Giles Critchley, Imogen Rogers and Anjum Memon

Introduction

Head injury is a major cause of morbidity and mortality in all age groups. Injury to the head can result in traumatic brain injury (TBI) of varying severity. TBI is common, with a self-reported lifetime prevalence of up to 40% in adults.[1] Currently, there is no effective treatment to reverse the effects of the primary brain injury sustained, and treatment is aimed at minimising the secondary brain injury that can occur due to the effects of ischaemia, hypoxia and raised intracranial pressure. This can occur immediately, within the following hours or days, or after a further head injury. An understanding of the epidemiology of head injury is essential for devising preventive measures, to plan population-based primary prevention strategies and to provide effective and timely treatment, including provision of rehabilitation facilities to those who have suffered a head injury. This information can then be used to improve TBI outcomes.

Definition and Classification of Traumatic Brain Injury

Whilst studying the epidemiology of TBI, it is important to realise that definitions, coding practices, inclusion criteria for patients and items of data collected have varied between studies. This has made it difficult to draw meaningful comparisons of incidence rates and risk factors between populations. TBI is usually considered an insult or trauma to the brain from an external mechanical force, leading to temporary or permanent impairments of physical, cognitive and psychosocial functions with an associated diminished or altered state of consciousness. The severity of TBI is usually classified according to the Glasgow Coma Scale (GCS) scores as mild (13–15), moderate (9–12) and severe (3–8). This classification may also be refined with data about pupillary response, age and CT findings, which further improves the prognostic and predictive value.[2,3] The International Classification of Diseases (ICD-10) codes for TBI are given in Table 1.1.

One of the problems of head injury research is case ascertainment. The majority of data collected will be from those who have presented to an accident and emergency (A & E) department, with subsequent admission to an observation or neurosurgical ward or a neurosurgical intensive care unit (Table 1.2). Following admission, they may not survive the injury or may be discharged home or to a rehabilitation facility or to long-term institutional care.

Burden of Traumatic Brain Injury

TBI is an important global public health problem. It is a major cause of disability. Survivors often suffer cognitive, mood and behavioural disorders. The societal cost of the disability

Table 1.1 List of ICD-10 codes which refer to traumatic brain injury

ICD code	Category
S06	Intracranial injury
S06.0	Concussion
S06.1	Traumatic cerebral oedema
S06.2	Diffuse brain injury
S06.3	Focal brain injury
S06.4	Epidural haemorrhage
S06.5	Traumatic subdural haemorrhage
S06.6	Traumatic subarachnoid haemorrhage
S06.7	Intracranial injury with prolonged coma
S06.8	Other intracranial injuries
S06.9	Intracranial injury, unspecified
S07	Crushing injury of head

Source: International Statistical Classification of Diseases and Related Health Problems, 10th Revision. Version for 2016 published by the WHO http://apps.who.int /classifications/icd10/browse/2016/en

Table 1.2 Sources of data on accidents and injury in the UK and on TBI

- Hospital record/statistics (including A & E departments): presentation to health services is dependent on severity of head injury and proximity/access to services.
- Mortality data: the most reliable and complete source of information on deaths due to external causes (www.statistics.gov.uk).
- HASS and LASS (Home and Leisure Accident Surveillance System): a reliable source of information on home and leisure accidents, dependent on data from A & E departments (www.hassandlass.org.uk).
- Health and Safety Executive: collects data on serious employment-related injuries and accidents (www.hse.gov.uk).
- TARN: the Trauma Audit and Research Network (www.tarn.ac.uk).
- CENTER-TBI: Collaborative European NeuroTrauma Effectiveness Research in TBI (www.center-tbi.eu).
- TRACK-TBI: Transforming Research and Clinical Knowledge in Traumatic Brain Injury (https://tracktbi.ucsf.edu).
- TBI-Prognosis Study (www.tbi-prognosis.ca/).
- InTBIR: International Initiative for Traumatic Brain Injury Research (https://intbir.nih.gov/).

following TBI can be substantial due to loss of years of productive life and a need for long-term or lifelong services. In the USA in 2009, there were 3.5 million TBI diagnoses, including 2 million A & E department visits, 300 000 hospitalisations and 53 000 deaths.[4] It has been estimated that 5.3 million people have some TBI-related disability, impairment, complaint or handicap in the USA. Similarly, it has been estimated that 6.2 million people in the European

Union (EU) have some form of TBI-related disability. The unemployment rate following TBI requiring inpatient rehabilitation has been reported as 60.4% at 2 years post-injury.[5]

Incidence of TBI

Incidence is a count of *new cases* of TBI in the population during a specified time period. The *incidence rate* is the number of *new cases* of TBI in a defined population within a specified time period (usually a calendar year), divided by the total number of persons in that population (usually expressed as per 100 000 population). Like most conditions, the incidence of TBI varies according to age, gender and geographic location. Most of the published reports are from developed countries in Europe and North America, and there is little information on epidemiology of head injury from most developing countries. The annual incidence rates of reported TBI range from a low of 47 per 100 000 population in Spain to a high of 811 per 100 000 in New Zealand (Table 1.3). Most rates are in the range of 150–450 new cases per 100 000 per year. The variation observed could be partly explained by differences in criteria used to define TBI or

Table 1.3 Incidence of traumatic head injury in different populations (selected studies)

Population	Annual incidence per 100 000 population	Male:female ratio
Africa		
South Africa, Johannesburg (Nell & Brown, 1991)	316	4.8:1
Asia		
Iran (Rahimi-Movaghar & Saadat 2011)	56	4.3:1
India (Gururaj et al. 2004)	160	NR
Taiwan, Taipei City (Chiu et al. 2007)	218	1.9:1
Europe		
Spain (Perez et al. 2012)	47[b]	2.0:1
Norway, Oslo (Andelic et al. 2008)	83[b]	1.8:1
Spain, Cantabria (Vazquez-Barquero et al. 1992)	91	2.7:1
Finland (Alaranta et al. 2000)	95	1.5:1
Finland (Koskinen & Alaranta, 2008)	101	1.5:1
Portugal (Santos et al. 2003)	137	1.8:1
Denmark (Engberg & Teasdale, 2001)	157	2.2:1
Italy, Northeast (Baldo et al. 2003)	212	1.6:1
Finland, Southeast (Numminen et al. 2011)	221[c]	1.2:1
Norway, Tromso (Ingebrigtsen et al. 1998)	229	1.7:1
UK, England (Tennant, 2005)	229	NR

Table 1.3 (cont.)

Population	Annual incidence per 100 000 population	Male:female ratio
Netherlands (Scholten et al. 2014)	242 males	1.4:1
	175 females	
Sweden (Kleiven et al. 2003)	259	2.1:1
UK, Staffordshire (Hawley et al. 2003)	280^a	1.8:1
France, Aquitaine (Tiret et al. 1990)	282	2.1:1
Italy, Romagna (Servadei et al. 2002)	297	1.6:1
Austria (Mauritz et al. 2014)	303^d	1.4:1
Italy, Trentino (Servadei et al. 2002)	332	1.8:1
Germany (Rickels et al. 2010)	332	1.4:1
Germany (Steudel et al. 2005)	337	NR
Germany (Firsching & Woischneck, 2001)	350	NR
Sweden, Northern (Styrke et al. 2007)	354	1.2:1
UK, Scotland (Shivaji et al. 2014)	446^b males	2.3:1
	195^b females	
UK, Southwest England (Yates et al. 2006)	453	1.6:1
Sweden, Western (Andersson et al. 2003)	546	1.4:1
North America		
USA, Alaska (Sallee et al. 2000)	105	2.3:1
USA, Utah (Thurman et al. 1996)	109	2.2:1
Canada, Ontario (Colantonio et al. 2010)	190^e males	1.9:1
	100^e females	
USA (Guerrero et al. 2000)	392	1.6:1
USA (Jager et al. 2000)	444	1.7:1
Oceania		
Australia, NSW (Tate et al. 1998)	100	NR
Australia, South (Hillier et al. 1997)	322	2.3:1
New Zealand, Hamilton and Waikato District (Feigin et al. 2013)	811^d	1.8:1
USA (Taylor et al. 2017)	890^d (2013)	1.2:1 (2013)
	625^d (2007)	

Note. This table is adapted from data reviewed by Tagliaferri et al.[6] with permission. NR = not reported. ^{a}In children aged ≤15 years. ^{b}Figures for hospital admissions. ^{c}Figures for all cases with symptoms of brain injury after head trauma collected from health centres and hospitals; excluding mild cases of TBI reduced incidence to 137. ^{d}Figures for hospital discharges, outpatients and deaths in and out of hospital. ^{e}Figures for hospital admissions and emergency department visits.

identify patients. In a recent study from England, the incidence rates of head injury varied by a factor of 4.6 across different health authorities (range 91–419 per 100 000). Similarly, in the USA, incidence rates of TBI vary from a low of 101 per 100 000 in Colorado to a high of 367 per 100 000 in Chicago. In a review of TBI epidemiology in the EU in 2006, an overall average rate of 235 per 100 000 per year was obtained. A review of TBI in Europe in 2015 reported an incidence rate of 262 per 100 000 for admitted TBI patients.

Association of TBI with Other Structures

It is important to consider TBI in the context of the skull and other structures above the neck, as well as to identify those with 'isolated' head injuries and those with multisystem polytrauma, where other injuries may contribute to secondary brain injury. In patients with a severe brain injury (GCS 8 or less), there is a 5% incidence of associated cervical spine fractures. About 50%–60% of severe TBI patients may have one or more other organ system injuries which may contribute to secondary insult.

Variation by Age

The median age in studies of TBI ranges from 29 to 45 years worldwide. In most studies, three distinct peaks in the incidence of TBI are noted: in children, young adults and the elderly population. The highest incidence reported now is in the elderly population. It is unclear whether this is a real increase or an improvement in reporting and case ascertainment. In the USA in 2013, more than 1 in 50 adults aged 75 years or older experienced a TBI resulting in A & E attendance, admission or death. In 2013, adults aged 75 years or older accounted for 31.4% of TBI-related hospitalisations and 26.5% of all TBI-related deaths. The next highest incidence is in children aged 0–4 years with an incidence rate of 1591 per 100 000. In one UK trauma centre, 80% of elderly patients admitted had a moderate or severe TBI with 78% survival and 57% having a good outcome.[10] In young adults, road traffic accidents (RTAs) are the most frequent cause of TBI.

Variation by Gender

Almost all studies show a male preponderance. Overall, males are about twice as likely as females to experience a TBI. For studies from Europe and North America, the male:female ratio varies from 1.2:1 in Sweden to 2.7:1 in Spain. Males in developing countries apparently have a much higher risk of TBI compared with those in developed countries. In a study from South Africa, the male:female ratio was 4.8:1 (Table 1.3). In the EBIC study of severe head injuries, 74% of the patients were males.[11] In the Traumatic Coma Data Bank of patients with severe head injury, about 77% were males.[12] In the CRASH study of the effect of corticosteroids on death within 14 days, which included 10 008 patients with clinically significant head injury, 81% were males.[13] The male excess of TBI is attributed to greater exposure and more risk-taking behaviour. At younger ages the exposure of males to violence and RTAs leads to a male:female ratio of head injury incidence of about 4:1.

Severity of TBI

The reported severity of TBI depends on the population studied and case ascertainment. In a systematic review of TBI over the world in 2016, including 60 reports, the severity levels were mild (GCS 13–15; 55%), moderate (GCS 9–12; 27.7%) and severe (GCS 3–8; 17.3%).[7]

In the pooled data from the CRASH and IMPACT studies, the severity levels were mild (20.8%), moderate (22.2%) and severe (57%).[2,3] In a study of TBI in Europe in 2015, the proportion of mild TBIs varied between 71% and 97.5%.[9]

In a study from the UK, a rate of 40 per 100 000 was found for moderate to severe (10.9%) head injuries with a Glasgow Coma Scale of ≤12. A figure of 4000 patients a year requiring neurosurgery in the UK has been reported. In the paediatric population aged 0–14 years, an incidence rate of 5.6 per 100 000 per year has been reported for admission to intensive care following a head injury.[14]

Mortality from TBI

The *mortality rate* is the number of deaths from TBI in a defined population within a specified time period (usually a calendar year) divided by the total number of persons in that population (usually expressed as per 100 000 population). The mortality rate varies considerably in different countries. In the UK, the mortality rate from head injury is 6–10 per 100 000 population per year. For France, a mortality rate of about 22 per 100 000 has been reported. In the EU, the mortality from TBI varies from a low of 9.4 per 100 000 in Germany to a high of 24.4 per 100 000 in Ravenna, Italy, with an overall average rate of 15 deaths per 100 000 population per year in 2006. In 2013 the mortality from TBI in Europe was reported as 10.5 per 100 000. In the USA, the overall mortality rate is 20–30 per 100 000, with half of the patients dying out of hospital. Amongst adults in Johannesburg, South Africa, a much higher mortality rate of 138 per 100 000 for males and 24 per 100 000 for females has been reported, with 20% of TBIs resulting in death. In the pooled data of 15 900 patients from the CRASH database and IMPACT database, the mortality was 23.8%.

Causes of Head Injury

The most common causes of TBI are falls, RTAs, assault/violence, 'struck by' or 'struck against' events and sporting or recreation activities (Figures 1.1 and 1.2). The majority of reports now show falls as the leading cause of TBI in developed countries (34.4%), whilst RTAs are the main cause in developing countries (42.4%).[7] In a review of studies from the EU in 2006, 21%–60% of TBIs were caused by RTAs (from a low of 21% in Norway and the UK to a high of 60% in Sweden and Spain) and 15%–62% were caused by falls (15% in Italy, 62% in Norway).[9] In a review of TBI in Europe in 2015, falls were the most common mechanism of injury in 14 out of 25 studies included.[9] One study from Glasgow, Scotland, reported violence/assault (28%) as the second most common cause after falls (46%). Overall, it has been estimated that in Europe, 40% of TBIs are caused by RTAs, 37% are caused by falls, 7% are caused by violence/assault and 16% result from other causes.[6]

It may be realised that the cause–effect relationships between the mechanisms of injury and TBI are confounded by age, gender, car ownership, urban residence and socioeconomic factors. Elderly people who have a relatively high incidence of falls are more likely than other age groups to be pedestrian victims of RTAs. The contributing factors may include side effects of medication, poor vision/hearing, slow reaction time and impairment of balance and mobility. In a study of TBI in children, the most common cause of injury was accidents involving children as pedestrians (36%), followed by falls (24%), cycling accidents (10%), motor vehicle occupants (9%) and assault (6%).[19] In a UK study of minor head injury in adults, the common causes of injury were assault (30%–50%), RTAs (25%) and falls (22%–43%).[10] In the USA, gunshot wound to the head is now a more frequent cause of serious head injury than RTA, with a case

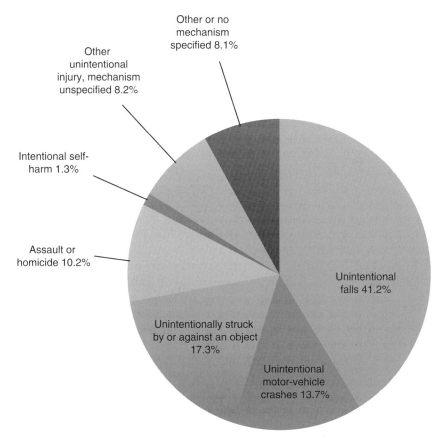

Figure 1.1 Percentage of TBI-related emergency department visits, hospitalisations and deaths by external cause in males in the USA, 2013. From Taylor et al.[8]

fatality of about 90%.[9] In a study from Canada, RTAs accounted for 43% and assault for 11% of head injuries. In the EBIC study of patients admitted to neurosurgical units (with GCS ≤ 12), 51% were involved in a RTA, 12% in a fall and 5% in an assault.[3] In the CRASH trial, RTAs accounted for 64% and falls for 13% of all head injuries.

Alcohol and TBI

It is reported that alcohol might be involved in 65% of adult head injuries. Alcohol intoxication was reported as being present in 32% of fatal motor vehicle accidents in the USA. In patients with TBI, 35%–81% are alcohol intoxicated and 42% of TBI patients were heavy drinkers before the injury. A history of alcohol abuse prior to TBI is also a strong predictor of heavy drinking after TBI.[15]

Sporting Head Injuries

The study of the epidemiology of TBI in sports is an area where significant advances in the prevention of head injuries by alteration of rules of participation and protective equipment

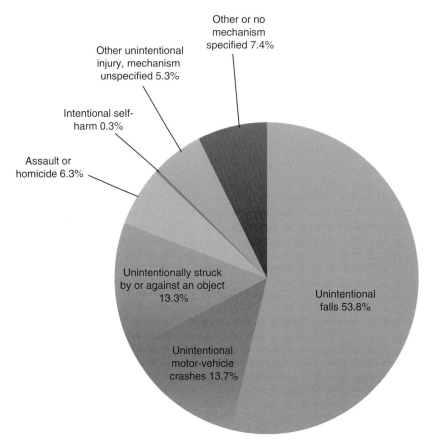

Figure 1.2 Percentage of TBI-related emergency department visits, hospitalisations and deaths by external cause in females in the USA, 2013. From Taylor et al.[8]

have been made. Media reporting of high-profile sports injuries may give the perception of a much higher incidence rate than actually occurs both within the sport and compared to other activities.

Overall, sports and recreation may account for up to 5%–10% of head injuries in studies of mechanism. Non-fatal TBIs from sports and recreational activities are reported for hospital emergency department presentations in the USA from 2001 to 2005 as part of the National Electronic Injury Surveillance System – All Injury Program. An estimated 207 830 patients with sports- and recreation-related TBIs accounted for 5.1% of sports-related emergency department visits. Approximately 10.3% of patients with sports-related TBIs required subsequent transfer to a specialist facility or hospitalisation. The most frequent causes of TBI were horse riding (11.7%), ice-skating (10.4%), riding all-terrain vehicles (8.4%), tobogganing/sledding (8.3%) and bicycling (7.7%). American football accounted for 5.7% and combative sports including boxing, wrestling, martial arts and fencing made up 4.8%.[16]

Much work has been done on the epidemiology of American football-related head injuries. The annual rate of non-fatal head-related catastrophic injuries in American football has averaged around 0.3 per 100 000 for high school and college participants. The rate of fatal injuries has stabilised at 0.32 per 100 000 per year.[17]

Prevention of Head Injury

Most TBI cases present with characteristic patterns of injury that are predictable and potentially preventable. Identification of risk factors is therefore a prerequisite for devising preventive measures and public health policy. Attempts at reducing trauma from all mechanisms will also have the effect of reducing TBI to varying degrees. The prevention programmes for TBI focus on RTA prevention, cessation of drinking and driving, minimising falls (particularly in the elderly), reducing sport injuries and decreasing violence and domestic abuse (particularly child abuse). Based on the standard principles of public health, William Haddon Jr, the first director of National Traffic Safety Bureau in the USA, proposed a conceptual model in the 1970s, the Haddon matrix, to address the problem of traffic safety.[18] The matrix illustrates the interaction of three factors – human, vehicle and environment – during three phases of an accident event – pre-accident, accident and post-accident. This concept can be successfully applied to the primary, secondary and tertiary prevention of RTAs and other types of accidents (Table 1.4). In the USA, the remarkable reduction in mortality attributed to RTAs has been hailed as one of the main public health achievements of the twentieth century.

Table 1.4 Haddon's matrix as applied to TBI in the elderly population

Phase	Factors		
	People	Cause	Environment
Pre-injury (accident prevention)	Co-morbidity Arrhythmia Dementia Balance Frailty Polypharmacy Visual impairment	Trip hazards Use of ladders Poor lighting	Awareness of risk of falls Handrails Non slip flooring Safe environment Footwear Balance aids
Injury (accident identification and limitation)	Associated reason for fall (e.g. MI, stroke) Anticoagulants	Lack of functional reserve Pre-injury conscious level may be impaired Injury severity may be greater in elderly	Hardness of floor Personal alarms Availability of emergency services
Post-injury (accident recovery)	Multidisciplinary care Balance classes/fall prevention Rehabilitation	Identification of causes of deterioration (e.g. haematoma expansion, chest infection, hyponatraemia, seizures)	Rehabilitation services Social support Occupational therapy Assessment of home environment before return

Legislative policy and enforcement to control motor vehicle accidents by making wearing of helmets compulsory for cyclists and motorcyclists and reducing legal permissible alcohol levels for driving have been shown to be associated with a reduction in RTA-associated head injuries.[19] Several studies have shown that the wearing of helmets by cyclists reduces the risk of head injury. In the Cochrane review of case-control studies, safety helmet use was associated with a 63%–88% reduction in the incidence of brain injury for all ages of cyclists. This protection was provided for crashes involving motor vehicles (69%) and all other causes (68%).[20] Evidence that wearing of helmets reduces injuries in skiers and snowboarders is also compelling.[21] Systematic reviews have shown that it is possible to reduce the incidence of falls by about 35% amongst older people.[22] Considering the wider determinants of public health, the role of health education and environmental engineering has been emphasised in the prevention of TBI.

References

1. Whiteneck GG, Cuthbert JP, Corrigan JD, Bogner JA. Prevalence of self-reported lifetime history of traumatic brain injury and associated disability: a statewide population-based survey. *J Head Trauma Rehabil* 2016;31:E55–E62.

2. Brennan PM, Murray GD, Teasdale GM. Simplifying the use of prognostic information in traumatic brain injury. Part 1: The GCS-Pupils score: an extended index of clinical severity. *J Neurosurg.* 2018;128:1612–620. DOI:10.3171/2017.12. JNS172780.

3. Murray GD, Brennan PM, Teasdale GM. Simplifying the use of prognostic information in traumatic brain injury. Part 2: Graphical presentation of probabilities. *J Neurosurg* 2018;128:1621–34. https://thejns.org/doi/abs/10.3171/2017.12.JNS172782

4. Coronado VG, McGuire LC, Sarmiento K, et al. Trends in traumatic brain injury in the US and the public health response: 1995–2009. *J Saf Res* 2012;43:299–307.

5. Cuthbert JP, Harrison-Felix C, Corrigan JD, Bell JM, Haarbauer-Krupa JK, Miller AC. Unemployment in the United States after traumatic brain injury for working-age individuals: prevalence and associated factors 2 years postinjury. *J Head Trauma Rehabil* 2015;30:160–74.

6. Tagliaferri F, Compagnone C, Korsic M, et al. A systematic review of brain injury epidemiology in Europe. *Acta Neurochir. (Wien)* 2006;148:255–68.

7. Li M, Zhao Z, Yu G, Zhang J. Epidemiology of traumatic brain injury over the world: a systematic review. *Austin Neurol. Neurosci.* 2016;1(2):id1007.

8. Taylor CA, Bell JM, Breiding MJ, Xu L. Traumatic brain injury-related emergency department visits, hospitalizations, and deaths – United States, 2007 and 2013. Morbidity and mortality weekly report. *MMWR Surveill. Summ.* 2017;66:1–16.

9. Peeters W, van den Brande R, Polinder S, Brazinova A, Steyerberg EW, Lingsma HF, Maas AIR. Epidemiology of traumatic brain injury in Europe. *Acta Neurochir.* 2015;157:1683–96.

10. Hawley C, Sakr M, Scapinello S, Alvo JS, Wrenn P. Traumatic brain injuries in older adults – 6 years of data for one UK trauma centre: retrospective analysis of prospectively collected data. *Emerg Med J* 2017;34:509–16.

11. Murray G, Teasdale G, Braakman R, Cohadon F, Dearden M, et al. The European Brain Injury Consortium survey of head injuries. *Acta Neurochir.* 1999;141:223–36.

12. Foulkes M, Eisenberg H, Jane J, Marmarou A, Marshall L, et al. The traumatic coma data bank: design, methods and baseline characteristics. *J Neurosurg* 1991;75:S8–14.

13. CRASH Trial Collaborators. Effect of intravenous corticosteroids on death within 14 days in 10 008 adults with clinically severe head injury (MRC CRASH Trial): randomised placebo controlled trial. *Lancet* 2004;364:1321–8.

14. Yates P, Williams W, Harris A, Round A, Jenkins R. An epidemiological study of head injuries in a UK population attending an emergency department. *J Neurol Neurosurg Psychiatry* 2006;77:699–701.

15. Opreanu RC, Kuhn D, Basson MD. The influence of alcohol on mortality in traumatic brain injury. *J Am Coll Surg.* 2010;210:997–1007.

16. Gilchrist J, Thomas K, Wald M, Langlois J. Nonfatal traumatic brain injuries from sports and recreation activities – United States 2001–2005. *Morbidity Mortality Weekly Rep* 2007;56:733–7.

17. Clarke K. The epidemiology of athletic head injuries. In: Cantu RC, ed. *Neurologic athletic head and spine injuries.* Philadelphia: WB Saunders; 2000.

18. Haddon W Jr. A logical framework for categorizing highway safety phenomena and activity. *J Trauma* 1972;12:193–207.

19. WHO. World report on road traffic injury prevention. WHO Report (Geneva) 2004.20.

20. Thompson DC, Rivara FP, Thompson R. Helmets for preventing head and facial injuries in bicyclists. *Cochrane Database of Systematic Reviews* 1999;4:Art. CD001855.

21. Hagel BE, Pless IB, Goulet C, Platt RW, Robitaille Y. Effectiveness of helmets in skiers and snowboarders: case-control and case crossover study. *Br Med J* 2005;330:281–3.

22. Gillespie L. Preventing falls in elderly people. *Br Med J* 2004;328:653–4.

The Neuropathology of Traumatic Brain Injury

David Hilton

Introduction

The neuropathological changes associated with head injuries are dependent on a number of factors, including both the type and severity of the injury, and the former can be divided into non-missile and missile types of injury. Non-missile injury (or blunt head injury) is usually due to rapid acceleration or deceleration of the head, with or without impact, or less commonly crushing of the head, and most often occur as the result of road traffic accidents or falls. Missile injuries are due to penetration of the skull by a rapidly moving external object, for example gunshot wounds, and result in a different pattern of brain injury. The neuropathology can be separated into focal (or localised) lesions such as contusions, haemorrhages, skull fractures, or diffuse changes such as diffuse axonal injury, diffuse vascular injury, brain swelling and ischaemia (see Table 2.1).

Although the lesions may develop at the time of the head injury (primary), many develop over a period of hours to days after the triggering event (secondary), and a significant minority of patients with severe head injury develop progressive neurological deterioration several years later. The pathological consequences of head injury are influenced by a number of factors including patient age, comorbidity such as alcohol,[1] other injuries (particularly if they result in ischaemia or hypoxia), sepsis and medical treatment. In addition there is now clear evidence that genetic polymorphisms for the apolipoprotein gene have a significant effect on both the pathological changes[2] and clinical outcomes from head injury.[3]

Table 2.1 Main types of injury following non-missile head injury

Focal	Diffuse
Scalp lacerations and contusions	Diffuse axonal injury
Skull fractures	Diffuse vascular injury
Haemorrhage (extradural, subdural, subarachnoid, parenchymal and intraventricular)	Brain swelling and ischaemic neuronal damage
Brain lacerations and contusions	
Brain stem and cranial nerve avulsion	
Arterial dissection	

Focal Injury

Scalp Injury

Focal injuries to the scalp such as abrasions and lacerations can be a useful indicator of the site of impact and may give some clues as to the type of object the brain came into contact with. Scalp lacerations may be an important route for infection and can result in excessive haemorrhage. Bruising may not always be a reliable indicator of impact location, for example periorbital bruising is often associated with fractures of the orbital roofs following a contracoup injury to the occiput, and mastoid bruising ('battle sign') can be caused by blood tracking from a fracture of the petrous temporal bone.

Skull Fractures

These are not always of clinical importance, although they do indicate that significant force was involved in the head injury, and are associated with intracranial injury such as haemorrhage.[4,5] Linear fractures are the most common type, and extend from the point of impact along lines of least resistance, although their direction is also dependant upon the anatomy of the skull. A significant force exerted over a larger area of the skull may result in a comminuted fracture with multiple fragments, whereas if the force is exerted over a relatively small area of skull a depressed fracture, with a fragment of skull being protruded inwards indenting the brain, results. Diastatic fractures, which follow suture lines, are more common in children. Compound fractures increase the likelihood of intracranial infection via the laceration to the overlying skin. Skull base fractures may result in CSF leakage and can extend into the air sinuses, causing aeroceles, and are also an important source of infection. Skull base fractures extending along both petrous ridges and through the pituitary fossa result in a 'hinge' fracture, which indicates severe side-to-side impact of the head, and are usually associated with fatal head injuries. A 'ring' fracture encircling the foramen magnum usually results from severe hyperextension of the neck, or falls from a height, where the individual landed on their feet. A common type of skull base fracture is that involving the orbital roofs due to contracoup injury when an individual falls backwards, hitting their occiput on a hard surface with the resulting shockwave passing through the skull and fracturing these relatively thin bones.

Brain Contusions and Lacerations

Tears to the pial membrane (lacerations) are often associated with underlying bruising (contusions). These may be of *coup* type, often associated with an overlying fracture (fracture contusion). More commonly contusions are due to *contracoup* injury and follow a stereotyped pattern occurring at the frontal poles, orbital surfaces of the frontal lobes, temporal poles and lateral surfaces of the temporal lobes. These *contracoup* contusions are due to continued movement of the brain within the cranial cavity, particularly following rapid deceleration such as when the moving head hits a solid surface, and occur at sites where the skull has an irregular internal surface. Contusions are relatively uncommon in young infants where the floor of the skull has a smoother contour. Contusions may also occur following herniation of brain, either internally where brain is compressed against a dural edge or externally via a craniectomy defect where brain is compressed against the skull edge. Contusions consist of areas of haemorrhage into brain parenchyma, often perpendicular to the cortical surface and on the crests of gyri, and may continue to bleed over a period of hours after the initial injury, making a significant contribution to raised intracranial pressure. Haemorrhage may extend to the subcortical white matter, or through the leptomeninges into the subdural space, resulting in a 'burst lobe', most often in the frontal and temporal poles. After a period of days to weeks the brain tissue will reabsorb resulting in a wedge-shaped area of cavitation at the crests of the gyri, which has an orange/brown colour due to the presence of blood breakdown products. Although contusions may be asymptomatic, they can be a cause of long-term epilepsy.

Intracranial Haemorrhage

Extradural Haemorrhage

Extradural haemorrhage results from direct impact and is uncommon at the extremes of age, but occurs in approximately 10% of severe head injury patients, most often in association with a fracture of the squamous temporal bone and tear in the underlying middle meningeal artery. However, particularly in children, where the bones are more flexible, a vascular tear may occur without a skull fracture. These are classically lens-shaped haematomas that accumulate over a period of hours as the dura is stripped from the skull, so that the patient may have an initial lucid interval. The volume of the haematoma is a predictor of outcome and most patients with more than 150 ml of blood have a poor prognosis.[6]

Subdural Haemorrhage

Subdural haemorrhage usually results from tearing of the bridging veins, particularly those adjacent to the superior sagittal sinus, in association with rapid acceleration or deceleration of the head, and does not require direct impact. It is more common in the elderly as brain atrophy results in an increased capacity for the brain to move within the cranial cavity. Rarely, subdural haemorrhage may be due to other causes such as arterial bleeding, including ruptured arteriovenous malformations and berry aneurysms.[7] Subdural haemorrhage may present shortly after the head injury (acute subdural haemorrhage), 1–2 weeks later (subacute subdural haemorrhage) or more than 2 weeks later (chronic subdural haemorrhage). Chronic subdural haematomas are particularly common in the elderly, alcoholics and patients with a low intracranial pressure, such as those shunted following hydrocephalus. In some of these patients (particularly the elderly) the head injury may be relatively trivial and not remembered by the patient. Clinical deterioration usually occurs if the volume of the haematoma exceeds around 40 ml, and death is common if there is more than 90 ml. Acute haematomas consist of soft clotted blood, often with a blackcurrant-jelly appearance. After several days this breaks down into serous fluid, and after a period of 1–2 weeks a membrane of granulation tissue with proliferating fibroblasts and capillaries develops, initially on the dural aspect of the haematoma, and later on the pial surface. Although the haematoma is usually eventually reabsorbed rebleeding is common, probably due to haemorrhage from the newly formed immature blood vessels[8] although a number of other factors including excessive fibrinolysis may be involved.[9]

Subarachnoid Haemorrhage

Small collections of subarachnoid blood are fairly common after head injury, particularly in association with contusions and lacerations. Subarachnoid haemorrhage may also complicate intraventricular haemorrhage due to a leakage of blood through the exit-foraminae of the fourth ventricle. Occasionally massive subarachnoid haemorrhage may occur around the ventral aspect of the brain stem due to laceration of a vertebral artery, basilar artery or one of the smaller arteries.[10,11] This type of haemorrhage often results from an impact to the head or neck in an assault, and causes immediate collapse, and is often fatal. Patients who survive significant subarachnoid haemorrhage may develop hydrocephalus as a chronic complication.

Intraventricular Haemorrhage

In the context of head injury, intraventricular haemorrhage is usually secondary to either deep haemorrhages in the region of the basal ganglia or contusions.[12]

Parenchymal Haemorrhage

Parenchymal haemorrhage may occur secondary to contusions or in association with diffuse axonal injury, when they are usually deep seated in the region of the basal ganglia, thalamus and parasagittal white matter.

Other Types of Focal Injury

Pituitary Infarction

This may result from traumatic transection of the pituitary stalk or severe elevation of intracranial pressure.

Brain Stem Avulsion

Severe hyperextension of the neck may result in brain stem avulsion and haemorrhage, usually at the pontomedullary junction or, less commonly, at the craniocervical junction, and unless incomplete, results in immediate death.

Cranial Nerve Avulsion

Olfactory bulb injury, resulting in anosmia, is common after head injury, but other avulsions including the optic, facial and auditory nerves also occur.

Focal Vascular Injury

Carotid cavernous fistula, resulting in pulsating exothalamus, and carotid or vertebral artery dissections also occur with head injuries.

Diffuse Injury

Traumatic Axonal Injury

The term diffuse axonal injury (DAI) indicates widespread axonal damage within the brain which may result from a number of insults, including a trauma, hypoxia, ischaemia and hypoglycaemia.[13,14] The neuropathological features of diffuse axonal injury following trauma differs from that seen after ischaemic injury.[15] Traumatic axonal injury (TAI) is caused by a rapid acceleration or deceleration of the head, particularly where there is rotational or coronal movement of the head.[16] TAI is particularly common following road traffic accidents, but may occur as a result of falls from a height and assaults[17] and is seen in the majority of patients with fatal head injury.[18] Patients with TAI are typically unconscious from the moment of injury and have a poor outcome, with death, severe disability and persistent vegetative state.[19] TAI is characterised by damage to axons, and in most cases, petechial haemorrhages. These haemorrhages which are 3–5 mm across occur instantaneously, and their presence determines the grade of TAI (see Table 2.2). They occur in the corpus callosum, often on either side of the midline, most extensively in the splenium, and also in the dorso-lateral quadrant of the upper brain stem, usually in the superior cerebellar peduncle and predominantly unilateral (Figure 2.1).

Axonal damage results in swollen tortuous and transected fibres throughout the white matter, including the corpus callosum, parasaggital subcortical fibres, deep grey matter, cerebellar folia and brain stem tracts.[20] The axonal swellings can be seen with silver preparations after several hours survival and have been termed 'axon retraction balls' (Figure 2.2). However, axonal damage can be detected histologically by the accumulation of β-amyloid precursor protein as early as 35 min after head injury.[21] After a period of several days to weeks there is accumulation of microglia around damaged axons followed by Wallerian degeneration of axons resulting in shrinkage and grey discolouration of hemispheric white matter, atrophy of the brain stem and ventricular dilatation (Figure 2.3). The axonal damage results from shearing forces exerted on long fibre tracts within the central nervous system causing damage to the axolemma, resulting in calcium influx and activation of calcium depended enzymes. Calpain activation results in damage to cytoskeletal

Table 2.2 Grading of traumatic axonal injury

Grade 1	Axonal damage
Grade 2	Axonal damage and haemorrhagic lesions in corpus callosum
Grade 3	Axonal damage and haemorrhagic lesions in corpus callosum and brain stem

Source: Adams et al.[19]

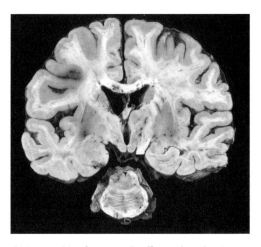

Figure 2.1 Traumatic axonal injury resulting from a road traffic accident showing petechial haemorrhages within the corpus callosum and dorso-lateral quadrant of the brain stem. Also note herniation contusion on parahippocampal gyrus indicating previous brain swelling.

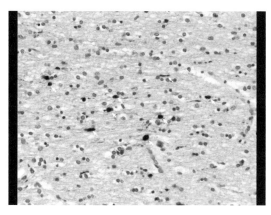

Figure 2.2 Following immunocytochemistry of β-amyloid precursor protein, swollen darkly stained axons can be seen.

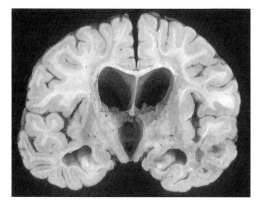

Figure 2.3 Patient who survived in a persistent vegetative state for 4 years after traumatic axonal injury showing extensive loss and cavitation of hemispheric white matter, with atrophy of the corpus callosum and hydrocephalus ex vacuo.

proteins,[22,23] disrupting axonal transport mechanisms and resulting in accumulation of proteins at the site of injury and eventual axotomy.[24,25] Deep grey matter and parasagittal haemorrhages ('gliding contusions'), which are often bilateral, may be associated with TAI.

Diffuse Vascular Injury

Some patients who die immediately following a severe acceleration or deceleration type of brain injury have widespread petechial haemorrhage throughout the brain due to shearing forces being exerted upon blood vessels. These patients do not survive long enough to develop any axonal changes.

Brain Swelling

Brain swelling is a common finding in patients with significant head injury, particularly in children and adolescents,[26] and may be due to a number of factors including the primary brain injury, intracranial haematomas, epilepsy and systemic complications such as hypoxia, ischaemia and sepsis. Following brain injury there may be an increase in cerebral blood volume due to vasodilation,[27] leakage of fluid due to incompetence of the blood-brain barrier (vasogenic oedema) and increased water content of cells within the central nervous system (cytotoxic oedema). Brain swelling results in raised intracranial pressure and a reduced cerebral perfusion pressure, causing ischaemic brain damage, which most marked in susceptible regions such as the watershed areas, particularly at the borders of the anterior and middle cerebral artery territories, and within the Sommer's sector of the hippocampus. Differential pressures between the intracranial compartments may result in herniation of brain and further more localised ischaemic injury; subfalcine herniation of the cingulate gyrus may result in compression of the anterior cerebral artery; transtentoral herniation (which is usually caudal, but may be rostral when there is a large posterior fossa haematoma) causes compression of the posterior cerebral artery, the parahippocampal gyrus and midbrain; transforaminal herniation of the brain stem (coning) causes ischaemia of vital brain stem functions and death.

Fat Embolism

Although not a direct result of head injury, fat embolism may be seen in patients with head injury who have long bone fractures. This syndrome classically causes dyspnoea, hypoxia and confusion 2–3 days after a traumatic incident with multiple petechial haemorrhages present in the white matter, and is due to lipid emboli released from the marrow lodging in lung and intracranial blood vessels.

Abusive Head Trauma in Childhood (Non-accidental Injury)

Abusive head trauma in children (also known as non-accidental head injury or the 'shaken baby syndrome') is important to recognise, and should be considered in young children and infants with unexplained head injuries. The relatively large head and weak neck together with an immature brain predispose infants and young children to brain injury resulting from shaking. Alertness to the syndrome should be raised by the presence of retinal haemorrhages, which are otherwise uncommon in infants more than a month after childbirth, and may be associated with other ocular injuries such as retinal tears, detachments, vitreous haemorrhage and retinal folds. These children often have a thin film of bilateral subdural haemorrhage, subarachnoid haemorrhage, haemorrhage into the optic nerve sheaths, cervical nerve roots and deep muscles of the neck. Traumatic axonal injury may be present, particularly in the lower medulla and upper cervical spinal cord.[28] There is usually marked brain swelling and, if an impact occurs, contusional tears within the white matter may occur in the orbital and temporal lobes. This constellation of injuries may occur as the result of severe shaking, with or without impact, although there is controversy as to the mechanisms causing these lesions.[29,30]

Missile Head Injury

Impact of the head by an external object may result in a depressed skull fracture or penetration into the cranial cavity and focal brain damage. Penetrating injuries are common with gunshot wounds but may also occur with knife stabs, particularly in the orbital and squamous temporal bones. Low-velocity penetrating injuries of this type cause damage by direct injury to blood vessels, nerves and brain tissue and the complications caused by persisting haemorrhage and infection. High-velocity bullets (such as from rifles) often exit the skull (perforating injury) and may result in extensive brain damage from the massive shockwave caused.

Progressive Neurological Degeneration and Chronic Traumatic Encephalopathy

The pathological consequences of head injury may continue for a considerable time,[31] there is evidence that an episode of head injury associated with loss of consciousness is a risk factor for the development of Alzheimer's disease[32] and approximately 15% of patients who survive severe head injury undergo progressive neurological decline 10–20 years later, especially if the head injury is repetitive, and was first described in boxers as 'punch drunk' syndrome or 'dementia pugilistica'. However, it is now recognised that this syndrome can occur in a wide variety of situations associated with repetitive mild head injury, including other contact sports such as American football, soccer, rugby and ice hockey, and is known as chronic traumatic encephalopathy.[33] Chronic traumatic encephalopathy may cause change in behaviour and mood, depression, memory loss, Parkinsonism and dementia. The neuropathology changes include a fenestrated septum pellucidum, degeneration of the substanta nigra and Alzheimer-type pathology in the cerebral cortex with neurofibrillary tangles and β-amyloid plaque deposition. β-amyloid deposition is seen in many head injury patients,[34] and the extent of deposition is determined by the apolipoprotein gene polymorphism.[35] Neurofibrillary tangle formation appears to be a relatively early event and has been seen in relatively young boxers[36] but, unlike Alzheimer's disease, is characteristically perivascular in distribution.[33]

Excitotoxicity and Nitric Oxide in Head Injury

The complex cascade of biochemical changes triggered by head injury is not fully understood, but some components may have a neuroprotective effect whilst others may contribute to cell injury and death. Key factors in these processes are glutamate-mediated excitotoxicity and nitric oxide production, which shall be briefly reviewed.

Widespread neuronal depolarisation occurs with severe head injury and leads to massive release of several excitatory amino acids, including glutamate, which is elevated in extracellular fluid in models of head injury[37] and in the CSF of head injury patients.[38] Glutamate is widely distributed in the brain and acts on a number of receptors, including N-methyl-D-aspartate (NMDA) receptors, kainate receptors, α-amino-3-hydroxy-5-methyl-4-isoxazole proprionic acid (AMPA) receptors and metabotropic receptors. Over stimulation of glutamate receptors causes massive calcium influx into neurons, which has been demonstrated in head injury,[39] and has a neurotoxic effect, particularly on dendrites,[40,41] and is more damaging in the developing brain.[42] A number of processes are triggered by calcium influx, including activation of calcium-dependent enzymes such as phospholipases, which cause cell membrane damage thus contributing to cerebral oedema[43,44] and calpains, which degrade a range of cytoskeletal and other proteins,[22,23] disrupting axonal function. Excitatory amino acids also contribute to the release of reactive oxygen species ('free radicals') which cause peroxidative damage to cell membranes, mitochondria, proteins and DNA.[45] Although the inflammatory response to head injury may contribute to tissue damage and release of reactive oxygen species,[46,47] inflammatory cytokines such as tumour necrosis factor, interleukin-1 and nerve growth factor also have neuroprotective properties.[48–51] Interestingly some inflammatory cytokines are chronically elevated in Alzheimer's disease and it has been suggested that head injury might trigger a 'cytokine cycle' in susceptible people that may in part explain the link between acute head injury and chronic neurodegeneration.[52] Another product of inflammatory cells is nitric oxide (NO), which is also synthesised by neurons and endothelial cells by the actions of endothelial and neuronal nitric oxide synthases (eNOS and nNOS). In the first few hours after head injury endothelial and neuronal NO production occurs, which have vasodilator[53,54] and neurotoxic effects[55] respectively. NO produced by inflammatory cells, due to activation of inducible nitric oxide synthase (iNOS), occurs several hours after injury and may have an overall beneficial effect.[56] NO has a number of effects in the brain, including increasing cerebral perfusion,[55] downregulating NMDA receptors thus attenuating excitotoxicity,[57] forming toxic peroxynitrite compounds with reactive oxygen species[58] and the inhibition of cell death mechanisms.[59] The location, timing and amount of NO production may alter the overall balance of these various actions, and determine whether there will be a neurotoxic or neuroprotective effect from NO.[60]

Many of these processes contribute to cell injury, triggering apoptosis, or 'programmed cell death', which occurs in both glia and neurons following head injury.[61] Cell death is associated with alterations in Bcl-2 gene expression, which is protective against apoptosis[62] and activation of caspases[63] which cleave cytoskeletal proteins,[64] and activate endonucleases which fragment DNA.[65] Many novel therapies are now being evaluated in animal and human trials, aimed at inhibiting the components of these processes that promote apoptosis, in order to improve outcome following head injury.

References

1. Tien HC, Tremblay LN, Rizoli SB, Gelberg J, Chughtai T, Tikuisis P, et al. Association between alcohol and mortality in patients with severe traumatic head injury. *Arch Surg* 2006;141:1185–91.

2. Smith C, Graham DI, Murray LS, Stewart J, Nicoll JA. Association of APOE e4 and cerebrovascular pathology in traumatic brain injury. *J Neurol Neurosurg Psychiatry* 2006;77:363–6.

3. Sorbi S, Nacmias B, Piacentini S, Repice A, Latorraca S, Forleo P, et al. ApoE as a prognostic factor for post-traumatic coma. *Nat Med* 1995;1:852.

4. Servadei F, Ciucci G, Morichetti A, Pagano F, Burzi M, Staffa G, et al. Skull fracture as a factor of increased risk in minor head injuries: indication for a broader use of cerebral computed tomography scanning. *Surg Neurol* 1988;30:364–9.

5. Mendelow AD, Teasdale G, Jennett B, Bryden J, Hessett C, Murray G. Risks of intracranial haematoma in head injured adults. *Br Med J (Clin Res Ed)* 1983;287:1173–6.

6. Rivas JJ, Lobato RD, Sarabia R, Cordobes F, Cabrera A, Gomez P. Extradural hematoma: analysis of factors influencing the courses of 161 patients. *Neurosurgery* 1988;23:44–51.

7. Tokoro K, Nakajima F, Yamataki A. Acute spontaneous subdural hematoma of arterial origin. *Surg Neurol* 1988;29:159–63.

8. Yamashima T, Yamamoto S. How do vessels proliferate in the capsule of a chronic subdural hematoma? *Neurosurgery* 1984;15:672–8.

9. Domenicucci M, Signorini P, Strzelecki J, Delfini R. Delayed post-traumatic epidural hematoma: a review. *Neurosurg Rev* 1995;18:109–22.

10. Coast GC, Gee DJ. Traumatic subarachnoid haemorrhage: an alternative source. *J Clin Pathol* 1984;37:1245–8.

11. Dolman CL. Rupture of posterior inferior cerebellar artery by single blow to head. *Arch Pathol Lab Med* 1986;110:494–6.

12. Fujitsu K, Kuwabara T, Muramoto M, Hirata K, Mochimatsu Y. Traumatic intraventricular hemorrhage: report of twenty-six cases and consideration of the

pathogenic mechanism. *Neurosurgery* 1988;23:423–30.

13. Dolinak D, Smith C, Graham DI. Global hypoxia per se is an unusual cause of axonal injury. *Acta Neuropathol (Berl)* 2000;100:553–60.

14. Dolinak D, Smith C, Graham DI. Hypoglycaemia is a cause of axonal injury. *Neuropathol Appl Neurobiol* 2000;26:448–53.

15. Reichard RR, Smith C, Graham DI. The significance of beta-APP immunoreactivity in forensic practice. *Neuropathol Appl Neurobiol* 2005;31:304–13.

16. Gennarelli TA, Thibault LE, Adams JH, Graham DI, Thompson CJ, Marcincin RP. Diffuse axonal injury and traumatic coma in the primate. *Ann Neurol* 1982;12:564–74.

17. Graham DI, Clark JC, Adams JH, Gennarelli TA. Diffuse axonal injury caused by assault. *J Clin Pathol* 1992;45:840–1.

18. Pilz P. Axonal injury in head injury. *Acta Neurochir Suppl (Wien)* 1983;32:119–23.

19. Adams JH, Doyle D, Ford I, Gennarelli TA, Graham DI, McLellan DR. Diffuse axonal injury in head injury: definition, diagnosis and grading. *Histopathology* 1989;15:49–59.

20. Strich SJ. Diffuse degeneration of the cerebral white matter in severe dementia following head injury. *J Neurol Neurosurg Psychiatry* 1956;19:163–85.

21. Hortobagyi T, Wise S, Hunt N, Cary N, Djurovic V, Fegan-Earl A, et al. Traumatic axonal damage in the brain can be detected using beta-APP immunohistochemistry within 35 min after head injury to human adults. *Neuropathol Appl Neurobiol* 2007;33:226–37.

22. Johnson GV, Litersky JM, Jope RS. Degradation of microtubule-associated protein 2 and brain spectrin by calpain: a comparative study. *J Neurochem* 1991;56:1630–8.

23. Kampfl A, Posmantur R, Nixon R, Grynspan F, Zhao X, Liu SJ, et al. Mu-calpain activation and calpain-mediated cytoskeletal proteolysis following traumatic brain injury. *J Neurochem* 1996;67:1575–83.

24. Povlishock JT. Traumatically induced axonal injury: pathogenesis and pathobiological implications. *Brain Pathol* 1992;2:1–12.

25. Maxwell WL, Graham DI. Loss of axonal microtubules and neurofilaments after stretch-injury to guinea pig optic nerve fibers. *J Neurotrauma* 1997;14:603–14.

26. Graham DI, Ford I, Adams JH, Doyle D, Lawrence AE, McLellan DR, et al. Fatal head injury in children. *J Clin Pathol* 1989;42:18–22.

27. Bouma GJ, Muizelaar JP, Fatouros P. Pathogenesis of traumatic brain swelling: role of cerebral blood volume. *Acta Neurochir Suppl* 1998;71:272–5.

28. Geddes JF, Hackshaw AK, Vowles GH, Nickols CD, Whitwell HL. Neuropathology of inflicted head injury in children. I. Patterns of brain damage. *Brain* 2001;124:1290–8.

29. Geddes JF, Tasker RC, Hackshaw AK, Nickols CD, Adams GG, Whitwell HL, et al. Dural haemorrhage in non-traumatic infant deaths: does it explain the bleeding in 'shaken baby syndrome'? *Neuropathol Appl Neurobiol* 2003;29:14–22.

30. Reece RM. The evidence base for shaken baby syndrome: response to editorial from 106 doctors. *BMJ* 2004;328:1316–7.

31. Smith DH, Chen XH, Pierce JE, Wolf JA, Trojanowski JQ, Graham DI, et al. Progressive atrophy and neuron death for one year following brain trauma in the rat. *J Neurotrauma* 1997;14:715–27.

32. Fleminger S, Oliver DL, Lovestone S, Rabe-Hesketh S, Giora A. Head injury as a risk factor for Alzheimer's disease: the evidence 10 years on; a partial replication. *J Neurol Neurosurg Psychiatry* 2003;7:857–62.

33. Maroon JC, Winkelman R, Bost J, Amos A, Mathyssek C, Miele V. Chronic traumatic encephalopathy in contact sports: a systematic review of all reported

pathological cases. *PloS ONE* 2015;10: e0117338.

34. Roberts GW, Gentleman SM, Lynch A, Graham DI. Beta A4 amyloid protein deposition in brain after head trauma. *Lancet* 1991;338:1422–3.

35. Nicoll JA, Roberts GW, Graham DI. Apolipoprotein E epsilon 4 allele is associated with deposition of amyloid beta-protein following head injury. *Nat Med* 1995;1:135–7.

36. Geddes JF, Vowles GH, Robinson SF, Sutcliffe JC. Neurofibrillary tangles, but not Alzheimer-type pathology, in a young boxer. *Neuropathol Appl Neurobiol* 1996;22:12–16.

37. Nilsson P, Hillered L, Ponten U, Ungerstedt U. Changes in cortical extracellular levels of energy-related metabolites and amino acids following concussive brain injury in rats. *J Cereb Blood Flow Metab* 1990;10:631–7.

38. Zhang H, Zhang X, Zhang T, Chen L. Excitatory amino acids in cerebrospinal fluid of patients with acute head injuries. *Clin Chem* 2001;47:1458–62.

39. Fineman I, Hovda DA, Smith M, Yoshino A, Becker DP. Concussive brain injury is associated with a prolonged accumulation of calcium: a 45Ca autoradiographic study. *Brain Res* 1993;624:94–102.

40. Olney JW, Rhee V, Ho OL. Kainic acid: a powerful neurotoxic analogue of glutamate. *Brain Res* 1974;77:507–12.

41. Olney JW, Ho OL, Rhee V. Cytotoxic effects of acidic and sulphur containing amino acids on the infant mouse central nervous system. *Exp Brain Res* 1971;14:61–76.

42. Ikonomidou C, Mosinger JL, Salles KS, Labruyere J, Olney JW. Sensitivity of the developing rat brain to hypobaric/ischaemic damage parallels sensitivity to N-methyl-aspartate neurotoxicity. *J Neurosci* 1989;8:2809–18.

43. Shohami E, Shapira Y, Yadid G, Reisfeld N, Yedgar S. Brain phospholipase A2 is activated after experimental closed head injury in the rat. *J Neurochem* 1989;53:1541–6.

44. Dhillon HS, Donaldson D, Dempsey RJ, Prasad MR. Regional levels of free fatty acids and Evans blue extravasation after experimental brain injury. *J Neurotrauma* 1994;11:405–15.

45. Dugan LL, Choi DW. Excitotoxicity, free radicals, and cell membrane changes. *Ann Neurol* 1994;35 Suppl:S17–S21.

46. Fee D, Crumbaugh A, Jacques T, Herdrich B, Sewell D, Auerbach D, et al. Activated/effector CD4+ T cells exacerbate acute damage in the central nervous system following traumatic injury. *J Neuroimmunol* 2003;136:54–66.

47. Feuerstein GZ, Wang X, Barone FC. Inflammatory gene expression in cerebral ischemia and trauma: potential new therapeutic targets. *Ann N Y Acad Sci* 1997;825:179–93.

48. Bruce AJ, Boling W, Kindy MS, Peschon J, Kraemer PJ, Carpenter MK, et al. Altered neuronal and microglial responses to excitotoxic and ischemic brain injury in mice lacking TNF receptors. *Nat Med* 1996;2:788–94.

49. Cheng B, Christakos S, Mattson MP. Tumor necrosis factors protect neurons against metabolic-excitotoxic insults and promote maintenance of calcium homeostasis. *Neuron* 1994;12:139–53.

50. DeKosky ST, Styren SD, O'Malley ME, Goss JR, Kochanek P, Marion D, et al. Interleukin-1 receptor antagonist suppresses neurotrophin response in injured rat brain. *Ann Neurol* 1996;39:123–7.

51. Mattson MP, Goodman Y, Luo H, Fu W, Furukawa K. Activation of NF-kappaB protects hippocampal neurons against oxidative stress-induced apoptosis: evidence for induction of manganese superoxide dismutase and suppression of peroxynitrite production and protein tyrosine nitration. *J Neurosci Res* 1997;49:681–97.

52. Griffin WS, Sheng JG, Royston MC, Gentleman SM, McKenzie JE, Graham DI, et al. Glial-neuronal interactions in

Alzheimer's disease: the potential role of a 'cytokine cycle' in disease progression. *Brain Pathol* 1998;1:65–72.

53. Huang Z, Huang PL, Ma J, Meng W, Ayata C, Fishman MC, et al. Enlarged infarcts in endothelial nitric oxide synthase knockout mice are attenuated by nitro-L-arginine. *J Cereb Blood Flow Metab* 1996;16:981–7.

54. Dewitt DS, Smith TG, Deyo DJ, Miller KR, Uchida T, Prough DS. L-arginine and superoxide dismutase prevent or reverse cerebral hypoperfusion after fluid-percussion traumatic brain injury. *J Neurotrauma* 1997;14:223–33.

55. Schulz JB, Matthews RT, Jenkins BG, Ferrante RJ, Siwek D, Henshaw DR, et al. Blockade of neuronal nitric oxide synthase protects against excitotoxicity in vivo. *J Neurosci* 1995;15:8419–29.

56. Sinz EH, Kochanek PM, Dixon CE, Clark RS, Carcillo JA, Schiding JK, et al. Inducible nitric oxide synthase is an endogenous neuroprotectant after traumatic brain injury in rats and mice. *J Clin Invest* 1999;104:647–56.

57. Lipton SA, Choi YB, Pan ZH, Lei SZ, Chen HS, Sucher NJ, et al. A redox-based mechanism for the neuroprotective and neurodestructive effects of nitric oxide and related nitroso-compounds. *Nature* 1993;364:626–32.

58. Beckman JS, Beckman TW, Chen J, Marshall PA, Freeman BA. Apparent hydroxyl radical production by peroxynitrite: implications for endothelial injury from nitric oxide and superoxide.

Proc Natl Acad Sci U S A 1990;87(4):1620–4.

59. Kim YM, Talanian RV, Billiar TR. Nitric oxide inhibits apoptosis by preventing increases in caspase-3-like activity via two distinct mechanisms. *J Biol Chem* 1997;272:31138–48.

60. Garry PS, Ezra M, Rowland MJ, Westbrook J, Pattinson KTS. The role of nitric oxide pathway in brain injury and its treatment – from bench to bedside. *Exp Neurol* 2015;263:235–43.

61. Newcomb JK, Zhao X, Pike BR, Hayes RL. Temporal profile of apoptotic-like changes in neurons and astrocytes following controlled cortical impact injury in the rat. *Exp Neurol* 1999;158:76–88.

62. Nakamura M, Raghupathi R, Merry DE, Scherbel U, Saatman KE, McIntosh TK. Overexpression of Bcl-2 is neuroprotective after experimental brain injury in transgenic mice. *J Comp Neurol* 1999;412:681–92.

63. Eldadah BA, Faden AI. Caspase pathways, neuronal apoptosis, and CNS injury. *J Neurotrauma* 2000;17:811–29.

64. Aikman J, O'Steen B, Silver X, Torres R, Boslaugh S, Blackband S, et al. Alpha-II-spectrin after controlled cortical impact in the immature rat brain. *Dev Neurosci* 2006;28:457–65.

65. Liu X, Zou H, Slaughter C, Wang X. DFF, a heterodimeric protein that functions downstream of caspase-3 to trigger DNA fragmentation during apoptosis. *Cell* 1997;89:175–84.

Experimental Models of Traumatic Brain Injury

Ciaran S. Hill and Hiren C. Patel

Introduction

The need for experimental traumatic brain injury (TBI) models comes from the drive to better understand TBI pathophysiology in order to improve outcome. Models are surrogates for human pathology, they can be cellular (*in vitro*) or whole organism (*in vivo*). Although no model can entirely replace the need for human studies, the use of cell cultures and animals offer unique advantages. There is uniformity of subjects, and the same injury can be repeatedly recreated. They allow for the creation of simple or complex injuries, whilst offering the ability to investigate global or focal change(s) from minutes to days following the insult, and there are no recruitment or loss of follow-up issues. The greatest advantages are possibly the ability to perform multiple and invasive sampling of tissues, measure fatal end points and trial widest range of drug doses which is precluded in clinical studies.

The value of models directly depends on their ability to reproduce different aspects of the human injury response in order to answer specific experimental questions. Therefore, when deciding which is the optimal model system, we must consider the ability of any given model to answer the posed experimental question. There are no intrinsically 'good' or 'bad' models. The two main variables when selecting a model system are the choice of species and the choice of biomechanical injury type. The cellular culture or species choice depends upon the scientific question posed – with different choices providing a different range of experimental tools. The biomechanical injury selected should be determined by the type of human TBI that the model is attempting to produce. This injury type can also be adjusted in terms of severity.

Cellular Models

There are two major variables that can be adjusted when selecting a cellular model of injury. The first is the cell type. Tissue can be directly derived from an animal – for example neurons from the brain or from autonomic or spinal dorsal root ganglion – dissociated and then cultured in a dish. Alternatively, tissue can be extracted whole as an explant and then cultured; this can include cortical or hippocampal brain slices which are supported until they recover from the initial injury and become 'organotypic' and hence are effectively living brain in dish. These organotypic cell cultures maintain neuronal and glial populations, tissue architecture, and electrical activity and circuits. Other important cell types include 'cell lines', which are immortalised cells, typically from an oncological precursor, that may display some neuronal-type characteristics, and neuronal cells derived from stem cells – these can be from animals or re-derived from other human cells such as fibroblasts.[1]

The second variable is the nature of the biomechanical injury applied. This may depend upon the tissue type used but can be broadly categorised as either a biochemical injury – including exposure inflammatory cytokines, toxins that mimic biochemical processes and ischaemia/metabolic derangements – or a physical injury. The latter can be subdivided into variations of biomechanical input type such as transection, stretch, shear strain or fluid shear stress, blast or contusional injuries.[1] Different biomechanical inputs are generally taken to correspond to different human brain injury types – for example a stretch injury is commonly used to model a diffuse axonal injury.

Benefits of using cellular models to investigate TBI include precise control of confounding factors, and direct access to living tissue for drug treatment, pharmacological screening or live imaging. These *in vitro* systems facilitate investigation of molecular mechanisms involved in response to injury, particularly secondary injury processes like excitotoxicity apoptosis, and reactive oxygen species.[1] Transfection of cells with plasmids allows genetic manipulation with either overexpression or knockdown of a target gene. There is also the opportunity to analyse genetic or protein level expression in response to injury, environmental changes or drug effects. Furthermore, *in vitro* models allow visualisation of morphological changes in subcellular components using antibody-based markers. The primary weaknesses of cellular models of injury are that they are even further removed from the human condition. Cells may act differently when studied in isolation or removed from their normal physiological environment. It is also not possible to investigate behavioural responses *in vitro*.

The combination of versatile experimental tools, allied to a wide variety of cellular and injury types, makes *in vitro* modelling a powerful device in TBI research.

Animal Models

The vast majority of *in vivo* traumatic brain injury models utilise mammals, particularly rodents – either mice or rats. These rodent models are generally well-characterised, widely available and are not prohibitively expensive. Rodent models have numerous experimental advantages including a wide range of available antibodies for immunohistological investigation and protein quantification, and transgenic animals that can be used to understand a range of genetic effects.[2]

Alternatives to rodent models include the modelling of TBI with large animals including pigs and primates. The major advantage of large animal models of TBI is their large gyrencephalic brains. These are anatomically more similar to human brains that the small smooth lissenchephalic brains of rodents. They also produce more representative structural deformation in response to biochemical forces. However, these benefits need to be weighed against the costs, ethical concerns and technical limitations – including lack of antibodies for immunohistochemical studies – inherent in larger animals. A large brain affords the opportunity to model acceleration forces, something that is severely limited with brains that have a small mass. A further benefit of larger animal models is they often have better developed myelination. Something that is poorly developed in the lissencephalic brains of many small animals.[3]

In the search for new ways to understand the pathological processes that are occurring in brain injury, other models include those in non-mammalian systems like the fruit fly *Drosophila melanogaster* or the zebrafish *Danio rerio* have been developed.[4,5] These versatile organisms offer methods of simple genetic modification with which to probe molecular mechanisms of injury responses. They also elicit less ethical constraints than mammals. However, non-mammalian models have greater evolutionary divergence from humans that may introduce unrecognised confounding variables. They may also pose additional challenges in reproducing injuries that is translatable to the human condition.

The remainder of this chapter concentrates on rodent TBI models as these are the most prevalent in the literature, we describe the methods and histopathological features of experimental injury, along with clinically relevant outcome measures.

Rodent Experimental Traumatic Brain Injury Models

Denny-Brown and Russell are credited with pioneering experimental head injury research using rodent models.[6] They classified injury models according to whether injury was induced by an acceleration or percussive force, and took these to be representative of a focal or diffuse injury.[6] As with human injuries, a 'focal' versus 'diffuse' classification is somewhat artificial and oversimplifies often heterogeneous injuries, but it remains a useful framework to broadly organise the injuries that a particular model characteristically produces.

There are several ways in which the application of an external force can be used to reproduce a TBI in animals. These include rapid loading forces – either as an impact or a deceleration injury, either with or without subsequent impact. The orientation of the applied force can alter the type of force the brain experiences and subsequent clinical findings.

Focal Traumatic Brain Injury Models

Weight Drop

The weight drop model (WDM) involves a direct impact, using a free falling weight onto the head of a restrained anaesthetised animal to cause brain injury.[7] The weight and height of release are varied to create a spectrum of injury. The weight is directed down a fixed track or tube to allow for reproducibility. A craniotomy is normally performed before injury, although this method has also been described with an intact skull. Injury results in a contusion with focal neuronal, glial and vascular cell death immediately under the area of impact – this is commonly in the region over lying the right parietal lobe and hippocampus. With severe injury, a deep haemorrhagic contusion and contralateral injury has been reported.[7]

Controlled Cortical Impact

The controlled cortical impact (CCI) model uses a pneumatic device to drive an impactor to deliver a blow to the head thereby producing injury.[8] Again, this is usually performed following a craniotomy in an anaesthetised animal, and as with the weight drop method, injury severity and site of the lesion can be altered, with the advantage that there is no risk of rebound injury.[3] The changes in the brain following the insult are similar to those with the WDM with evidence of contusional injury with neuronal and glial cell loss combined with a reactive microglial and astrocytic response. There is also some evidence of pericapillary haemorrhage within the lesion as well as petechial haemorrhages consistent with diffuse axonal injury in distant white matter tracts.

Overall both these methods induce pathology consistent with cerebral contusions and some associated axonal injury. Both are relatively simple, quick to perform and produce a wide spectrum of injury severity in a reproducible manner. The weight drop method has its critics mainly because there may be double injury caused by bouncing of the weight following initial impact.

Acute Subdural Haematoma

Clinically, acute subdural haematomas are related to either a contusion or laceration, or are a result of ruptured bridging veins, with underlying cerebral ischaemia and/or cerebral swelling driving poor outcome. Acute subdural haemorrhage may be induced by CCI, and impact acceleration injury (see below), but they are not seen consistently. A more reliable and reproducible method is to introduction 300–400 µl of autologous blood into the rat subdural space following a small craniotomy.[9,10] This results in a zone of brain damage underneath the subdural collection that is a result of ischaemia induced by the presence of the blood.[9] In order to mimic the brain swelling/diffuse injury that often accompanies acute subdural haemorrhage in humans, autologous blood injection has been combined with the impact acceleration model. Other associated injuries like hypoxia can also be co-applied.[10] This paradigm of injury has resulted in both ischemic injury as well as increased cerebral swelling and is thought to be a more clinically relevant model.[10,11]

Epidural Haematoma

In extradural haemorrhage models, compression can be mimicked by inflating a balloon in the extradural compartment following a craniotomy.[11] Injury severity is controlled by changing either the volume of balloon inflation (0.1–0.4 ml) or the rate of inflation, and can be guided intracranial pressure monitoring. Criticism of the model comes from the lack of blood in the extradural space. However, the model replicates radiological features including midline shift and basal cistern effacement, and physiological features including Cushing's response and anisocoria. Disturbances associated with brain stem compression in the rat also occur, supporting the suggestion that this model may be representative of the pathology found in the human condition.[11]

Diffuse Injury Models

The focal models described above all have components of 'diffuse axonal injury' but contusional injury predominates. The inertial acceleration and impact acceleration models representing Denny-Brown and Russell's acceleration concussion injury, more consistently produce diffuse injury without overt focal lesions.

Inertial Acceleration

The inertial acceleration model was the first model of diffuse axonal injury and was described for non-human primates.[12] The injury is induced by the rapid deceleration of a moving frame to which the primate body is attached. This results in a whiplash motion, initial coma and subcortical white matter injury consistent with diffuse axonal injury.[12] The forces needed to induce this injury are dependent on the weight of the brain, with lighter brains requiring exponentially high rotational forces. Therefore, this method had been mainly limited to use in large animals with greater cortical mass, although there have been limited attempts to replicate this injury in rodents.[13] The anaesthetised rodent head is fixed to a rotation device that requires a head clip with fixation achieved using a tooth hole and ear pins. The release of a spring results in the rapid rotation (2 ms) of the head from anywhere from 15° to 90°. No contusional injury or subarachnoid haemorrhage was seen, and petechial haemorrhage in the temporal lobe and ventrolateral pons was the only observed macroscopic change. Axonal swellings and retraction balls characteristic of diffuse axonal injury were seen from 6 hours and increased over time. These were initially only observed in the midbrain, medulla and upper cervical cord, although by 24 hour these changes were also observed in the corpus callosum, internal capsule and optic tracts. The authors acknowledged problems of mechanical fatigue in the apparatus and the strict standardisation of rat weight within experiments to achieve consistent injury.[13]

Impact Acceleration

The more conventional method to induce diffuse injury in rats is to use the impact acceleration model.[14] Injury is induced in a similar fashion to the weight drop method. Instead of a direct injury to the cerebrum, the weight is allowed to drop onto a steel plate that is glued onto the skull whilst the anaesthetised rat is supported on a foam bed of a known spring constant. Injury severity is altered by changing the height of release, weight and/or the spring constant of the foam.[14] The pathological changes were dependent on the injury severity and ranged from traumatic subarachnoid haemorrhage in the basal cisterns with mild injury to extensive subarachnoid and intraventricular haemorrhage with frequent petechial haemorrhages in more severe injury. The main pathology observed was axonal swelling, the magnitude of which was related to the severity of the injury. Axonal swelling was seen as early as 6 hours after injury and reached a maximum after 24 hours. Injury was seen throughout the white matter with predominance in the optic tracts, cerebral peduncles and the pyramidal decussation in the medulla oblongata. Axonal injury was also observed to a lesser extent in the internal capsule and the corpus callosum without any evidence of focal contusion.[15] This model has been modified by Cernak et al. by the addition of a laser to more precisely target the steel disc. It is suggested that this system results in more consistent site of injury and hence a more consistent injury pattern.[16]

Focal Axonal Injury

The optic nerve stretch injury model representing diffuse axonal injury, first described in guinea pigs and then modified for mice is a pure experimental traumatic brain injury paradigm.[17,18] The injury is produced by the application of a transient (20 ms) traction force on the optic nerve exposed by detaching the conjunctiva from the sclera and then detaching the extraocular muscles from their attachment around the optic nerve. The application of a transient force results in the rapid elongation of the optic nerve; depending on the degree of force applied, this may cause primary axotomy or initiate a pathological cascade resulting in secondary axotomy. This is characterised by the hallmarks of axonal injury such as the presence of axonal swellings and retraction balls, neurofilament and microtubule disruption, disruption of axonal transport and accumulation of transported proteins. There is also a progressive increase in axonal damage over time that may lead to deafferentation of the neuronal cell body.[17,18]

Other Animal Models of Traumatic Brain Injury

Lateral Fluid Percussion

Many severe human brain injuries are heterogenous and may contain both focal and diffuse injury. The focal models of experimental injury described above all result in some degree of diffuse injury, but this is small. Changing the severity or site of injury can lead to more diffuse injury as typified by the midline injury caused by CCI of moderate or severe intensity. This results in axonal injury in the corpus callosum and internal capsule in addition to distant hippocampal and thalamic degeneration below the contusion site.[19] A more widely accepted model of combined injury is the lateral fluid percussion (LFP) model in which injury is induced by releasing a weighted-pendulum from a known height onto a saline filled reservoir that results in the impact of a fluid bolus against the dura on the side of the head of an anaesthetised experimental animal. The injury severity is controlled by the height from which the pendulum is released resulting in a mixed injury typically consisting of a focal contusion at the site of impact, subdural haematoma, subarachnoid haemorrhage, white matter tears, as well as selective neuronal damage in the hippocampus and thalamus. LFP injury also consistently results in bilateral damage with diffuse white matter damage distant from the site of injury.[20]

Blast Injury Models

The increasing recognition of TBI consequences of military blasts has led to a proliferation of related models. The commonest form is the use of a shock tube that mimics a pressure wave.[6] The way in which a rodent is placed within the tube determines whether the injury is isolated to the head, or also affects the rest of the body. These non-impact blasts cause widespread white matter injury, brain oedema and functional deficits. They have also been used to model chronic neurodegenerative pathologies.[7]

Outcome Measurements in Experimental TBI Models

If experimental models are to be used as preclinical trials and direct clinical studies, then outcome measures need to be clinically relevant. *In vivo* experimental studies can use a range of outcome measures including functional/behavioural and histopathological measures. Outcome measures need to be tailored to the experimental question in order to avoid inappropriate inferences.

In general, outcomes assessment may include a global measure of outcome such as mortality, a functional measure such as cognition or behavioural response, motor and/or sensory assessments, as well as more specific measures that are implicated in influencing outcome in human head injury such as cerebral perfusion, cerebral blood flow, cerebral oedema, blood-brain barrier disruption or intracranial pressure monitoring. Detailed pathological and molecular assessments may also be relevant depending on the experimental hypothesis. Careful consideration and selection of appropriate outcomes are vital to ensure that research is as valid and clinically relevant as possible.

Behavioural Assessment

Behavioural assessment typically encompasses a series of tests that have been carefully designed and validated. They can include quantification of motor function (strength and reflex behaviours), cognitive (memory and learning) and neurological function. Motor assessment tests may include strength (forelimb reflex, lateral pulsion, akinesa), reflex behaviours (Von Frey hair test, forelimb placing) and fine motor coordination (activity monitoring, grid walking tests).[21] Motor assessments have been widely applied in experimental TBI studies, with motor deficits observed following CCI (Bracing rigidity test, Von Frey hair test, beam walk and balance test), inertial acceleration (beam walk and balance tests, inclined plane test, rotarod tests) and LFP injury (forelimb reflex test, lateral pulsion test, beam walk and balance test, rotating pole test).[21]

Cognitive tests, which assess memory and learning, have been used as correlates of post-traumatic and retrograde amnesia which are reliable predictors of outcome following human TBI.[22] The most commonly used measure is the Morris water maze which comprises a circular water tank with a submerged platform.[23] To test memory, animals are trained to find the submerged platform before exposure to an experimental injury. Post-injury, the time taken and consistency with which the platform is found are taken as markers for memory function. For the learning test paradigm, the time taken for the rats to find the platform from a fixed point is taken as a marker of new learning. Deficits in both short- and long-term memory and learning have been reported following CCI, LFP and impact acceleration injury in rodents.[21]

Cerebral Blood Flow and Cerebral Oedema

Although temporally and spatially variable, cerebral ischaemia following TBI in humans is common and negatively influences outcome.[24] For focal injury most studies in rodents have reported a reduction in the cerebral blood flow to up to 50% of baseline within 4 hours of the injury.[25,26] The reduction in cerebral blood flow is observed up to 7 days post-injury in autoradiography studies in the rat and is related to injury severity.[25] A reduction in cerebral blood flow is also noted with the autologous blood injection model of acute subdural haemorrhage which is further compromised by additional diffuse injury and reduced by early decompression of the surgical lesion.[27] Cerebral oedema assessed using MRI-based techniques and wet dry methods and through the quantification of the extravasation of Evans blue dye – for vasogenic oedema – have all confirmed that brain water content increases following injury to a maximum at 24 hours, and persists for at least 1 week.[25,28] As in the clinical setting, blood-brain barrier opening occurs transiently, and cerebral oedema is significantly worsened by secondary insults such as experimental hypoxia and hypotension in the rat.[28,29]

Intracranial Pressure and Cerebral Perfusion Pressure

Currently intracranial pressure (ICP) and cerebral perfusion pressure (CPP) studies are limited either to an immediate assessment of the injury severity or short-term monitoring. As with brain tissue oxygen monitoring in the ambulant rodent, probe size and fixation for long-term use are currently being explored.[8,9] Telemetry-based solutions with implantable probes offer a potential route for long-term monitoring, but this has not yet been fully characterised.

Summary

The use of animals, and animal-derived tissue, to experimentally model TBI remains controversial. Critics have cited the failure of experimental TBI research to translate into clinical gains, and concerns about animal suffering. It can be argued that there are funda-mental biological differences between species and the modelled injuries that prevent mean-ingful extrapolation of the data to humans.[30,31] Similar criticisms have been levelled at cellular culture injury models, with detractors pointing to differences in biology between cells derived from tumours, animals or stem cells. Furthermore, cellular culture conditions may be vastly different from that found in the living body. Others have contested that the failure in translation does not necessarily equate to an inadequacy of the models but may be a consequence of poor experimental design – including a failure to consider pathological processes that often co-exist with TBI in humans but are not represented in most models – for example hypoxia, hypotension and polytrauma, and that findings from small mammals required confirmation in large animal models.[3,10] Despite these criticisms, many commen-tators remain confident in the use of models and support their use. Despite the lack of translation they have contributed to the understanding of core molecular pathways and biomechanical responses.[2]

It is widely accepted that human and experimental TBI will always be different, and no experimental model can completely replicate the human condition. However, there are now well-characterised histopathologically accurate experimental correlates of human TBI with robust methods of assessing clinically relevant acute pathophysiological events and cognitive outcomes. There has also been a realisation that, in common with human head injury, there is a considerable heterogeneity in experimental TBI, including variability in injuries between laboratories and lack of standardisation of outcome measures. It is also increasingly accepted that outcome following brain injury cannot be based on a single, often histopathological assessment. This increased understanding of the tools available and potential pitfalls of *in vitro* and *in vivo* models may lead to more effective translation of preclinical studies in order to improve clinical outcomes.

References

1. Morrison B, Elkin BS, Dolle JP. In vitro models of traumatic brain injury. *Annu Rev Biomed Eng* 2011;13:91–126.

2. Hill CS, Coleman MP, Menon DK. Traumatic axonal injury: mechanisms and translational opportunities. *Trends Neurosci* 2016;39(5):311–24.

3. Morales DM, Marklund N, Lebold D, Thompson HJ, Pitkanen A, Maxwell WL, et al. Experimental models of traumatic brain injury: do we really need to build a better mousetrap? *Neuroscience* 2005;136(4):971–89.

4. Katzenberger RJ, Loewen CA, Wassarman DR, Petersen AJ, Ganetzky B, Wassarman DA. A Drosophila model of closed head traumatic brain injury. *PNAS* 2013;110(44):E4152–9.

5. McCutcheon V, Park E, Liu E, Sobhebidari P, Tavakkoli J, Wen XY, Baker AJ. A novel model of traumatic brain injury in adult zebrafish demonstrates response to injury and treatment comparable with mammalian models. *J Neurotrauma* 2017;34(7):1382–93.

6. Denny-Brown DR, Ritchie Russell W. Experimental cerebral concussion. *Brain* 1941;64:93–164.

7. Feeney DM, Boyeson MG, Linn RT, Murray HM, Dail WG. Responses to cortical injury: I. Methodology and local effects of contusions in the rat. *Brain Res* 1981;211(1):67–77.

8. Dixon CE, Clifton GL, Lighthall JW, Yaghmai AA, Hayes RL. A controlled cortical impact model of traumatic brain injury in the rat. *J Neurosci Methods* 1991;39(3):253–62.

9. Miller JD, Bullock R, Graham DI, Chen MH, Teasdale GM. Ischemic brain damage in a model of acute subdural

hematoma. *Neurosurgery* 1990;27(3):433–9.

10. Tomita Y, Sawauchi S, Beaumont A, Marmarou A. The synergistic effect of acute subdural hematoma combined with diffuse traumatic brain injury on brain edema. *Acta Neurochir Suppl* 2000;76:213–16.

11. Burger R, Bendszus M, Vince GH, Roosen K, Marmarou A. A new reproducible model of an epidural mass lesion in rodents. Part I: Characterization by neurophysiological monitoring, magnetic resonance imaging, and histopathological analysis. *J Neurosurg* 2002;97(6):1410–18.

12. Gennarelli TA, Thibault LE, Adams JH, Graham DI, Thompson CJ, Marcincin RP. Diffuse axonal injury and traumatic coma in the primate. *Ann Neurol* 1982;12(6):564–74.

13. Xiao-Sheng H, Sheng-Yu Y, Xiang Z, Zhou F, Jian-ning Z. Diffuse axonal injury due to lateral head rotation in a rat model. *J Neurosurg* 2000;93(4):626–33.

14. Marmarou A, Foda MA, van den Brink W, Campbell J, Kita H, Demetriadou K. A new model of diffuse brain injury in rats. Part I: Pathophysiology and biomechanics. *J Neurosurg* 1994;80(2):291–300.

15. Foda MA, Marmarou A. A new model of diffuse brain injury in rats. Part II: Morphological characterization. *J Neurosurg* 1994;80(2):301–13.

16. Cernak I, Vink R, Zapple DN, Cruz MI, Ahmed F, Chang T, et al. The pathobiology of moderate diffuse traumatic brain injury as identified using a new experimental model of injury in rats. *Neurobiol Dis* 2004;17(1):29–43.

17. Gennarelli TA, Thibault LE, Tipperman R, Tomei G, Sergot R, Brown M, et al. Axonal injury in the optic nerve: a model simulating diffuse axonal injury in the brain. *J Neurosurg* 1989;71(2):244–53.

18. Saatman KE, Abai B, Grosvenor A, Vorwerk CK, Smith DH, Meaney DF. Traumatic axonal injury results in biphasic calpain activation and retrograde transport impairment in mice. *J Cereb Blood Flow Metab* 2003;23(1):34–42.

19. Hall ED, Sullivan PG, Gibson TR, Pavel KM, Thompson BM, Scheff SW. Spatial and temporal characteristics of neurodegeneration after controlled cortical impact in mice: more than a focal brain injury. *J Neurotrauma* 2005;22(2):252–65.

20. Thompson HJ, Lifshitz J, Marklund N, Grady MS, Graham DI, Hovda DA, et al. Lateral fluid percussion brain injury: a 15-year review and evaluation. *J Neurotrauma* 2005;22(1):42–75.

21. Fujimoto ST, Longhi L, Saatman KE, Conte V, Stocchetti N, McIntosh TK. Motor and cognitive function evaluation following experimental traumatic brain injury. *Neurosci Biobehav Rev* 2004;28(4):365–78.

22. Povlishock JT, Hayes RL, Michel ME, McIntosh TK. Workshop on animal models of traumatic brain injury. *J Neurotrauma* 1994;11(6):723–32.

23. Morris RG, Garrud P, Rawlins JN, O'Keefe J. Place navigation impaired in rats with hippocampal lesions. *Nature* 1982;297(5868):681–3.

24. Graham DI, Ford I, Adams JH, Doyle D, Teasdale GM, Lawrence AE, et al. Ischaemic brain damage is still common in fatal non-missile head injury. *J Neurol Neurosurg Psychiatry* 1989;52(3):346–50.

25. Kochanek PM, Marion DW, Zhang W, Schiding JK, White M, Palmer AM, et al. Severe controlled cortical impact in rats: assessment of cerebral edema, blood flow, and contusion volume. *J Neurotrauma* 1995;12(6):1015–25.

26. Shen Y, Kou Z, Kreipke CW, Petrov T, Hu J, Haacke EM. In vivo measurement of tissue damage, oxygen saturation changes and blood flow changes after experimental traumatic brain injury in rats using susceptibility weighted imaging. *Magn Reson Imaging* 2007;25(2):219–27.

27. Sawauchi S, Marmarou A, Beaumont A, Signoretti S, Fukui S. Acute subdural hematoma associated with diffuse brain injury and hypoxemia in the rat: effect of surgical evacuation of the

hematoma. *J Neurotrauma* 2004;21
(5):563–73.

28. Shapira Y, Setton D, Artru AA,
Shohami E. Blood-brain barrier permeability,
cerebral edema, and neurologic function
after closed head injury in rats. *Anesth Analg*
1993;77(1):141–8.

29. Unterberg AW, Stover J, Kress B,
Kiening KL. Edema and brain trauma.
Neuroscience 2004;129(4):1021–9.

30. Croce P. *Vivisection or science? An
investigation into testing drugs and
safeguarding health.* London: Zed Books;
1999.

31. Perel P, Roberts I, Sena E,
Wheble P, Briscoe C, Sandercock
P, et al. Comparison of treatment
effects between animal experiments
and clinical trials: systematic
review. *BMI* 2007;334(7586):
197.

Chapter 4

Clinical Assessment of the Head-Injured Patient

Amr H. Mohamed, Peter C. Whitfield and Deva S. Jeyaretna

Introduction

The rapid and accurate clinical assessment of a head-injured patient is crucial. The initial management should be governed by attention to the airway, breathing and circulation according to the principles of the Advanced Trauma Life Support (ATLS) care system. This is vital not only to identify immediately life-threatening injuries but also to prevent secondary cerebral insults. The cervical spine should be immobilised, since patients with a head injury may also harbour a cervical spine injury.[1] The level of consciousness and pupil size and reaction should be determined early and at regular intervals when managing patients with TBI.

History

The clinical history should be obtained from the patient, witnesses and paramedical staff as appropriate. History-taking should include details of the mechanism of the injury and status of the patient at the accident scene in addition to the following: past medical history, medications, allergies, smoking, alcohol or drug use and social circumstances. Symptoms depend upon the severity of the injury. In conscious patients, headache due to somatic pain from a scalp injury is common. The headache caused by raised ICP is exacerbated by coughing, straining or bending and is associated with nausea, vomiting and impaired consciousness. Deterioration can be extremely rapid, highlighting the low threshold required to undertake imaging investigations looking for intracranial mass lesions. Amnesia, repetitive speech and disorientation are very common early features, even after relatively minor trauma. Focal neurological deficits affecting any part of the brain and cranial nerves can occur. Anosmia due to disruption of the olfactory pathways is perhaps the most common focal symptom. CSF rhinorrhoea and otorrhoea occasionally may be reported by the patient at this early stage. Witnessed seizures should be noted.

Examination

Neurological examination of the head-injured patient begins with an assessment of the level of consciousness and pupillary reactions. An external examination of the cranium and a tailored formal examination of cranial nerve and peripheral nerve function should their follow.

Glasgow Coma Scale (GCS) Assessment

The GCS is the most extensively used grading system for assessing the level of consciousness.[2] It is reproducible with high levels of interobserver agreement.[3] The scale is based on the best motor, verbal and eye-opening responses of the patient (Table 4.1) and is used to classify injury severity as minor (GCS 13–15), moderate (GCS 9–12) and severe (GCS 3–8). Repeated assessment of the

GCS is of importance in monitoring the condition of the patient. Although other factors such as alcohol and iatrogenic administration of sedating drugs can affect the level of consciousness, they should not be assumed to be the cause of impaired consciousness. If the patient is unarousable, a central painful stimulus is applied. Supraorbital pressure is most commonly used. In clinical practice documentation of the motor score causes most difficulty. Localisation to pain is noted if the patient raises the hand above the clavicle in response to central pain or tries to remove the stimulus in response to a sternal rub. Flexion is characterised by flexion at the elbow with the forearm in a supinated position and the wrist held in a neutral or flexed position. Abnormal flexion is observed when flexion occurs at the elbow but the forearm is pronated with a flexed wrist posture. Extension occurs when the elbow extends and the arm rotates into a pronated position. Again, the wrist is usually flexed. A GCS of 3 represents no eye-opening to pain, no verbal response and no motor response to pain. This is usually annotated as E1,V1,M1 in the medical records. A GCS of 15 represents spontaneous eye opening, orientated (who they are, where they are, why they are where they are) and obeying commands; E4,V5,M6. If the patient is intubated or has a tracheostomy, the verbal response should be marked 'T'. This enables the eye opening and motor parameters to continue to be used to assess the level of consciousness. Sometimes severe periorbital swelling precludes accurate eye-opening responses. High spinal cord injury makes motor assessment difficult. However, the itemised GCS continues to provide useful information within these constraints. When recording the GCS, the scores of individual components should be noted rather than just the total, as patients with the same total GCS but with different component scores may have differing outcomes.[4] The motor component is generally regarded as the most accurate predictor of outcome.

Table 4.1 Glasgow Coma Scale

Eye opening	
Eyes open spontaneously	4
Eyes opening to verbal stimuli	3
Eyes opening to painful stimuli	2
No eye opening	1
Verbal response	
Orientated	5
Confused	4
Inappropriate words	3
Incomprehensible sounds	2
No verbal response	1
Motor response	
Obeys commands	6
Localising pain	5
Normal flexion to pain	4
Abnormal flexion to pain	3
Extension to pain	2
No motor response	1

Source: From Teasdale and Jennett.[2] Reproduced with permission from Elsevier. Copyright © 1974.

The GCS has been modified for children less than 5 years of age and is called the Paediatric GCS. The eye-opening response remains the same, but the verbal response is different in under 5 s. It is described as follows.

Verbal response in children < 5 years	
Alert, babbles, coos, words or sentences to usual ability	5
Less than usual ability, irritable cry, inconsolable cries	4
Cries to pain	3
Moans to pain	2
No verbal response	1
Motor response in children < 5 years	
Normal spontaneous movements	6
Localising pain	5
Normal flexion to pain	4
Abnormal flexion to pain	3
Extension to pain	2
No motor response	1

Source: Jennett and Bond.[4]

Pupillary Reflexes

Examination of the pupillary reflexes provides critical information about the integrity of the optic and oculomotor pathways. Shining a light into one eye causes direct contraction of the ipsilateral pupil and consensual contraction of the contralateral pupil. Light-sensitive afferent fibres travel via the optic nerve into both optic tracts synapsing in the pretectal nuclei of the midbrain. These project bilaterally to the Edinger–Westphal nuclei, which supply parasympathetic fibres to the oculomotor nerves.[5,6] The oculomotor nerves emerge from the midbrain and travel anteriorly in the interpeduncular cistern and then along the ipsilateral free edge of the tentorium cerebelli before entering the cavernous sinus through its roof and going through the lateral wall of the cavernous sinus to emerge in the orbit via the superior orbital fissure. The parasympathetic fibres cause contraction of the sphincter pupillae. In a patient with an expanding mass lesion, herniation of the medial temporal lobe (uncus) causes compression of the ipsilateral oculomotor nerve. The fibres to the ipsilateral sphincter pupillae cease to function, causing unopposed dilatation of the pupil, which fails to contract on direct or consensual testing.

External Examination

Inspect the scalp for signs of injury including bruising and lacerations; these are commonly found in cases of assault with direct impact injuries. Sometimes depressed skull fractures can be palpated.

Subconjunctival haemorrhages and bleeding from the external auditory meatus may occur with skull base fractures. Otoscopy may reveal a haemotympanum. Other features associated with skull base fractures include periorbital and postauricular ecchymoses (Battle's sign), CSF rhinorrhoea and CSF otorrhoea.

The face should be examined for asymmetry, localised tenderness and fractures. Log-rolling enables a careful examination of the posterior aspect of the head and whole spine to be conducted.

When examining the eyes, pulsatile proptosis associated with orbital pain, ophthalmo-plegia, reduced vision, chemosis and a bruit over the globe are the classical signs of a traumatic cavernous carotid fistula (CCF). Fundoscopy may reveal ocular injuries such as sub-retinal or vitreal haemorrhages.

Cranial Nerves

If the patient is conscious and cooperative, the cranial nerves should be examined systematically.

In unconscious patients the brain stem reflexes (pupillary, corneal and gag) and gaze palsies should be noted. Oculocephalic and vestibulo-ocular reflexes are not normally conducted unless ascertaining the presence of any brain stem function when undertaking brain stem tests.

Anosmia may occur due to tearing of the olfactory nerves at the cribiform plate. Patients with anosmia often report a change in the quality of taste sensation. Formal testing for sense of smell is performed using test bottles of peppermint solution and clove oil. Visual acuity, fields and pupillary reflexes are tested. Diplopia may be reported with impaired eye movements (Figure 4.1). A complete oculomotor (III) nerve palsy results in a ptosis, ipsilateral pupillary dilatation unreactive to light directly or consensually, and the eye in the 'down and out' position. Trochlear (IV) and abducent (VI) nerve palsies result in vertical and lateral gaze diplopia, respectively. Superior orbital fissure fractures can result in cranial nerves III, IV, VI and the ophthalmic division of the trigeminal (V) nerve being injured. The trigem-inal nerve is examined by testing sensation over the face and anterior scalp and the strength

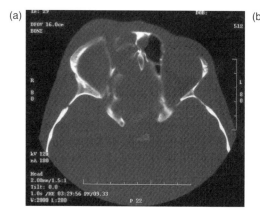 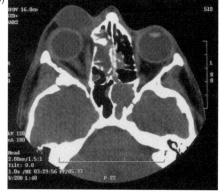

Figure 4.1 Axial CT scans showing complex anterior fossa skull fractures. The patient had anosmia, no perception of light in the right eye and a visual field defect in the left eye. These injuries were consistent with trauma to the olfactory nerves and both optic nerves. The fractures were also complicated by a CSF rhinorrhoea.

of the muscles of mastication. Branches can be injured distally by facial fractures or more proximal nerve injury can occur at the petroclinoid ridge near Meckel's cave.[7] The facial nerve (VII) supplies the muscles of facial expression and can be disrupted by fractures of the petrous temporal bone causing a complete lower motor neurone type of facial palsy. The corneal reflex, elicited by lightly touching the lateral aspect of each cornea and inspecting for bilateral blinking, tests the integrity of the trigeminal and facial nerve pathways. Hearing loss should be characterised as either sensorineural or conductive; both commonly occur after head trauma. The gag reflex is tested by touching the soft palate or pharynx with a stick or tongue depressor and observing elevation of the uvula. The afferent limb of the reflex tests the integrity of the glossopharyngeal (IX) nerve, whilst the vagus (X) causes contraction of the palatal musculature. Changes in the quality of voice are related to vagal injuries causing altered phonation. The spinal accessory nerve (XI) supplies the sternocleidomastoid and trapezius muscles. The hypoglossal nerve (XII) is rarely injured but does course through the anterior condylar canal and may be disrupted in fractures of the foramen magnum.

Peripheral Nervous System

A thorough examination of the peripheral nervous system may be impaired by a depressed level of consciousness and limb injuries. Furthermore, injuries of the brachial plexus, rarely the lumbosacral plexus and the peripheral nerves, can complicate the interpretation of abnormal findings. Observation of movement is important in assessing spinal cord function and corticospinal tract injury. Any asymmetry is documented. Unilateral motor signs (e.g. hemiplegia) may occur with an intracranial mass lesion and warrant further investigation.

False Localising Signs

The concept of false localising signs was first described in 1904 by James Collier based on his examination and post-mortem study of 161 patients with intracranial tumours.[8] A false localising sign occurs when the neurological signs elicited are a reflection of pathology distant from the expected anatomical locus.[9] The most common example is a VI nerve palsy presumably occurring due to traction of the nerve at the petroclinoid ligament, remote from the brain stem origin of the nerve. An intracranial mass lesion is usually associated with a contralateral hemiplegia due to either cortical dysfunction or compression of the ipsilateral cerebral peduncle. However, a supratentorial mass lesion can cause shift of the midbrain to the opposite side. The contralateral cerebral peduncle can then impinge on the tentorium cerebelli, causing the unexpected finding of an ipsilateral hemiplegia. At post-mortem this can be visualised as the Kernohan–Woltman notch indenting the midbrain.[10]

Raised Intracranial Pressure

In 1783 Alexander Monro noted that the cranium was a rigid box containing a nearly incompressible brain. He observed that any increase in one of the component contents (brain, blood and CSF) required accommodation by displacement of the other elements. During the initial stages of rising intracranial pressure due to a mass lesion, cerebrospinal fluid and venous blood are displaced from the cranium buffering the change in pressure.[11,12] However, once the point of compensatory reserve has been reached, rapid elevation of the ICP occurs (Figure 4.2). This may manifest as a decreased level of consciousness and an oculomotor nerve palsy secondary to temporal lobe herniation.

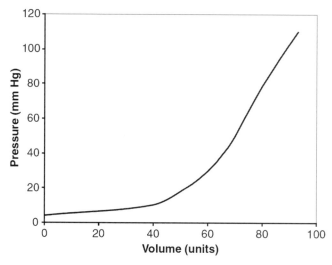

Figure 4.2 Pressure–volume curve of the cerebrospinal fluid space based on work by Lofgren et al. in canine models.[11,12]

Intracranial Herniation

Intracranial herniation is the pathological process of brain shifting from one compartment to another as a result of differential pressure gradients (Figure 4.3). The dural folds normally minimise movement within the cranium. The falx cerebri is a sickle-shaped midline structure that separates the cerebral hemispheres and decreases lateral movement. Anteriorly, it is attached to the crista galli and frontal crest. Posteriorly, it attaches to the internal occipital protuberance and the midline of the tentorium cerebelli suspending the latter structure. Supratentorial masses may cause displacement of the cingulate gyrus under the falx cerebri resulting in subfalcine herniation. This can cause compression of the anterior cerebral artery and subsequent ischaemia and infarction. The tentorium cerebelli supports the occipital lobes and separates them from the cerebellar hemispheres. The midbrain passes through the opening in the tentorium; the tentorial incisura. A supratentorial mass lesion commonly causes the uncus of the medial temporal lobe to herniate from the middle cranial fossa medially and downwards through the tentorial incisura compressing the oculomotor nerve and the midbrain. An oculomotor nerve palsy and contralateral hemiparesis usually occur and require urgent intervention. Compromise of the reticular activating system of the midbrain contributes to the impairment of consciousness. Uncal herniation can also compress the posterior cerebral artery leading to occipital lobe infarction and obstruction to the flow of cerebrospinal fluid through the aqueduct of Sylvius causing hydrocephalus.[13] Transtentorial herniation may also stretch perforating branches of the basilar artery causing secondary 'Duret' haemorrhages in the brain stem.[14]

This coronal view shows an extradural haematoma causing (1) subfalcine herniation of the cingulate gyrus (2) herniation of the uncus of the medial temporal lobe through the tentorial hiatus leading to compression of the ipsilateral oculomotor nerve, the posterior

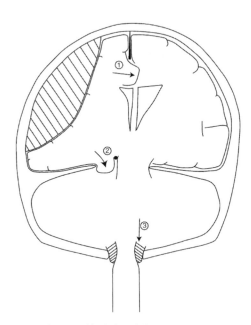

Figure 4.3 Intracranial pressure gradients and brain herniation.

cerebral artery and the midbrain and (3) herniation of the cerebellar tonsils through the foramen magnum leading to compression of the cervicomedullary junction.

Tonsillar herniation is the downward descent of the cerebellar tonsils through the foramen magnum. Mass lesions of the posterior fossa are more likely to cause tonsillar herniation, although any supratentorial mass can cause severe elevations of ICP throughout the cranial cavity leading to tonsil herniation. As the cerebellar tonsils descend, they compress the medulla and the fourth ventricle and efface the cisterna magna. Fourth ventricular compromise leads to obstructive hydrocephalus, compounding the situation. Direct compression of the medulla depresses the cardiac and respiratory centres leading to hypertension, bradycardia, ventilatory compromise and death.

Non-accidental Traumatic Brain Injury

Non-accidental traumatic brain injury is an important condition to consider when assessing a young child with a head injury. The neurosurgeon should engage in the management of the acute injury and enlist the assistance of an experienced paediatrician in determining the cause of the injury. Diagnostic errors are well recognised.[15] The terms 'battered baby' and 'shaken baby syndrome' imply specific mechanisms of injury and have been surpassed with the term 'non-accidental paediatric trauma'. The classical triad of features that strongly suggest a diagnosis of non-accidental traumatic brain injury comprise subdural haematomas, retinal haemorrhages and brain injury (encephalopathy). In addition, the injuries are inflicted unwitnessed by a sole carer and the history is inconsistent with the clinical findings. Corroborative evidence includes features of previous trauma.

Mechanical experiments show that severe non-accidental head injury is most likely to be caused by the combination of shaking and impact rather than shaking alone. Scottish cases of suspected non-accidental head injury have identified four patterns of presentation.[16]

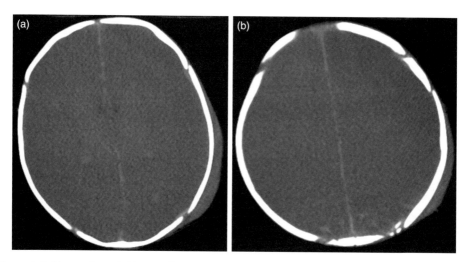

Figure 4.4 CT scan of a probable case of non-accidental head injury.

The scan of this 1-month-old child showed a partly comminuted fracture of the left parietal bone with an overlying scalp swelling. This was consistent with extensive bruising on clinical examination. The brain appeared homogenous with a loss of grey–white differentiation, generalised brain swelling and ventricular effacement. Small subdural collections were present within the interhemispheric cleft and overlying the tentorium cerebelli. Some preservation of hyperdensity in the basal ganglia suggests diffuse hypoxic injury.

1   The cervicomedullary syndrome results from hyperflexion and hyperextension of the neck disrupting the integrity of the brain stem resulting in rapid death. At post-mortem, severe brain swelling due to hypoxia is evident with axonal disruption in the brain stem and trivial subdural haematomas.

2   Acute encephalopathy. This common mode of presentation is characterised by coma, seizures, apnoea and widespread retinopathy. There may be associated signs of impact trauma to the scalp (Figure 4.4).

3   Subacute non-encephalopathic presentation. The depression of conscious level is less severe without brain swelling and parenchymal hypodensities on CT scanning. Subdural haematomas and retinal haemorrhages may be seen.

4   Chronic subdural haematoma presentation. The child may present with features of an isolated chronic subdural haematoma. These include expanding head circumference, vomiting, failure to thrive, drowsiness and fits. Retinal haemorrhages are usually absent. The features develop a few weeks after primary trauma and an adequate explanation may not be found.

Geddes et al. postulated that hypoxia and ischaemia are important factors in causing the neuropathological changes of non-accidental head injury rather than the widespread traumatic axonal injury seen in adult head injury. They hypothesised that thin subdural haematomas may be consequential to venous or arterial hypertension rather than due to bridging vein disruption.[17,18] Others have emphasised the uncertainty of diagnostic accuracy if 'pathognomic' diagnostic criteria such as ocular haemorrhages and subdural haematomas are used in isolation.[19,20] In some cases other explanations of the trauma or insult (e.g. choking, vomiting, birth trauma) may be valid, although this is hotly contested by many paediatricians.[21] Corroborative evidence must be sought to identify the aetiology of the presentation in any individual case.

The management of paediatric traumatic brain injury is discussed in Chapter 21.

References

1. Mercer SJ, Guha A. Assessing the implementation of guidelines for the management of the potentially injured cervical spine in unconscious trauma patients in England. *J Trauma* 2010 Jun;68(6):1445–50.

2. Teasdale G, Jennett B. Assessment of coma and impaired consciousness: a practical scale. *Lancet* 1974 Jul 13;2(7872):81–4.

3. Fischer M, Rüegg S, Czaplinski A, Strohmeier M, Lehmann A, Tschan F, et al. Inter-rater reliability of the Full Outline of UnResponsiveness score and the Glasgow Coma Scale in critically ill patients: a prospective observational study. *Crit Care* 2010;14(2):R64.

4. Jennett B, Bond M. Assessment of outcome after severe brain damage. *Lancet* 1975 Mar 1;1(7905):480–4.

5. Campbell WW, DeJong RN, Haerer AF. *DeJong's the neurologic examination: incorporating the fundamentals of neuroanatomy and neurophysiology.* 6th edn. Philadelphia, PA: Lippincott, Williams & Wilkins; 2005.

6. Sinnatamby CS, Last RJ. *Last's anatomy: regional and applied.* Edinburgh: Elsevier/Churchill Livingstone; 2006.

7. Feldman JS, Farnoosh S, Kellman RM, Tatum SA. Skull base trauma: clinical considerations in evaluation and diagnosis and review of management techniques and surgical approaches. *Semin Plast Surg* 2017 Nov;31(4):177–88.

8. Collier J. The false localising signs of intracranial tumour. *Brain* 1904;27:490–508.

9. Larner AJ. False localising signs. *J Neurol Neurosurg Psychiatry* 2003;74:415–18.

10. Kernohan JW, Woltman HW. Incisura of the crus due to contralateral brain tumor. *Arch Neurol Psychiatry* 1929;21:274–87.

11. Lofgren J, von Essen C, Zwetnow NN. The pressure–volume curve of the cerebrospinal fluid space in dogs. *Acta Neurol Scand* 1973;49(5):557–74.

12. Lofgren J, Zwetnow NN. Cranial and spinal components of the cerebrospinal fluid pressure-volume curve. *Acta Neurol Scand* 1973;49(5):575–8.

13. Rhoton AL Jr. Tentorial incisura. *Neurosurgery* 2000;47(3 Suppl):S131–53.

14. Parizel PM, Makkat S, Jorens PG, et al. Brainstem hemorrhage in descending transtentorial herniation (Duret hemorrhage). *Intens Care Med* 2002;28(1):85–8.

15. Wheeler DM, Hobbs CJ. Mistakes in diagnosing non-accidental injury: 10 years' experience. *Br Med J* 1988 296:1233–6.

16. Minns RA, Busuttil A. Four types of inflicted brain injury predominate. *Br Med J* 2004;328:766.

17. Geddes JF, Vowles GH, Hackshaw AK, Nichols CD, Scott IS, Whitwell HL. Neuropathology of inflicted head injury in children I. Patterns of brain damage. *Brain* 2001;124:1290–8.

18. Geddes JF, Vowles GH, Hackshaw AK, Nichols CD, Scott IS, Whitwell HL. Neuropathology of inflicted head injury in children II. Microscopic brain injury in infants. *Brain* 2001;124:1299–306.

19. Lantz PE, Sinal SH, Stanton CA, Weaver RG Jr. Perimacular retinal folds from childhood head trauma. *Br Med J* 2004;328:754–6.

20. Squier W. Shaken baby syndrome: the quest for evidence. *Dev Med Child Neurol* 2008;50:10–14.

21. Reece RM. The evidence base for shaken baby syndrome: response to editorial from 106 doctors. *Br Med J* 2004;328:1316–17.

Neuroimaging in Trauma

Won Hyung A. Ryu, Jonathan Coles and Clare N. Gallagher*

Introduction

Traumatic brain injury (TBI) is one of the leading causes of morbidity and mortality with an estimated annual incidence of 295 per 100 000.[1] Injury severity is broad and can range from mild, difficult to detect cognitive effects to profound disturbances of consciousness with prolonged coma and persistent vegetative state. The optimal modality and utility of neuroimaging depends not only on the mechanism and severity of injury but also the time since injury occurred and the information that is being sought out. The purpose of imaging patients with TBI includes guiding immediate treatment decisions, and prognostication of health outcome in the acute setting along with research into head injury pathophysiology. Indeed, recent advances in imaging techniques have allowed greater understanding of both structural and functional changes that occur after TBI. This review will briefly outline the techniques available for TBI and their usefulness in both clinical and research settings.

Acute Imaging

An estimated 2.2 million visits to the emergency departments in the USA stem from TBI leading to 280 000 hospitalisations.[2] The arrival of an injured patient in the emergency department often necessitates the decision whether to obtain imaging of the head. This decision is, for the most part, clear when substantial neurological deficits are observed or if there is considerable suspicion of possible head injury. In addition, extensive research has led to establishment of multiple imaging guidelines to guide clinicians in this decision process. Acute imaging is directed at identifying lesions which need urgent surgical intervention or stabilisation to prevent further injury. The full extent of the sustained injuries is determined after the patient has been resuscitated and stabilised.

CT

Computed Tomography (CT) scanning, now widely available in the emergency departments of most hospitals, has replaced the use of skull X-rays as the modality of choice in assessing patients with acute TBI.[3] Its ability to rapidly image trauma patients has made it invaluable for use in the acute phase following neurotrauma. A non-contrast CT can rapidly identify space occupying haematomas requiring immediate removal. With examination of both the soft tissue, and bony windows, and 3D reconstruction, calvarial and skull base fractures are equally easily identified. CT also has the advantage of being able to rapidly

* The authors acknowledge V. Newcombe, Wolfson Brain Imaging Centre, University of Cambridge, and P. Al-Rawi, University of Cambridge.

image the neck, chest, abdomen and pelvis in cases of polytrauma. As time is important in appropriately managing the trauma patient, there is no other imaging technique which is more appropriate in the acute phase.[4] Indeed, the use of multidetector helical CT has reduced acquisition time to within 30 s[5] and image slices that are degraded by motion artefact can easily be repeated. Over the last 20 years, the development, validation and refinement of imaging guidelines for evaluating trauma patients resulted in increased efficiency and efficacy in the use of CT scans.[6–8] For example, the adoption of guidelines developed by The National Institute for Health and Clinical Excellence (NICE) in the UK has changed the way CT is used (Table 5.1).[9] Similar guidelines were also developed in North American, such as the Canadian CT Head Rule (Table 5.2)[10] and the American College of Emergency Physicians/Centers for Disease Control and Prevention (ACEP/CDC) joint practice guideline (Table 5.3).[3] Overall the guidelines have proved cost effective with admission rates decreased from 9% to 4%. A decrease in skull X-rays use from 37% to 4% of patients with minor head injury and an increase in CT use from 3% of patients to 7% were shown.[9] In mild TBI the risk of deterioration in patients with injuries on CT can be predicted by several risk factors.[11] These include age, anticoagulant status, type of injury and initial GCS.[11]

Primary head injury lesions seen on CT include acute extradural haematoma, subdural haematoma, subarachnoid haemorrhage, contusions, intracerebral haematoma and diffuse axonal injury (Figure 5.1). However, initial CT scans with diffuse axonal injury (DAI) will be abnormal in only 20%–50% of cases.[4] Lesions that are visible are commonly located in the hemispheric subcortical lobar white matter, centrum semiovale, corpus callosum, basal ganglia, brain stem and cerebellum.[4] Due to the high percentage of normal scans in diffuse axonal injury (DAI), prognosis is difficult with these patients. Some factors seen on initial scans do

Table 5.1 NICE guidelines for CT scanning in adults with minor head injury

CT scan if any of the following are present:
• GCS less than 13 at any point since the injury
• GCS less than 15 at 2 hours after the injury on assessment in emergency department
• Suspected open or depressed skull fracture
• Any sign of basal skull fracture
• Post-traumatic seizure
• Focal neurological deficit
• More than one episode of vomiting since head injury
• Currently on warfarin treatment
• Loss of consciousness or amnesia since head injury + any of the following
• Age equal or greater than 65
• History of bleeding or clotting disorder
• Dangerous mechanism of injury (pedestrian or cyclist struck by motor vehicle or fall from height of 1 m or 5 stairs)
• Greater than 30 min of retrograde amnesia of events immediately before head injury

Table 5.2 Canadian CT head rule

CT scan for patients with minor head injury and any one of the following:

High risk

- GCS score <15 at 2 hours after injury
- Suspected open or depressed skull fracture
- Any sign of basal skull fracture (haemotympanum, 'racoon eyes', cerebrospinal fluid otorrhoea/rhinorrhoea, Battle's sign)
- Vomiting ≥ two episodes
- Age ≥ 65 years

Medium risk

- Amnesia before impact > 30 min
- Dangerous mechanism (pedestrian struck by motor vehicle, occupant ejected from motor vehicle, fall from height > 3 feet or five stairs)

Table 5.3 American College of Emergency Physicians/Centers for Disease Control and Prevention (ACEP/CDC) joint practice guideline

Non-contrast CT scan indicated for patients older than 16 years of age with no multisystem trauma and initial GCS of 14–15 with a history of loss of consciousness or post-traumatic amnesia only if one or more of the following is present:

- Headache
- Vomiting
- Older than 60 years of age
- Drug or alcohol intoxication
- Short-term memory loss
- Signs of trauma above the clavicle
- Post-traumatic seizure
- GCS less than 15
- Focal neurologic deficit
- Coagulopathy

seem to correlate. Those which correlate with persistent vegetative state include: number of lesions, lesions in the supratentorial white matter, corpus callosum and corona radiata.[12] While acute CT scans serve an essential role in the initial trauma management, other imaging modalities may provide additional insight in the subacute setting especially for prognostication. Specifically, a study by Bigler et al.[13] has indicated that there is poor correlation between acute CT and prognosis, apart from those patients with brain stem injury.

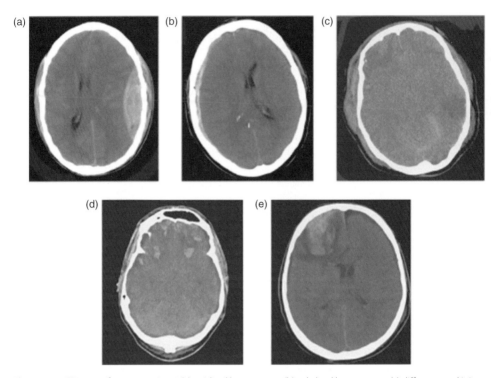

Figure 5.1 CT scans of trauma patients: (a) epidural haematoma, (b) subdural haematoma, (c) diffuse axonal injury, (d) multiple bifrontal contusions and (e) haemorrhagic right frontal contusion.

Subacute Imaging

MRI

Magnetic Resonance Imaging (MRI) is not routinely used in the acute phase of traumatic brain injury due to the technical difficulties of transporting critically ill patients and equipment compatibility. After the patient has been stabilised MRI can be used to obtain a clearer picture of the extent of injury and information about prognosis while the patient is in an intensive care unit (ICU) setting. Advances in imaging have relied on the use of MRI over all other modalities. While CT is superior to MRI in detecting acute haematoma and bony abnormalities, in the acute phase MRI has a much higher sensitivity for detecting diffuse axonal injury (DAI).[14] DAI is characterised by acceleration-deceleration inertial forces.[15] Although regarded as a widespread injury, DAI is predominately found in the parasagittal white matter, corpus callosum and pontine-mesencephalic junction.[15] In the acute phase this is seen as punctate haemorrhages; however, true extent of DAI is often underestimated. In general, T1 and T2 sequences used for morphological studies have largely been replaced by FLAIR (fluid attenuated inversion recovery). FLAIR sequences show T2 weighting but with hypo-intense CSF. These images show better cortical and periventricular lesions.[5] T2 and FLAIR produce hyper-intense areas associated with non-haemorrhagic shear injury. T2*-weighted gradient recalled echo (GRE) has been shown to

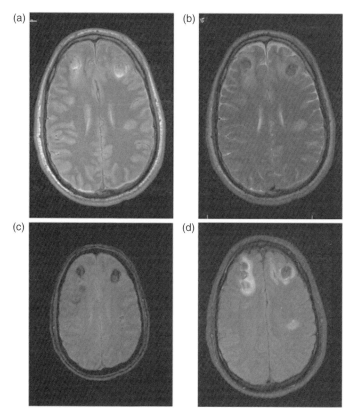

Figure 5.2 MRI of trauma patient with DAI using several different sequences: (a) proton density, (b) T2, (c) gradient echo, (d) FLAIR. Frontal contusions are apparent on all the sequences with the GE showing the highest sensitivity. Images courtesy of V. Newcombe, Wolfson Brain Imaging Centre, University of Cambridge.

be sensitive to blood breakdown products increasing the sensitivity for DAI. Local magnetic field inhomogeneities, caused by the paramagnetic properties of haemosiderin, result in lesions of low intensity following haemorrhage within the brain (Figure 5.2). In addition to T2* GRE the use of ultra-fast sequences such as turbo-Proton Echo Planar Spectroscopic Imaging (t-PEPSI) have shown promise for assessment of DAI.[16] Other gradient echo imaging methods have further improved the detection of haemorrhagic shearing injury. One such sequence, susceptibility weighted imaging (SWI) also utilises the paramagnetic properties of haemorrhagic blood products.[17] SWI has also been shown to be more sensitive for evaluating TBI than conventional MRI,[18] and the outcome of paediatric patients imaged with SWI has been shown to correlate with the number of lesions and numbers of locations affected.[19] MRI is increasingly being used to develop prognostic tools for both adult and paediatric patients. By determining the anatomic locations of visualised injuries, a more informed picture of outcomes can be determined. Brain stem injuries are often not evident on CT scans. Mannion et al.[20] used MRI to classify brain stem injury and determine outcome. They classified injury into three types: I, secondary to supratentorial herniation; II, Severe diffuse brain injury; III, Isolated/remote brain stem injury. Outcome for types I and II were found to be poor while outcome from type III was relatively good. Smitherman et al.[21] have used lesion location and volume to predict outcome in children. Measuring FLAIR lesion volume in three different brain zones was used to predict long-term neurological outcome in the paediatric population. These zones were divided into A: cortical structures; B: basal ganglia, corpus callosum, internal capsule and thalamus; C: brain stem. Findings from this study indicated that lesion volume, multiple zones of injury and anatomic areas correlated with outcome. There was also age-specific findings. Hamdeh et al.[22] have also determined that the lesions in substantia nigra and mesencephalic tegmentum are indicative of poor outcome.

DWI/DTI

Diffusion-weighted imaging (DWI) has been used extensively for various neurological disorders such as stroke and traumatic brain injury. This technique relies upon the difference in diffusion of water molecules in normal and injured brain. Diffusion within the brain is affected by many factors and its measurement has been utilised following ischaemic stroke where a reduction in diffusion is an early sign of tissue injury consistent with cytotoxic oedema. It is thought that the increased intracellular concentration of water associated with cytotoxic oedema is more restricted in movement than the water which was initially extra cellular. In addition, brain regions with vasogenic oedema and an increase in extra-cellular water demonstrate an increase in diffusion.[23] Images of such diffusion are generally displayed as maps of apparent diffusion coefficient (ADC) since signal on DWI images can be affected by T2 and T2* effects. Using ADC maps, regions of restricted diffusion appear dark, while bright regions represent increased diffusion. While not used as commonly as for the investigation of acute stroke, DWI has been used in trauma imaging.[23] DAI imaged by DWI does not have the same sensitivity for haemorrhagic lesions as T2* but does identify additional lesions to those found with T2* and FLAIR.[24-26] Schaefer et al.[27] have shown that signal intensity on DWI correlates with modified Rankin score and that lesions in the corpus callosum also had a strong correlation with Rankin score, although a poor correlation with initial Glasgow Coma Scale. This also applied to other MRI images. The combination of DWI with other MRI sequences may provide additional information about extent of injury and should be included in initial MRI imaging (Figure 5.3). Bradley and Menon[28] have outlined in some detail the diffusion- and perfusion-weighted imaging associated with traumatic brain injury (TBI) and its complex interpretation. Moen et al.[29] have used the burden of lesions in the corpus callosum, brain stem and thalamus on both DWI and FLAIR to predict outcome. Severe injury was highly correlated with DWI lesions in the corpus callosum. Cortical contusions on the other hand were more predictive in moderate injury.

Measurements of water diffusion vary across the brain depending on the direction in which the tissue is examined. Due to the structure of white matter fibre tracts, water diffusion will appear less restricted along fibre tracts compared with perpendicular to the fibre tract. The directionality of diffusion is called anisotropy and is measured by Diffusion Tensor Imaging (DTI)[30,31] (Figure 5.3). DTI has found a role in the imaging of brain tumours and in anatomical studies with mapping of myelinated fibres as they are distorted by space occupying lesions or in the development of immature brain. As with DWI and other MRI techniques its value in trauma is related to DAI. A growing number of researchers have shown that DTI has the capacity to detect white matter changes in TBI that are not seen on conventional scans and give some information regarding prognosis both in severe

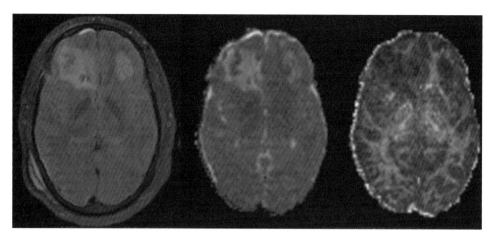

Figure 5.3 MRI of trauma patient using diffusion-weighted imaging. The FLAIR image (left panel) demonstrates a large right frontal and smaller left frontal contusion. The ADC image (middle panel) in the region of the right frontal contusion is composed of tissue with mixed diffusion signal. The bright signal of increased diffusion and the darker signal of restricted diffusion are consistent with vasogenic and cytotoxic oedema, respectively. The fractional anisotropy image (right panel) demonstrates high signal consistent with white matter, with reduced signal within the frontal regions consistent with disruption of the white matter tracts. Images courtesy of V. Newcombe, Wolfson Brain Imaging Centre, University of Cambridge.

and mild TBI.[32–36] Specifically, post-traumatic alteration of white matter organisation and integrity is inferred from fractional anisotropy. Commonly DTI is used to look at regions of interest in injured brain including the corona radiata, fronto-occipital fasciculus, corpus callosum and fornix. Both at the whole brain level and at specific regions of interest, studies have found signs of myelin and axonal injury leading to reduced white matter integrity.[33,37] Furthermore, these changes are predictive of cognitive deficits in executive function, memory and attention.[33,38] Similarly, in the paediatric population DTI has also been correlated with deficits in cognitive processing after injury.[39,40] White matter damage in mild TBI has an association with neuropsychological impairment.[41] Nakayama et al.[42] have been able to show disruption of the corpus callosum and fornix even without lesions identified by other radiological methods, in a severely injured patients with cognitive impairment. The use of DTI and other clinical markers such as GCS and Rankin score also shows correlation.[43] Voss et al.[44] have used DTI in combination with PET to examine two patients in a minimally conscious state. Years after the initial traumatic brain injury clinical improvement was noted with subsequent examination with both DTI and PET suggesting axonal regrowth. The Track-TBI study which examined MRI and CT in mTBI was able to demonstrate prediction of worse outcome measured with Glasgow Outcome Scale-Extended Score.[45]

Functional MRI

Along with research in structural imaging, there is a growing emphasis in characterising and quantifying the effects of TBI in brain function and neuronal connectivity. One such imaging modality to assess cortical function is functional MRI (fMRI). Specifically, it allows assessment of neuronal activity based on the changes in blood flow during a specified action.[46] This is achieved by measuring task-associated changes in blood-oxygen-level-dependent (BOLD) signals which corresponds to changes in metabolic demands of neurons in certain brain regions. In the context of TBI, fMRI studies have revealed altered neuronal activity after injury in various regions such as frontal lobe, anterior cingulate, temporal lobe, cerebellum, insula and parietal lobe.[47] These changes in specific functional networks are shown to correlate with neuropsychological impairments.[48]

A newer form of fMRI called resting-state fMRI utilises BOLD signal acquisition without behavioural task performance. The oscillating patterns of BOLD signals at various regions of the brain are analysed to determine intrinsic functional connections and networks.[49] Studies of TBI patients utilising resting-state fMRI have revealed significant alterations in functional connectivity, specifically the default mode network (DMN) consisting of ventromedial prefrontal cortex, posterior cingulate cortex, lateral parietal cortex and precuneus, after injury.[50–53] Moreover, increase in functional connectivity in the DMN and other networks may reflect the process of brain recovery after TBI.[51] For example, Palacio et al. found greater functional connectivity in regions near the frontal node of the DMN in patients after diffuse TBI which is hypothesised to be a compensatory mechanism against post-traumatic loss of structural connectivity seen in DTI imaging.[53]

PET

Positron emission tomography measures the accumulation of positron-emitting radio-isotopes within the brain.[54,55] These positron-emitting isotopes can be administered via the intravenous or inhalational route, and for imaging of the brain, 15-oxygen (^{15}O) is employed to measure cerebral blood flow (CBF), blood volume, oxygen metabolism (CMRO$_2$) and oxygen extraction fraction (OEF), while 18-fluorodeoxyglucose (^{18}FDG) is used to measure cerebral glucose metabolism (CMRgluc). The emitted positrons are annihilated in a collision with an electron resulting in the release of energy in the form of two photons (gamma rays) released at an angle of 180° to each other. This annihilation energy can be detected externally using coincidence detectors, and the region of each reaction localised within the object by computer algorithms. The images obtained are then generally co-registered with CT or MR to obtain anatomic relationships. Combining this information with other clinical parameters can be used to detect whether blood flow is sufficient to meet the needs of the injured brain. PET is very expensive and time consuming and requires extensive interventional expertise. PET in TBI is used mainly for research, and its use is restricted to a few centres due to its dependence on a co-located cyclotron to produce the short half-life radioisotopes required. However, the technique has proved valuable in the identification of regional ischaemia following head injury. In response to a reduction in blood flow the injured brain increases oxygen extraction to meet energy requirements. Previous ^{15}O PET studies have shown regional pathophysiological derangements consistent with regional ischaemia, especially within the first day post–head injury (Figure 5.4).[56,57] Indeed, using ^{15}O PET the volume of ischaemic brain can be calculated based on the measurement of brain regions which demonstrate a critically high OEF.[56,57] This same research group has shown that regions of ischaemia and hyperaemia can be found within the same patient, demonstrating the heterogeneous nature of derangements in flow metabolism coupling following TBI. In addition, brain regions which are unable to increase oxygen unloading through an increase in OEF may demonstrate tissue hypoxia due to microvascular collapse and perivascular oedema.[57,58] These data suggest that the injured brain may not be able to increase its oxygen extraction

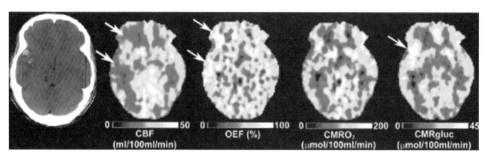

Figure 5.4 Positron emission tomography imaging of regional cerebral ischaemia. CT, PET cerebral blood flow (CBF), oxygen extraction fraction (OEF) and glucose metabolism (CMRgluc) images obtained following early head injury. Note the right temporal haemorrhagic contusion with surrounding rim of hypodensity on the CT. The pericontusional cerebral hemisphere displays a reduction in CBF (white arrows). The slight fall in CMRO$_2$ and large increase in OEF (white arrows) are suggestive of regional cerebral ischaemia. In addition, the increase in CMRgluc surrounding the contusion (white arrow) implies a switch to non-oxidative metabolism of glucose in order to meet underlying metabolic need.

in response to a decrease in blood flow.[59] Numerous reports on cerebral ischaemia and abnormal metabolism following TBI have been published indicating that significant interest remains in improving our understanding of head injury pathophysiology using such research techniques.[56,57,60–63] Recent studies of mTBI have used PET to investigate chronic changes in mTBI after blast injury showing decreased metabolic rates.[64] New techniques have targeted neuroinflammation after injury using ligands for 18 kDa translocator protein.[64] Inflammation was demonstrated months to years after injury.[65,66] There has been considerable work with PET in the area of sport concussion particularly National Football League players.[64]

SPECT/Xe-CT

Single Photon Emission Computed Tomography (SPECT) is a nuclear medicine imaging technique for the evaluation of cerebral blood flow. A radionucleotide is bound to a compound that crosses the blood-brain barrier and is trapped for at least the length of time required to image the patient. Xenon-133 is the most commonly used marker in neuroimaging along with 99 m Tchexamethylpropylene amine oxide (HMPAO), Tc99 m-ethylcysteinate dimer and DatScan for use in different neuronal systems.[67] The uptake of the radiopharmaceutical is imaged by using a gamma camera. SPECT images are of a lower sensitivity than PET, are very sensitive to motion and require a longer imaging time than for MRI. In addition, in the clinical setting SPECT does not provide additional information to MRI for the management of severe traumatic brain-injured patients. In view of these limitations SPECT has largely been replaced by MRI and Xenon CT. However, it has found application in the investigation of mild traumatic brain injury. Mild injury generally does not show structural abnormalities on conventional CT or MRI. In these cases, it is sometimes hard to reconcile residual symptoms such as post-concussive syndrome with the lack of imaging abnormalities. Several studies have demonstrated the presence of SPECT abnormalities in mild injury even without CT abnormality.[67,68] These abnormalities have been found to correlate with loss of consciousness, post-traumatic amnesia and post-concussive syndrome. Software that allow statistical parametric mapping in analysing

SPECT scans to increase objective evaluation may also lead to further development of this technique.[69] By combining results from SPECT scans with neuropsychological impairments further information can be obtained in both mTBI and DAI.[64,70,71]

Xenon-CT is a technique to quantify cerebral blood flow. Its usefulness in imaging traumatic brain injury is important in those cases where CBF is compromised. It does however have the advantage of being both simple and quick to perform (Figure 5.5). Xenon-CT can be used with other techniques to determine the effect of loss of autoregulation during injury and its effect on cerebral perfusion and ICP.[72] This enables interventions to be taken to decrease hyperaemia leading to high ICP. Changes in cerebral blood flow have been correlated with outcome. Several studies have shown correlation of CBF with lowered GOS.[73–75] In one study patient outcome at 6 months could be predicted by quantitative CBF at <6 hours and <12 hours.[75]

For the clinical management of brain injury, CT and MRI are now standards for both acute and subacute care. New techniques are giving us more information about the extent of injury, underlying physiological changes and anatomy. By combining neuroimaging techniques with functional testing, the changes seen on imaging become more relevant. Each of these areas provides ongoing feedback to the other to give us more information about prognosis which even with our best efforts is still not predictable for many patients. Research tools are also providing us with more information about the physiological changes leading to secondary injury, which will hopefully lead to better treatment of this devastating condition. Advances in imaging of mTBI have changed the way we look at mild injury and

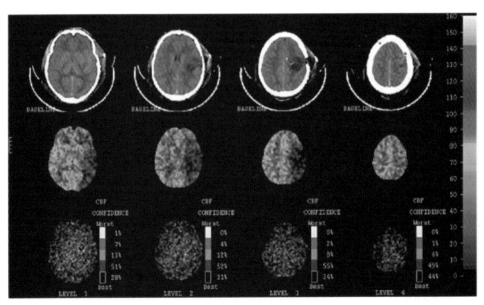

Figure 5.5 Xenon CT of trauma patient. This scan was done to evaluate regional perfusion in a patient with persistent elevated ICP. The patient shows reduced perfusion under a compound depressed skull fracture which had been lifted at surgery. The first row consists of CT images of various levels in the injured brain. Second row is images of corresponding CBF values from 0 to 160 ml/100 g/min according to the colour scale at the right. The third row indicates image quality, with black being highest and white the lowest quality. Courtesy of P. Al-Rawi, University of Cambridge.

have led to a greater understanding of functional changes. By using imaging techniques which rely not just on structural changes but on metabolic and connectivity, we are beginning to understand what injury really means.

References

1. Nguyen R, et al. The international incidence of traumatic brain injury: a systematic review and meta-analysis. *Can J Neurol Sci* 2016;43(6):774–85.

2. Centers for Disease Control and Prevention. *Report to Congress on traumatic brain injury in the United States: epidemiology and rehabilitation*. Atlanta: Centers for Disease Control and Prevention; 2015.

3. Jagoda AS, et al. Clinical policy: neuroimaging and decisionmaking in adult mild traumatic brain injury in the acute setting. *Ann Emerg Med* 2008;52(6): 714–48.

4. Toyama Y, et al. CT for acute stage of closed head injury. *Radiat Med* 2005;23 (5):309–16.

5. Teasdale E, Hadley DM. *Imaging the head injury*. 2nd edn. London: Hodder Educational; 2005.

6. Stiell IG, et al. Comparison of the Canadian CT Head Rule and the New Orleans Criteria in patients with minor head injury. *JAMA* 2005;294(12):1511–18.

7. Smits M, et al. External validation of the Canadian CT Head Rule and the New Orleans Criteria for CT scanning in patients with minor head injury. *JAMA* 2005;294(12):1519–25.

8. Sultan HY, et al. Application of the Canadian CT head rules in managing minor head injuries in a UK emergency department: implications for the implementation of the NICE guidelines. *Emerg Med J* 2004;21(4):420–5.

9. Hassan Z, et al. Head injuries: a study evaluating the impact of the NICE head injury guidelines. *Emerg Med J* 2005;22 (12):845–9.

10. Stiell IG, et al. Canadian CT head rule study for patients with minor head injury: methodology for phase II (validation and economic analysis). *Ann Emerg Med* 2001;38(3):317–22.

11. Marincowitz C, et al. The risk of deterioration in GCS13-15 patients with traumatic brain injury identified by computed tomography imaging: a systematic review and meta-analysis. *J Neurotrauma* 2018;35 (5):703–18.

12. Lee B, Newberg A. Neuroimaging in traumatic brain imaging. *NeuroRx* 2005;2 (2):372–83.

13. Bigler ED, et al. Day-of-injury computerized tomography, rehabilitation status, and development of cerebral atrophy in persons with traumatic brain injury. *Am J Phys Med Rehabil* 2006;85 (10):793–806.

14. Bradley WG Jr. MR appearance of hemorrhage in the brain. *Radiology* 1993;189(1):15–26.

15. Meythaler JM, et al. Current concepts: diffuse axonal injury-associated traumatic brain injury. *Arch Phys Med Rehabil* 2001;82(10):1461–71.

16. Giugni E, et al. Fast detection of diffuse axonal damage in severe traumatic brain injury: comparison of gradient-recalled echo and turbo proton echo-planar spectroscopic imaging MRI sequences. *AJNR Am J Neuroradiol* 2005;26 (5):1140–8.

17. Sehgal V, et al. Clinical applications of neuroimaging with susceptibility-weighted imaging. *J Magn Reson Imaging* 2005;22(4):439–50.

18. Ashwal S, Holshouser BA, Tong KA. Use of advanced neuroimaging techniques in the evaluation of pediatric traumatic brain injury. *Dev Neurosci* 2006;28(4–5): 309–26.

19. Ashwal S, et al. Susceptibility-weighted imaging and proton magnetic resonance spectroscopy in assessment of outcome after pediatric traumatic brain injury.

Arch Phys Med Rehabil 2006;87(12 Suppl 2):S50–8.

20. Mannion RJ, et al. Mechanism-based MRI classification of traumatic brainstem injury and its relationship to outcome. *J Neurotrauma* 2007;24(1):128–35.

21. Smitherman E, et al. Predicting outcome after pediatric traumatic brain injury by early magnetic resonance imaging lesion location and volume. *J Neurotrauma* 2016;33(1):35–48.

22. Abu Hamdeh S, et al. Extended anatomical grading in diffuse axonal injury using mri: hemorrhagic lesions in the substantia nigra and mesencephalic tegmentum indicate poor long-term outcome. *J Neurotrauma* 2017;34(2):341–52.

23. Huisman TA. Diffusion-weighted imaging: basic concepts and application in cerebral stroke and head trauma. *Eur Radiol* 2003;13(10):2283–97.

24. Huisman TA, et al. Diffusion-weighted imaging for the evaluation of diffuse axonal injury in closed head injury. *J Comput Assist Tomogr* 2003;27(1): 5–11.

25. Kinoshita T, et al. Conspicuity of diffuse axonal injury lesions on diffusion-weighted MR imaging. *Eur J Radiol* 2005;56(1):5–11.

26. Ezaki Y, et al. Role of diffusion-weighted magnetic resonance imaging in diffuse axonal injury. *Acta Radiol* 2006;47 (7):733–40.

27. Schaefer PW, et al. Diffusion-weighted MR imaging in closed head injury: high correlation with initial Glasgow Coma Scale score and score on modified Rankin Scale at discharge. *Radiology* 2004;233 (1):58–66.

28. Bradley PG, Menon DK. *Diffusion, perfusion weighted MR imaging in head injury.* 1st edn. Cambridge: Cambridge University Press; 2005.

29. Moen KG, et al. Traumatic axonal injury: the prognostic value of lesion load in corpus callosum, brain stem, and thalamus in different magnetic resonance imaging

sequences. *J Neurotrauma* 2014;31 (17):1486–96.

30. Chan JH, et al. Diffuse axonal injury: detection of changes in anisotropy of water diffusion by diffusion-weighted imaging. *Neuroradiology* 2003;45(1):34–8.

31. Lee JW, Choi CG, Chun MH. Usefulness of diffusion tensor imaging for evaluation of motor function in patients with traumatic brain injury: three case studies. *J Head Trauma Rehabil* 2006;21(3):272–8.

32. Mayer AR, et al. A prospective diffusion tensor imaging study in mild traumatic brain injury. *Neurology* 2010;74(8):643–50.

33. Kraus MF, et al. White matter integrity and cognition in chronic traumatic brain injury: a diffusion tensor imaging study. *Brain* 2007;130(Pt 10):2508–19.

34. Ling JM, et al. Biomarkers of increased diffusion anisotropy in semi-acute mild traumatic brain injury: a longitudinal perspective. *Brain* 2012;135(Pt 4):1281–92.

35. Hulkower MB, et al. A decade of DTI in traumatic brain injury: 10 years and 100 articles later. *AJNR Am J Neuroradiol* 2013;34(11):2064–74.

36. Betz J, et al. Prognostic value of diffusion tensor imaging parameters in severe traumatic brain injury. *J Neurotrauma* 2012;29(7):1292–305.

37. Inglese M, et al. Diffuse axonal injury in mild traumatic brain injury: a diffusion tensor imaging study. *J Neurosurg* 2005;103 (2):298–303.

38. Salmond CH, et al. Diffusion tensor imaging in chronic head injury survivors: correlations with learning and memory indices. *Neuroimage* 2006;29 (1):117–24.

39. Wilde EA, et al. Diffusion tensor imaging in the corpus callosum in children after moderate to severe traumatic brain injury. *J Neurotrauma* 2006;23(10):1412–26.

40. Ewing-Cobbs L, et al. Corpus callosum diffusion anisotropy correlates with neuropsychological outcomes in twins disconcordant for traumatic brain injury.

AJNR Am J Neuroradiol 2006;27 (4):879–81.

41. Veeramuthu V, et al. Diffusion tensor imaging parameters in mild traumatic brain injury and its correlation with early neuropsychological impairment: a longitudinal study. *J Neurotrauma* 2015;32(19):1497–509.

42. Nakayama N, et al. Evidence for white matter disruption in traumatic brain injury without macroscopic lesions. *J Neurol Neurosurg Psychiatry* 2006;77(7):850–5.

43. Huisman TA, et al. Diffusion tensor imaging as potential biomarker of white matter injury in diffuse axonal injury. *AJNR Am J Neuroradiol* 2004;25(3):370–6.

44. Voss HU, et al. Possible axonal regrowth in late recovery from the minimally conscious state. *J Clin Invest* 2006;116(7):2005–11.

45. Yuh EL, et al. Diffusion tensor imaging for outcome prediction in mild traumatic brain injury: a TRACK-TBI study. *J Neurotrauma* 2014;31(17):1457–77.

46. Logothetis NK, et al. Neurophysiological investigation of the basis of the fMRI signal. *Nature* 2001;412(6843):150–7.

47. Eierud C, et al. Neuroimaging after mild traumatic brain injury: review and meta-analysis. *Neuroimage Clin* 2014;4:283–94.

48. Irimia A, Van Horn JD. Functional neuroimaging of traumatic brain injury: advances and clinical utility. *Neuropsychiatr Dis Treat* 2015;11:2355–65.

49. Lang S, Duncan N, Northoff G. Resting-state functional magnetic resonance imaging: review of neurosurgical applications. *Neurosurgery* 2014;74 (5):453–64; discussion 464–5.

50. Hannawi Y, et al. Resting brain activity in disorders of consciousness: a systematic review and meta-analysis. *Neurology* 2015;84(12):1272–80.

51. Sharp DJ, et al. Default mode network functional and structural connectivity after traumatic brain injury. *Brain* 2011;134(Pt 8):2233–47.

52. Bonnelle V, et al. Default mode network connectivity predicts sustained attention deficits after traumatic brain injury. *J Neurosci* 2011;31(38):13442–51.

53. Palacios EM, et al. Resting-state functional magnetic resonance imaging activity and connectivity and cognitive outcome in traumatic brain injury. *JAMA Neurol* 2013;70(7):845–51.

54. Baron JC, et al. Use of PET methods for measurement of cerebral energy metabolism and hemodynamics in cerebrovascular disease. *J Cereb Blood Flow Metab* 1989;9(6):723–42.

55. Coles JP. Imaging after brain injury. *Br J Anaesth* 2007;99(1):49–60.

56. Coles JP, et al. Incidence and mechanisms of cerebral ischemia in early clinical head injury. *J Cereb Blood Flow Metab* 2004;24 (2):202–11.

57. Menon DK, et al. Diffusion limited oxygen delivery following head injury. *Crit Care Med* 2004;32(6):1384–90.

58. Stein SC, et al. Association between intravascular microthrombosis and cerebral ischemia in traumatic brain injury. *Neurosurgery* 2004;54(3):687–91; discussion 691.

59. Pickard JD, et al. Imaging of cerebral blood flow and metabolism in brain injury in the ICU. *Acta Neurochir Suppl* 2005;95:459–64.

60. Cunningham AS, et al. Physiological thresholds for irreversible tissue damage in contusional regions following traumatic brain injury. *Brain* 2005;128 (Pt 8):1931–42.

61. Wu HM, et al. Selective metabolic reduction in gray matter acutely following human traumatic brain injury. *J Neurotrauma* 2004;21(2):149–61.

62. Vespa P, et al. Metabolic crisis without brain ischemia is common after traumatic brain injury: a combined microdialysis and positron emission tomography study. *J Cereb Blood Flow Metab* 2005;25 (6):763–74.

63. Menon DK. Brain ischaemia after traumatic brain injury: lessons from 15O2 positron emission tomography. *Curr Opin Crit Care* 2006;12(2):85–9.

64. Shin SS, et al. Structural imaging of mild traumatic brain injury may not be enough: overview of functional and metabolic imaging of mild traumatic brain injury. *Brain Imaging Behav* 2017;11(2):591–610.

65. Folkersma H, et al. Widespread and prolonged increase in (R)-(11)C-PK11195 binding after traumatic brain injury. *J Nucl Med* 2011;52(8):1235–9.

66. Ramlackhansingh AF, et al. Inflammation after trauma: microglial activation and traumatic brain injury. *Ann Neurol* 2011;70 (3):374–83.

67. Raji CA, Henderson TA. PET and Single-Photon Emission Computed Tomography in Brain Concussion. *Neuroimaging Clin N Am* 2018;28 (1):67–82.

68. Gowda NK, et al. Technetium Tc-99 m ethyl cysteinate dimer brain single-photon emission CT in mild traumatic brain injury: a prospective study. *AJNR Am J Neuroradiol* 2006;27(2):447–51.

69. Shin YB, et al. Voxel-based statistical analysis of cerebral blood flow using Tc-99 m ECD brain SPECT in patients with traumatic brain injury: group and individual analyses. *Brain Inj* 2006;20 (6):661–7.

70. Romero K, et al. Old wine in new bottles: validating the clinical utility of SPECT in predicting cognitive performance in mild traumatic brain injury. *Psychiatry Res* 2015;231(1):15–24.

71. Uruma G, Hashimoto K, Abo M. A new method for evaluation of mild traumatic brain injury with neuropsychological impairment using statistical imaging analysis for Tc-ECD SPECT. *Ann Nucl Med* 2013;27(3):187–202.

72. Poon WS, et al. Cerebral blood flow (CBF)-directed management of ventilated head-injured patients. *Acta Neurochir Suppl* 2005;95:9–11.

73. Inoue Y, et al. Changes in cerebral blood flow from the acute to the chronic phase of severe head injury. *J Neurotrauma* 2005;22 (12):1411–18.

74. Fridley J, Robertson C, Gopinath S. Quantitative lobar cerebral blood flow for outcome prediction after traumatic brain injury. *J Neurotrauma* 2015;32(2):75–82.

75. Kaloostian P, et al. Outcome prediction within twelve hours after severe traumatic brain injury by quantitative cerebral blood flow. *J Neurotrauma* 2012;29(5):727–34.

Scoring Systems for Trauma and Head Injury

Laura White, Antoinette Edwards and Fiona Lecky

Trauma care systems deal with patients who have an infinite variety of injuries requiring complex treatment. The assessment of such systems is a major challenge in clinical measurement and audit. Which systems are most effective in delivering best outcomes? Implementing recommendations for improved procedures will often incur additional costs – will the expense be worthwhile? Clearly, case-mix-adjusted outcome analysis must replace anecdote and dogma. Outcome prediction in trauma is a developing science that enables the assessment of trauma system effectiveness. This chapter will review some of the commonly used scoring systems and their particular applications in patients with traumatic brain injury.

The effects of injury can be defined in terms of *input* an anatomical component, the physiological response, and *outcome* – mortality and morbidity. These must be coded numerically to enable measurement before we can comment with confidence on the quality of treatment or process of care. Older people survive trauma less well than children and younger adults; therefore age and comorbidity must be taken into account and the association between gender and age is also considered to be important. Most recent work has been concerned with the measurement of injury severity and its relation to mortality.

Input Measures

Severity of injury is assessed through the anatomical component and the physiological response. These two elements are scored separately.

Anatomical Scoring System

The abbreviated injury scale (AIS), first published in 1969, is anatomically based. There is a single AIS severity score – threat to life – for each injury a patient may sustain. Scores range from 1 (minor) to 6 (incompatible with life) (Table 6.1).

There are more than 2000 injuries listed in both the AIS 2005 (update 08) and 2015 dictionaries.[1] The AIS 2015 dictionary was released in 2017 and is the sixth edition. Intervals between the scores are not always consistent – for example the difference between AIS3 and AIS4 in terms of threat to life is not necessarily the same as that between AIS1 and AIS2. (Copies of the booklet are available from www.aaam.org.)

Patients with multiple injuries are scored by adding together the squares of the three highest AIS scores in three predetermined regions of the body. This is the injury severity score (ISS; Table 6.2). Scores of 7 and 15 are unattainable because these figures cannot be obtained from summing squares. The maximum score is 75 (25 + 25 + 25). By convention, a patient with an AIS6 in one body region is also given an ISS of 75. The injury severity score

Table 6.1 Examples of injuries scored by the Abbreviated Injury Scale[1]

Injury	Score
Shoulder pain (no injury specified)	Not coded
Wrist sprain	1 (Minor)
Closed distal tibial fracture	2 (Moderate)
>3 ribs fractured	3 (Serious)
Laceration of thoracic aorta with blood loss <20%	4 (Severe)
Complex (grade V) liver laceration	5 (Critical)
Laceration of the brain stem	6 (Incompatible with life)

Table 6.2 Injury severity score (ISS)

To obtain this:
- Use the AIS05 (update 08) dictionary to score every injury
- Identify the highest AIS score in each of the following six areas of the body:

1 head, neck and cervical spine
2 face
3 chest and thoracic spine
4 abdomen, lumbar spine and pelvic contents
5 bony pelvis and extremities
6 external injuries

- Add together the squares of the highest AIS scores in three body areas

is non-linear, and there is pronounced variation in the frequency of different scores; 9 and 16 are common, 14 and 22 unusual.[2]

Case Study

A man is injured in a fall from a ladder while at work. He is disorientated on arrival; his mandible appears unstable and he has difficulty breathing. There is no external haemorrhage. There are abrasions around the left temple, left shoulder, left side of the chest and left knee. After a rapid sequence intubation, a CT brain scan shows a large subdural haematoma.

Radiographic examination of the cervical spine suggests no abnormality. There is a comminuted fracture of the body of the mandible. There are also fractures of the left wrist, and left ribs (4–9) with a flail segment (Table 6.3).

For the purpose of the analysis described here, the ISS should be calculated only from injuries described by operative findings, imaging investigations or post-mortem reports. The ISS is an ordinal scale; therefore the overall score for a cohort of patients should be described by the median value and the interquartile range, rather than the mean. As 30% of patients with severe traumatic brain injury will have significant other injuries, a global anatomical scoring system needs to be used as extracranial injuries will have a significant bearing on outcome.

Table 6.3 Case study

Injury	AIS score
Comminuted fracture of body of mandible	2
Fracture of distal radius (not further specified)	2
Fracture of ribs 4–9 with flail segment	4
Abrasions (all sites)	1
Subdural haematoma (>1 cm thickness)	5
AIS05 (update 08), abbreviated injury scale ISS = $5^2 + 4^2 + 2^2 = 45$	

There are other ways of combining AIS values such as A Severity Characterization Of Trauma (ASCOT) and the New Injury Severity Score (NISS).[3,4] International Classification of Disease codes can be adapted to ISS scores but, in general, lack sufficient clinical detail, particularly for brain injury. ISS therefore remains the gold standard for scoring the anatomical severity of injury in multiply injured patients.

Physiological Scoring Systems

Historically, the physiological responses of an injured patient have been assessed by the revised trauma score (RTS). The physiological parameters that make up the RTS are respiratory rate, systolic blood pressure and Glasgow Coma Scale (GCS). The RTS was developed following statistical analysis of a large North American database to determine the most predictive independent outcome variables. Selection of variables was also influenced by their ease of measurement and clinical opinion. In practice the RTS is a complex calculation combining coded measurements of the three physiological values multiplied by a weighting factor, for each variable, derived from regression analysis of the database.

After injury, the patient's physiological response is constantly changing but for the purposes of injury scoring, and by convention, the first measurements, when the patient arrives at hospital, are used. If the patient is intubated before arrival, a RTS cannot be measured.

Current Practice

European research has shown the GCS to be the most valuable physiological predictor in trauma patients at the time of Emergency Department presentation.[5,12] If the patient is intubated before arrival, a GCS measured at the scene of the incident can be used. Most trauma predictive models use the full GCS on arrival at the Emergency Department as physiological predictors.[6] TBI predictive models have been reviewed and used either the full GCS or the motor value of the GCS; however, the timing of the latter is variable.[7–9] Various modifications of the scale have been suggested for use in small children. Some doctors reduce the maximum score to that which is consistent with neurological maturation. A more useful clinical device, which ensures more accurate communication and simplifies epidemiological research, is to retain the maximum score of 15 but redefine the descriptions.[10]

Trauma Outcome Prediction Methodology

The degree of physiological derangement and the extent of anatomical injury are measures of the threat to life. Mortality will also be affected by the age, gender and comorbid status of the patient.

Traditionally, the 'TRISS methodology' combined four elements – the revised trauma score (RTS), the injury severity score (ISS), the patient's age and whether the injury was blunt or penetrating – to provide a measure of the probability of survival.[11] From the database of the Trauma Audit & Research Network (TARN) the outcome prediction model has evolved[12] to reflect the characteristics of the European trauma population and specifically includes:

- outcome (survival or death) measured both at 30 days or discharge (whichever is soonest) and 'true 30 day' outcome, based on ONS (Office of National Statistics) data linkage.
- GCS is now the only physiological marker used, where GCS is missing intubation is used (in intubated patients) with an appropriate weighting. Where both GCS and presence of intubation are missing, GCS is imputed; imputation is based on patients with a similar profile on the TARN database. The addition of imputation means that all patients are now included in the outcome prediction model.
- as the age-related increases in mortality are more pronounced for males, the model incorporates an age/gender interaction.
- comorbidities are included and a modified version of the Charlson Comorbidity Index (mCCI) was developed to assign weightings to certain medical conditions.

In order to achieve the best statistical model, there must be a balance between accurate prediction rates and clinical 'face validity'. The data used for the model's development must also reflect 'real-world' data. Over the years, the statistical modelling work at TARN has reflected these concerns.

The probability of survival (**Ps**) of each injured patient is calculated using the following six factors:

· Age · Gender · Age Gender interaction · Glasgow Coma Scale · Injury Severity Score · Co-morbidities

It is important to realise that **Ps** is a mathematical calculation; it is not an absolute measure of mortality but only an indication of the probability of survival. If a patient with a **Ps** of 80% dies, the outcome is unexpected because four out of five patients with such a **Ps** would be expected to survive. However, the fifth would be expected to die – and this could be the patient under study. The **Ps** is used as a filter for highlighting patients for study in multidisciplinary trauma audit rather than a categoric identification of an 'unexpected death implying poor care'.

Outcome Prediction in Traumatic Brain Injury (TBI)

It is clearly possible to use this approach to create a prognostic model for brain-injured patients. Guidelines for appraising the quality of prognostic models in health care are published elsewhere.[13] The anatomical, physiological and demographic variables used in a TBI model will depend on the setting and functional requirements of the model. For example, if a prognostic model is to be used for clinical audit and benchmarking, then it is

Table 6.4 Common 'independent' prognostic variables in published traumatic brain injury outcome prediction models (predicting outcome)

	Comments
Age	Present in more accurate models, predicting death or death and disability
GCS or motor GCS	Present in all accurate models
Blood pressure	Present in recent models
Hypoxaemia	Present in recent models
Pupillary reactivity	Present in all models
Pupillary size	Present in one European model
Oculocephalic reflex	Present infrequently
Mechanism of Injury	Present infrequently
ISS	Present in most models
CT classification	Present in models not using AIS/ISS
Intracranial haematoma	Present infrequently
Subarachnoid haemorrhage	Present as separate variable in models using CT classification
Midline shift	Present infrequently

Note: Most models have studied only patients with moderate and severe TBI, lesser injuries are incorporated in general trauma models such as TARN.
Source: Summarised from Perel et al.[7]

reasonable to include the ISS as the prognosis is calculated once all the specific injury details are known. The same model is more difficult to use early in the patient's clinical course when the full injury descriptions from imaging and surgery, needed for ISS derivations, may not be available.

The utility of clinical variables will vary depending on the setting in which they are used, for example the GCS provides good discrimination and outcome prediction when applied to the whole population of patients with head injury presenting to an emergency department.[14] The motor GCS is likely to be more useful and indeed more reliably measured if the subset of TBI patients to be studied are those ventilated on intensive care units. Table 6.4 summarises the factors that have been found to have some prognostic ability for outcome after TBI in a systematic review of prognostic models.[7] These factors have also been incorporated into more recent studies of TBI prognosis[15] and have informed the current large studies of TBI occurring worldwide such as the Collaborative European Neurotrauma Effectiveness Research in Traumatic Brain Injury study (www.center-tbi.eu).

Comparing Systems of Trauma Care

Comparison of the probabilities of survival of all patients seen at a particular hospital with the observed outcome can be used as an index of overall performance. Probabilities of survival are combined in the 'standardised W statistic' (**Ws**) to assess a group of patients.[16]

This provides a measure of the number of excess survivors, or deaths, for every 100 patients treated at each hospital accounting for different mixes of injury severity, age and other factors in the model. The 95% confidence limits of Ws provide a measure of its statistical significance.

A positive **Ws** is desirable as this indicates that more patients are surviving than would be predicted from the patient profile (Ps model factors) of a hospital over a given time period methodology. Conversely, a negative **Ws** signifies that the system of trauma care has fewer survivors than expected from the Ps model predictions. Consequently, hospitals have the opportunity to evaluate their trauma care systems through comparative national audit and improve care provided where needed (www .tarn.ac.uk/performance). Clearly data quality is key to the reliability of these measures of excess survival rates

Applications of Trauma Outcome Prediction

The outcome prediction method developed by TARN is now used in England, Wales, Northern and the Republic of Ireland to audit the effectiveness of systems of trauma care and the management of individual patients. The model has been applied to TBI patients with the addition of a pupillary response variable. A recent TARN/Society of British Neurosurgeons Publication demonstrated consistent outcomes within English Neuroscience centres.[17] The probability of survival methodology is currently applied in all patients with trauma who are admitted to hospital for 3 days or more managed in an intensive care area (for any time period), referred for specialist care or who die in hospital. Additional information is sought on the process and timing of care interventions and length of stay.

It is important that an evolving outcome prediction model reflects the changing trauma and TBI patient demographic. Comorbidities are included in the current TARN model; however, with evidence of an increasingly ageing trauma population, other factors such as frailty need to be considered (www.tarn.ac.uk/Content.aspx?c=3793).

TARN provides a valuable method of comparing patterns of care in different parts of the country. It is reliant on careful collection of data in a consistent format to allow collation and comparison of results. Deaths caused by trauma are too varied, too complicated and too important to be discussed in isolation in individual hospitals.

The wider perspective of TARN is increasingly recognised as a valid approach to trauma audit and has been adopted by regional and national bodies. However, identification of deficiencies is valuable only if a mechanism exists to correct them. Local & Network wide audit meetings and national comparisons must be used to stimulate appropriate changes in systems of trauma care.

The original development of the TRISS and latterly the probability of survival methodologies have been a major advance in the benchmarking of trauma care. The detailed structure of the scales and the method of developing a single number to represent threat to life are under constant review.

European trauma registries have collaborated through the EuroTARN initiative to compare crude outcomes (percentage mortality) in similar groups of patients[18] followed by the development of the Utstein Template for uniform reporting of data following major trauma.[19] Measurement of outcome in terms of survival or death is, however, a crude yardstick.

Further progress is required in measuring disability as little is known about the long-term outcome and quality of life of both adults and children following injury. Most life-threatening visceral injuries leave the patient with little disability. Disability after musculoskeletal and brain injury is more common; however, many studies of disability suffer from losses to follow-up. Furthermore, it is uncertain whether the Glasgow Outcome Scale, commonly used in brain injury studies, adequately addresses the impact of extracranial injury on disability outcome.[20]

Patient Reported Outcome Measures (PROMs) is a method of collecting patient's views on their functional outcome and health-related quality of life. Collected at different time points, PROMs is traditionally used to measure long-term recovery after elective procedures.[21] Commissioned by NHS England, TARN have developed a PROM specifically for trauma and are currently collecting 6 month outcomes of patients treated at Major Trauma Centres (both adults and children including those with brain injuries). Although findings are yet to be published, patient response rates are encouraging and hospitals now receive routine reports that highlight patients that report severe to extreme problems in their quality of life at 6 months. Refinement of the PROMs process continues; however, measuring long-term outcomes after trauma is certainly achievable.

Summary

Scoring systems for trauma have been developed which have facilitated the development of outcome prediction models, case mix adjustment and trauma system benchmarking. For trauma in England, Wales, Northern and Republic of Ireland, there is consensus that a TRISS or TRISS-like model such as the TARN Ps should be used. These models should contain measurement of host vulnerability (age, gender, comorbidities), anatomical severity of injury (ISS) and physiological derangement (GCS).

There are many traumatic brain injury prognostic models in the literature that use different combinations of variables. The gold standard is work in progress, but seems likely to include the types of scoring systems and variables used in general trauma models plus assessment of pupillary reactivity.

Further details of TARN can be obtained from www.tarn.ac.uk

References

1. Committee on Injury Scaling, Association for the Advancement of Automotive Medicine. The Abbreviated injury scale 2005 revision (2008 update). Des Plaines, IL; 2005.

2. Baker SP, O'Neill B. The injury severity score: an update. *J Trauma* 1976;16:882–5.

3. Champion HR, Copes WS, Sacco WJ, et al. Improved predictions from A Severity Characterization of Trauma (ASCOT) over Trauma and Injury Severity Score (TRISS): results of an independent evaluation. *J Trauma* 1996;40:42–9.

4. Osler TMD, Baker SPMPH, Long WMD. A modification of the Injury Severity Score that both improves accuracy and simplifies scoring. *J Trauma* 1997;43:922–6.

5. Bouamara O, Wrotchford AS, Hollis S, Vail A, Woodford M, Lecky FE. A new approach to outcome prediction in trauma: a comparison with the TRISS model. *J Trauma* 2006;61: 701–10.

6. Champion HR, Sacco WJ, Copes WS, Gann DS, Gennarelli TA, Flanagan ME. A revision of the Trauma Score. *J Trauma* 1989;29:623–9.

7. Perel P, Edwards P, Wentz R, Roberts I. Systematic review of prognostic models in traumatic brain injury. *BMC Med Inform Decision Making* 2006;6:38.

8. Jennett B, Teasdale G. Aspects of coma after severe head injury. *Lancet.* 1977;1:878–81.

9. Healey C, Osler T, Rogers F, et al. Improving the Glasgow Coma Score scale: motor score alone is a better predictor. *J Trauma* 2003;54:671–80.

10. Teasdale J. The Child's Glasgow Coma Scale has evolved from adaptations to Jennett and Teasdale's Glasgow Coma Scale. *Lancet* 1977;1:878–81.

11. Champion HC, Copes WS, Sacco WJ, et al. The Major Trauma Outcome Study: establishing national norms for trauma care. *J Trauma* 1990;30:1356–65.

12. Bouamra O, Jacques R, Edwards A, Yates DW, Lawrence T, Jenks T, Woodford MI, Lecky F. Prediction modelling for trauma using comorbidity and 'true' 30-day outcome. *Emerg Med J* 2015;32(12):933–8.

13. Altman DG, Royston P. What do we mean by validating a prognostic model? *Stat Med* 2000;19:453–73.

14. Stiell IG, Wells GA, Vandemheen K, et al. The Canadian CT head rule for patients with minor head injury. *Lancet* 2001;357:1391–6.

15. Roozenbeek B, Lingsma HF, Lecky FE, Lu J, Weir J, Butcher I, McHugh GS, Murray GD, Perel P, Maas AIR, Steyerberg EW. Prediction of outcome after moderate and severe traumatic brain injury: external validation of the IMPACT and CRASH prognostic models *Crit Care Med* 2012;40(5):1609–17.

16. Hollis S, Yates DW, Woodford M, Foster P. Standardised comparison of performance indicators in trauma: a new approach to case-mix variation. *J Trauma* 1995;38:763–6.

17. Lawrence T, Helmy A, Bouamra O, Woodford M, Lecky F, Hutchinson, PJ. *Traumatic brain injury in England and Wales Epidemiology: complications and standardised mortality BMJ Open* 2016;6: e01219718.

18. EuroTARN Writing Committee on behalf of the EuroTARN Group. A comparison of European Trauma Registries: the first report from the EuroTARN Group. *Resuscitation* 2007;75:286–97.

19. Ringdal KG, Coats TJ, Lefering R, Di Bartolomeo S, Steen PA, Røise O, Handolin L. Hans Morten Lossius and Utstein TCD expert panel: the Utstein template for uniform reporting of data following major trauma: a joint revision by SCANTEM, TARN, DGU-TR and RITG. *Scand J Trauma Resuscitation Emerg Med* 2008;16:7.

20. Jennett B, Bond M. Assessment of outcome after severe brain damage: a practical scale. *Lancet* 1975;1: 480–4.

21. Black N. Patient reported outcome measures could help transform healthcare. *BMJ* 2013;346:f167.

Early Phase Care of Patients with Mild and Minor Head Injury

Anthony Kehoe

Introduction

Mild traumatic brain injury (mTBI) is a common presentation to the Emergency Department (ED). In most cases patients can be assessed and discharged the same day with reassurance that within a short period any residual symptoms will resolve. However, for a sizeable minority of patients diagnosed with mTBI, the term can seem a cruel misnomer. Many will suffer with a constellation of debilitating symptoms including fatigue, irritability, lability of mood, inability to concentrate, headache, dizziness, sensitivity to noise and light, depression and anxiety.[1] Although in most, these symptoms will subside within 3 months; in up to 30% of patients with mTBI, they can persist well beyond 6 months.[2] The consequences for quality of life, relationships and employment can be devastating.

This 'silent epidemic' of mTBI is slowly starting to be tackled. Advances in our understanding of the underlying pathophysiology at microscopic level offer the tantalising prospect of novel pharmacological targets in the near future.[3] The development of new diagnostic strategies involving advanced imaging and serum biomarkers of tissue injury should soon allow better identification of individuals at risk.[4,5] Meanwhile, raising awareness of mTBI amongst front-line clinicians in primary care and emergency departments will improve screening for those with established problems, although better resourcing of multi-disciplinary clinics where their specific needs can be addressed will also be required.

Definition of mTBI

Patients are traditionally categorised as having mTBI (as opposed to moderate or severe TBI) if they have:

- A period of initial unconsciousness ranging from transient to less than 30 min
- No Glasgow Coma Scale (GCS) score thereafter of less than 13
- No anterograde post-traumatic amnesia lasting longer than 24 hours

The simplicity of this definition is attractive; however, there are inherent problems with this functional definition. GCS score does not reflect the anatomical severity of injury uniformly across all age groups. Older patients with TBI seem able to accommodate a greater volume of intracranial haematoma before GCS becomes impaired, a finding most likely to be explained by increasing cerebral atrophy.[5] Thus a definition that does not include macroscopic injury identified during initial CT scan may fail to identify patients with an increased risk of long-term complications.

Box 7.1 Mayo Traumatic Brain Injury (TBI) Classification System

A. Classify as *Moderate–Severe (Definite) TBI* if one or more of the following criteria apply:

1. Death due to this TBI
2. Loss of consciousness of 30 min or more
3. Post-traumatic anterograde amnesia of 24 hours or more
4. Worst Glasgow Coma Scale full score in first 24 hours < 13
   (unless invalidated upon review, e.g. attributable to intoxication, sedation, systemic shock)
5. One or more of the following present:

   i. Intracerebral haematoma
   ii. Subdural haematoma
   iii. Epidural haematoma
   iv. Cerebral contusion
   v. Haemorrhagic contusion
   vi. Penetrating TBI (dura penetrated)
   vii. Subarachnoid haemorrhage
   viii. Brain stem injury

B. If none of Criteria A apply, classify as *Mild (Probable) TBI* if one or more of the following criteria apply:

1. Loss of consciousness momentarily to less than 30 min
2. Post-traumatic anterograde amnesia momentarily to less than 24 h
3. Depressed, basilar or linear skull fracture (dura intact)

C. If none of Criteria A or B apply, classify as *Symptomatic (Possible) TBI* if one or more of the following symptoms are present:

1. Blurred vision
2. Confusion (mental state changes)
3. Daze
4. Dizziness
5. Focal neurological symptoms
6. Headache
7. Nausea

The Mayo classification of traumatic brain injury incorporates intracranial findings on CT alongside clinical features and categorises patients into definite, probable and suspected TBI categories (Box 7.1).[6]

Under this classification, patients with initial GCS score of 13–15 and resolution of post-traumatic amnesia within 24 hours but who have macroscopic evidence of intracranial injury on CT would be classified as having moderate-severe (definite) TBI. This group of patients is sometimes referred to as having 'complicated mTBI'. Patients in this group are more likely to benefit from admission to hospital for a period of observation and should ideally be cared for in a suitable setting where a full assessment of rehabilitation needs can be completed. In major trauma centres this may be a neurosurgical ward, but for patients presenting to other hospitals, suitable facilities often exist on stroke units.

Patients identified by the Mayo classification as having mild (probable) TBI or symptomatic (possible) TBI are likely to be discharged home once GCS score has returned to 15 and any post-traumatic amnesia has resolved. It is rare for patients in these groups to have any specific follow-up arranged, yet a significant proportion will go on to develop disabling symptoms. It is therefore in this group that improved diagnostic strategies may yield the greatest benefits.

Epidemiology of mTBI

It is difficult to be exact about the incidence of head injury as many patients at the milder end of the injury spectrum will present to primary care surgeries or minor injury units. In the UK it was estimated that in the 1970s there were around 1 million attendances to emergency departments with head injury per year.[7] More recently NICE have quoted a figure of around 700 000 attendances per year in England and Wales which corresponds to 1200 attendances per 100 000 population[8] with even higher rates in other European countries.[9] The overwhelming majority of such injuries, around 90%, will be classified as mild.

Since the advent of major trauma networks in England in 2012, the accuracy of national trauma data collection has improved markedly.[10] Most noticeably, there has been a surge in the reporting of major trauma in the elderly. Patients from 75 to 100 years now represent the age group most commonly recorded as sustaining major trauma and falls from standing height have recently overtaken road traffic collisions as the most frequently occurring mechanism of injury.[11] Around 75% of older patients with major trauma have TBI.[12] Compared with younger patients, older patients are less likely to receive care in a neurosciences centre, average time to initial CT increases with age and outcomes are much worse.[12] However presenting GCS in older patients with TBI can be surprisingly high. A recent study using the UK trauma registry found that the median presenting GCS in older patients with anatomically severe TBI (Abbreviated injury scale 5 (out of 6) usually indicating a large mass lesion with midline shift) was 14.[13] Such patients meet the standard definition of mTBI.

TBI is also a significant problem in children. A national confidential report from 2012 published findings from an analysis of the records of children (age under 15 years) presenting to UK hospitals with head injury over a 6 month period.[14] More than half of the cases were of children less than 5 years old, with a peak incidence in infancy. Just over 60% were boys and the male:female ratio increased with age. The incidence of head injury was associated with increasing social deprivation. Falls accounted for 60% of all presentations with head injury with sports and recreational injuries the next largest group at 13.7%. The high rate of brief hospital admission (88%) and low rate of CT scanning (30%) reflect a suitably cautious approach to managing head injuries in children and a desire to minimise potentially harmful radiation exposure.

Pathophysiology

In mTBI, the primary injury may result from direct impact or from acceleration/deceleration or rotational shearing forces. As in other severities of TBI, secondary injury then develops, driven by local inflammation.[15,16] In animal studies, the penumbra around the primary injury is rich in signalling molecules which activate inflammatory and immunomodulatory cascades.[17] Within hours, local oedema and endothelial dysfunction develop and coagulopathy can occur which contribute to the haemorrhagic progression of small contusions.[18] Microglial activation drives further inflammation and apoptosis occurs. Demyelination is detectable from myelin breakdown products within the first 3 days, which contributes to damage in the white-matter tracts.[19]

Animal models suggest that the first few hours represent the window in which pharmacological intervention to prevent damaging neuroinflammation is most likely to be beneficial.[20] Numerous agents have been tested, both novel compounds and existing drugs such as statins, erythropoietin analogues and angiotensin-receptor blockers repurposed for their putative neuroprotective properties.[20–23] While several have shown benefits in reducing inflammation and lesion size and even improving functional outcomes in animal models of mTBI, none have yet proved beneficial in clinical trials involving humans. One of the largest ongoing studies, CRASH-3, which is investigating tranexamic acid in TBI, will shortly complete recruitment.[24] The inclusion criteria have allowed the recruitment of many patients meeting the definition of complicated mTBI, enabling analysis of outcomes in this subgroup.

Clinical Evaluation and Diagnostic Strategies

Mild TBI can be a difficult diagnosis to make with certainty. It is rare for patients to present at hospital within 30 min of injury, so by definition unconsciousness should have resolved in mTBI before arrival. In some cases, an element of 'concussion' will persist. This may be manifest as confusion, disorientation, repetitive speech and sometimes agitation, but in many cases clinical signs will have largely resolved on arrival at the emergency department. Common presenting symptoms include headache, nausea and dizziness.[25]

The diagnostic strategy could be considered to have two principal components, one relatively straightforward, the other much more challenging and nuanced. The initial priority is to rapidly identify patients with a neurosurgically important TBI or those with the highest risk of neurological deterioration. Subsequently, the much greater challenge is to identify those patients with few or no abnormalities detected on initial imaging who have a higher risk of developing long-term problems.[26] This is a developing area and there are emerging techniques using specialist MRI[27] and serum biomarkers of injury[28] that have not yet made it into routine clinical practice, alongside cognitive screening tools that can be employed currently.

Clinical Evaluation

On arrival in the emergency department, a full history and examination will be undertaken, with particular emphasis on the mechanism of injury and a detailed neurological examination. An eye-witness account is invaluable to understand the impact forces and details of any subsequent period of unconsciousness. A thorough examination to detect associated injuries should be undertaken, particularly of the cervical spine. When required, resuscitation should follow standard principles and particular attention should be paid to avoiding hypotension and hypoxia.[29]

Serial neurological observations comprising GCS, pupil size and reactivity, limb movements, pulse rate, respiratory rate and blood pressure, temperature and blood oxygen saturations should be undertaken at regular intervals. National Institute of Clinical Excellence (NICE) guidance recommends half-hourly until GCS 15 is achieved and then half-hourly for a further 2 hours, hourly for the next 4 hours and 2 hourly thereafter.[8]

Imaging Strategy

Validated tools such as NICE head injury guidance[8] or the Canadian CT rules[30] are used in most emergency departments to identify patients who require prompt imaging. CT is a rapid and widely available imaging modality and will identify nearly all patients with significant intracranial bleeding. Extradural haematoma, subdural haematoma, subarachnoid haemorrhage and brain contusion are relatively easy to detect. Patients with these injuries have the highest risk of clinical deterioration within the acute period and should be admitted to a suitable area for frequent neurological observations.[31] Special consideration should be given to patients on anticoagulant or anti-platelet therapy with a careful assessment of the risks and benefits of reversal tailored to each case.[32]

In most acute clinical situations, patients with no abnormality detected on CT scanning will not undergo further neuroimaging. The diagnostic goal is to identify patients with an injury that might require neurosurgical intervention rather than to diagnose mTBI *per se*. Conventional mode MRI investigation adds little additional information to CT and is therefore seldom used acutely, due to the additional cost and time involved. However, the increased recognition of the subsequent burden of disease in patients with mTBI and a negative initial CT scan has provided some impetus to develop diagnostic strategies to identify those patients at the highest risks of long-term complications during their acute presentation. Specialist MRI techniques such as Diffusion Tensor Imaging (DTI), functional MRI (fMRI) and susceptibility weighted imaging (SWI) may have a role in identifying subtle axonal and vascular injuries that are invisible to CT yet correlate with worse outcome.[33]

It has been postulated that frontal areas of the brain are particularly susceptible to damage in mTBI.[34] Meta-analyses of results reported in advanced MRI imaging studies have revealed some consistent changes that are correlated with short- and long-term outcomes.[35] Changes in cerebral blood flow during the acute phase can be detected by fMRI.[36] Reduced activity is consistently reported in areas of the frontal region involved in higher cognitive functions, including working memory. Meanwhile, increased activity is demonstrated in some areas of the cerebellum which are also important for working memory, executive functions, behavioural control and postural balance.[37]

Perhaps the most promising MRI technique is DTI which can give an indication of disruption to the microstructure of axonal tracts in the white matter.[34] During the acute phase of injury increased anisotropy can be detected, most commonly in frontal areas, whereas more chronically, decreased anisotropy is revealed.[38] These techniques have yet to become part of routine assessment of patients with mTBI in the emergency department, but many already advocate that they should represent the standard of care.[33]

Serum Biomarkers

Tissue damage occurring at a microscopic level in mTBI is likely to drive local secondary injury processes like inflammation, oedema and vascular changes.[16] Such damage may be revealed by serum injury biomarkers which may help to identify patients at higher risk of short- and long-term complications.[5]

S100B is a calcium-binding peptide found in glial cells and is the most comprehensively studied serum biomarker in patients with mTBI. Glial fibrillary acidic protein (GFAP) and ubiquitin C-terminal hydrolase L1 (UCH-L1) are also emerging as candidate serum biomarkers in mTBI. All are detectable within the first few hours of injury and acute elevations reliably predict the presence of intracranial lesions on CT.[39,40] The 6 hour concentration of S100B can also help to predict the likelihood of developing post-concussive symptoms at 1 month,[41] and an elevated GFAP within the first 24 hours is associated with failure to return to baseline function at 6 months.[42]

TRACK-TBI[43] and CENTER-TBI,[44] from the USA and Europe, respectively, are landmark studies due to report their main findings in the near future. Part of their objectives will be to correlate serial imaging and serum biomarker findings with outcomes across the spectrum of severity in TBI. This should help to define what role, if any, serum biomarkers should play in the clinical management of mTBI in the emergency department. Although biomarkers have considerable promise for case identification and prognostication, they remain a long way from routine clinical use at present.

Neurocognitive Screening

There are numerous, validated neurocognitive testing tools available to clinicians. They are most commonly employed a period of weeks or months following initial injury with patients in whom post-concussive symptoms have already developed. However, there is considerable research interest in identifying screening tools that can predict higher-risk patients before they have been discharged from the emergency department. The Galveston Orientation Amnesia Test (GOAT) and Rivermead Post Concussion Survey Questionnaire (RPCSQ) have both been studied in this acute setting. The GOAT consists of questions within 11 domains. Any errors are summed and then subtracted from 100 to derive the final score. Scores of less than 75 indicate the presence of post-traumatic amnesia. The RPCSQ is a 30 question instrument that generates scores from 0 to 65. In one study lower GOAT scores in the ED were significantly associated with the need for hospitalisation and the development of post-concussive symptoms at late follow-up, while higher RPCSQ scores were associated with hospitalisation and the development of early symptoms.[45]

Computer-based neurocognitive assessment tools also show promise for screening patients in the ED. Many have been developed from sports medicine where they have been used to monitor the severity of concussion in athletes and provide an objective assessment of when it is safe to return to contact sport, often using a pre-injury assessment of the individual athlete as a baseline. One such, the Immediate Post-concussion Assessment and Cognitive Test (ImPACT™), combines demographic data with a survey of post-concussive symptoms and six neuropsychological tests to derive a composite score reported in five domains. This test has been applied to a sample of children presenting to an ED within 12 hours of a head injury and the results compared to existing normative data. There was a strong correlation between the results of initial testing and ImPACT results obtained at follow-up across three of the reported domains: reaction time, processing speed and verbal memory.[46] The test is sufficiently brief and convenient to administer that it could very reasonably form part of routine ED assessment and may detect subtle deficits in performance that predict individuals at higher risk of delayed recovery who would otherwise be missed. The routine use of neurocognitive screening in emergency department patients with mTBI is now advocated by some experts.[47]

Discharge Advice and Follow-Up

There is considerable variation between institutions in selecting which patients should have routine follow-up arranged, which may well reflect differences in local commissioning arrangements. In neurosurgical hospitals participating in the CENTER-TBI study, only 10% offered routine follow-up for patients who present with mTBI and just over half arranged follow-up even for patients who had required hospital admission.[48]

In the absence of clear consensus guidance on follow-up strategy, a pragmatic approach is required. Where local facilities allow, patients with mTBI who have been identified as being at greater risk of delayed recovery should be offered routine follow-up. This may be through the confirmation of anatomical brain injury by neuro-imaging or from the identification of patients with greater functional deficit by neuro-cognitive screening in the ED. This will not capture all patients who go on to suffer prolonged concussive problems and so the most important element of discharge planning is that patients are given clear written guidance outlining the symptoms they are likely to experience and a sensible time-frame within which they can antici-pate resolution. The same written guidance should contain instructions on what to do in the event that symptoms do not resolve, both for the patient and for the primary care physician to whom they will most likely present in the first instance. There are excellent discharge advice leaflets compiled by head injury charities such as Headway which are freely available to emergency departments.[49] Patients should also be offered general advice on the gradual re-introduction of normal activity. It is believed that physical and mental stress should be avoided initially with a slow and progressive increase in activity over subsequent days provided symptoms are improving.[50] Where mTBI has occurred in a sporting context or the patient is an active participant in contact sports, specific return to play advice is vital to avoid suffering a second impact while the recovering brain is still vulnerable. Although the scientific basis of the so-called second impact syndrome remains controversial,[51] this rare condition is reported to have devastating consequences, particularly in the young. The Rugby Football Union website and other sporting bodies offer excellent return to play advice general-izable to other contact sports.[52]

Conclusion

In the past mTBI has been a rather neglected condition. It has been difficult to diagnose using the imaging techniques available in most emergency departments, treatment options are limited and there remains confusion and some controversy about the diagnosis and nature of post-concussive problems which overlap with and sometimes co-exist with psychiatric conditions such as post-traumatic stress disorder. However, in the last decade research has unlocked rapid progress in our under-standing of the condition at a molecular and microscopic level and a greater appre-ciation of the functional problems that can ensue, along with a willingness to establish clinical pathways to address them. The next decade should see these scientific advances translated into routine clinical practice with advanced imaging and serum biomarkers available in the ED able to clearly establish the presence and location of anatomical injury in mTBI alongside computer-aided neurocognitive testing to identify patients with early functional problems. The surge in interest in mTBI from military conflicts and contact sports is likely to result in better general facilities for the care of patients in the wider population with established problems, and we remain hopeful that the elusive drug intervention to improve outcomes will finally be revealed.

References

1. Hou R, Moss-Morris R, Peveler R, Mogg K, Bradley BP, Belli A. When a minor head injury results in enduring symptoms: a prospective investigation of risk factors for postconcussional syndrome after mild traumatic brain injury. *J Neurol Neurosurg Psychiatry* 2012;83(2):217–23.

2. Stulemeijer M, van der Werf S, Borm GF, Vos PE. Early prediction of favourable recovery 6 months after mild traumatic brain injury. *J Neurol Neurosurg Psychiatry* 2008;79(8):936–42.

3. Loane DJ, Stoica BA, Faden AI. Neuroprotection for traumatic brain injury. *Handb Clin Neurol* 2015;127:343–66.

4. Khong E, Odenwald N, Hashim E, Cusimano MD. Diffusion tensor imaging findings in post-concussion syndrome patients after mild traumatic brain injury: a systematic review. *Front Neurol* 2016;7:156.

5. Kulbe JR, Geddes JW. Current status of fluid biomarkers in mild traumatic brain injury. *Exp Neurol* 2016;275(Pt 3):334–52.

6. Malec JF, Brown AW, Leibson CL, Flaada JT, Mandrekar JN, Diehl NN, Perkins PK. The mayo classification system for traumatic brain injury severity. *J Neurotrauma* 2007;24(9):1417–24.

7. Kay A, Teasdale G. Head injury in the United Kingdom. *World J Surg* 2001;25(9):1210–20.

8. Hodgkinson S, Pollit V, Sharpin C, Lecky F. National Institute for H, Care Excellence Guideline Development G: early management of head injury: summary of updated NICE guidance. *BMJ* 2014;348:g104.

9. Majdan M, Plancikova D, Brazinova A, Rusnak M, Nieboer D, Feigin V, Maas A. Epidemiology of traumatic brain injuries in Europe: a cross-sectional analysis. *Lancet Public Health* 2016;1(2):e76–83.

10. Kanakaris NK, Giannoudis PV. Trauma networks: present and future challenges. *BMC Med* 2011;9(121):1–10.

11. Kehoe A, Smith JE, Edwards A, Yates D, Lecky F. The changing face of major trauma in the UK. *Emerg Med J* 2015;32(12):911–15.

12. Trauma Audit Research Network. Major trauma in older people. Press release (2017).

13. Kehoe A, Smith JE, Bouamra O, Edwards A, Yates D, Lecky F. Older patients with traumatic brain injury present with a higher GCS score than younger patients for a given severity of injury. *Emerg Med J* 2016;33(6):381–5.

14. Trefan L, Houston R, Pearson G, Edwards R, Hyde P, Maconochie I, Parslow RC, Kemp A. Epidemiology of children with head injury: a national overview. *Arch Dis Child* 2016;101(6):527–32.

15. Fehily B, Fitzgerald M. Repeated mild traumatic brain injury: potential mechanisms of damage. *Cell Transplant* 2017;26(7):1131–55.

16. Lozano D, Gonzales-Portillo GS, Acosta S, de la Pena I, Tajiri N, Kaneko Y, Borlongan CV. Neuroinflammatory responses to traumatic brain injury: etiology, clinical consequences, and therapeutic opportunities. *Neuropsychiatr Dis Treat* 2015;11:97–106.

17. Perez-Polo JR, Rea HC, Johnson KM, Parsley MA, Unabia GC, Xu G, Infante SK, Dewitt DS, Hulsebosch CE. Inflammatory consequences in a rodent model of mild traumatic brain injury. *J Neurotrauma* 2013;30(9):727–40.

18. Juratli TA, Zang B, Litz RJ, Sitoci KH, Aschenbrenner U, Gottschlich B, Daubner D, Schackert G, Sobottka SB. Early hemorrhagic progression of traumatic brain contusions: frequency, correlation with coagulation disorders, and patient outcome: a prospective study. *J Neurotrauma* 2014;31(17):1521–7.

19. Flygt J, Djupsjo A, Lenne F, Marklund N. Myelin loss and oligodendrocyte pathology in white matter tracts following traumatic brain injury in the rat. *Eur J Neurosci* 2013;38(1):2153–65.

20. Timaru-Kast R, Wyschkon S, Luh C, Schaible EV, Lehmann F, Merk P, Werner C, Engelhard K, Thal SC. Delayed inhibition of angiotensin II receptor type 1 reduces secondary brain damage and improves functional recovery after experimental brain trauma. *Crit Care Med* 2012;40(3):935–44.

21. Peng W, Yang J, Yang B, Wang L, Xiong XG, Liang Q. Impact of statins on cognitive deficits in adult male rodents after traumatic brain injury: a systematic review. *Biomed Res Int* 2014;2014:261409.

22. Lesniak A, Pick CG, Misicka A, Lipkowski AW, Sacharczuk M. Biphalin protects against cognitive deficits in a mouse model of mild traumatic brain injury (MTBI). *Neuropharmacology* 2016;101:506–18.

23. Robertson CS, Garcia R, Gaddam SS, Grill RJ, Cerami Hand C, Tian TS, Hannay HJ. Treatment of mild traumatic brain injury with an erythropoietin-mimetic peptide. *J Neurotrauma* 2013;30(9):765–74.

24. Dewan Y, Komolafe EO, Mejia-Mantilla JH, Perel P, Roberts I, Shakur H, Collaborators C. Crash-3 – tranexamic acid for the treatment of significant traumatic brain injury: study protocol for an international randomized, double-blind, placebo-controlled trial. *Trials* 2012;13 (87):1–14.

25. Julien J, Tinawi S, Anderson K, Frenette LC, Audrit H, Ferland MC, Feyz M, De Guise E. Highlighting the differences in post-traumatic symptoms between patients with complicated and uncomplicated mild traumatic brain injury and injured controls. *Brain Inj* 2017;31(13–14):1846–55.

26. van der Naalt J, Timmerman ME, de Koning ME, van der Horn HJ, Scheenen ME, Jacobs B, Hageman G, Yilmaz T, Roks G, Spikman JM. Early predictors of outcome after mild traumatic brain injury (upfront): an observational cohort study. *Lancet Neurol* 2017;16 (7):532–40.

27. Delouche A, Attye A, Heck O, Grand S, Kastler A, Lamalle L, Renard F, Krainik A. Diffusion MRI: pitfalls, literature review and future directions of research in mild traumatic brain injury. *Eur J Radiol* 2016;85(1):25–30.

28. Topolovec-Vranic J, Pollmann-Mudryj MA, Ouchterlony D, Klein D, Spence J, Romaschin A, Rhind S, Tien HC, Baker AJ. The value of serum biomarkers in prediction models of outcome after mild traumatic brain injury. *J Trauma* 2011;71(5 Suppl 1):S478–86.

29. Spaite DW, Hu C, Bobrow BJ, Chikani V, Barnhart B, Gaither JB, Denninghoff KR, Adelson PD, Keim SM, Viscusi C, Mullins T, et al. The effect of combined out-of-hospital hypotension and hypoxia on mortality in major traumatic brain injury. *Ann Emerg Med* 2017;69(1):62–72.

30. Stiell IG, Laupacis A, Wells GA, Canadian CTH. Cervical-Spine Study G: indications for computed tomography after minor head injury. Canadian CT head and cervical-spine study group. *N Engl J Med* 2000;343(21):1570–1.

31. Kreitzer N, Hart K, Lindsell CJ, Betham B, Gozal Y, Andaluz NO, Lyons MS, Bonomo J, Adeoye O. Factors associated with adverse outcomes in patients with traumatic intracranial hemorrhage and Glasgow Coma Scale of 15. *Am J Emerg Med* 2017;35(6):875–80.

32. Peck KA, Calvo RY, Schechter MS, Sise CB, Kahl JE, Shackford MC, Shackford SR, Sise MJ, Blaskiewicz DJ. The impact of preinjury anticoagulants and prescription antiplatelet agents on outcomes in older patients with traumatic brain injury. *J Trauma Acute Care Surg* 2014;76(2):431–6.

33. Fox WC, Park MS, Belverud S, Klugh A, Rivet D, Tomlin JM. Contemporary imaging of mild TBI: the journey toward diffusion tensor imaging to assess neuronal damage. *Neurol Res* 2013;35(3):223–32.

34. Hellstrom T, Westlye LT, Kaufmann T, Trung Doan N, Soberg HL, Sigurdardottir S, Nordhoy W, Helseth E, Andreassen OA, Andelic N. White matter microstructure is associated with functional, cognitive and emotional symptoms 12 months after mild traumatic brain injury. *Sci Rep* 2017;7(1):13795.

35. Oehr L, Anderson J. Diffusion-tensor imaging findings and cognitive function following hospitalized mixed-mechanism mild traumatic brain injury: a systematic review and meta-analysis. *Arch Phys Med Rehabil* 2017;98(11):2308–19.

36. Mayer AR, Bellgowan PS, Hanlon FM. Functional magnetic resonance imaging of mild traumatic brain injury. *Neurosci Biobehav Rev* 2015;49:8–18.

37. Eierud C, Craddock RC, Fletcher S, Aulakh M, King-Casas B, Kuehl D, LaConte SM. Neuroimaging after mild traumatic brain injury: review and meta-analysis. *Neuroimage Clin* 2014;4:283–94.

38. Mayer AR, Mannell MV, Ling J, Gasparovic C, Yeo RA. Functional connectivity in mild traumatic brain injury. *Hum Brain Mapp* 2011;32(11):1825–35.

39. Heidari K, Vafaee A, Rastekenari AM, Taghizadeh M, Shad EG, Eley R, Sinnott M, Asadollahi S. S100b protein as a screening tool for computed tomography findings after mild traumatic brain injury: systematic review and meta-analysis. *Brain Inj* 2015;29:1–12.

40. Posti JP, Takala RS, Runtti H, Newcombe VF, Outtrim J, Katila AJ, Frantzen J, Ala-Seppala H, Coles JP, Hossain MI, Kyllonen A, et al. The levels of glial fibrillary acidic protein and ubiquitin C-terminal hydrolase-L1 during the first week after a traumatic brain injury: correlations with clinical and imaging findings. *Neurosurgery* 2016;79(3):456–64.

41. Heidari K, Asadollahi S, Jamshidian M, Abrishamchi SN, Nouroozi M. Prediction of neuropsychological outcome after mild traumatic brain injury using clinical parameters, serum S100B protein and findings on computed tomography. *Brain Inj* 2015;29(1):33–40.

42. Okonkwo DO, Yue JK, Puccio AM, Panczykowski DM, Inoue T, McMahon PJ, Sorani MD, Yuh EL, Lingsma HF, Maas AI, Valadka AB, et al. GFAP-BDP as an acute diagnostic marker in traumatic brain injury: results from the prospective transforming research and clinical knowledge in traumatic brain injury study. *J Neurotrauma* 2013;30(17):1490–7.

43. Yue JK, Vassar MJ, Lingsma HF, Cooper SR, Okonkwo DO, Valadka AB, Gordon WA, Maas AI, Mukherjee P, Yuh EL, Puccio AM, et al. Transforming research and clinical knowledge in traumatic brain injury pilot: multicenter implementation of the common data elements for traumatic brain injury. *J Neurotrauma* 2013;30(22):1831–44.

44. Maas AI, Menon DK, Steyerberg EW, Citerio G, Lecky F, Manley GT, Hill S, Legrand V, Sorgner A, Participants C-T. Investigators: collaborative European neurotrauma effectiveness research in traumatic brain injury (center-TBI): a prospective longitudinal observational study. *Neurosurgery* 2015;76(1):67–80.

45. Ganti L, Daneshvar Y, Ayala S, Bodhit AN, Peters KR. The value of neurocognitive testing for acute outcomes after mild traumatic brain injury. *Mil Med Res* 2016;3:23.

46. Thomas DG, Collins MW, Saladino RA, Frank V, Raab J, Zuckerbraun NS. Identifying neurocognitive deficits in adolescents following concussion. *Acad Emerg Med* 2011;18(3):246–54.

47. Hartwell JL, Spalding MC, Fletcher B, O'Mara MS, Karas C. You cannot go home: routine concussion evaluation is not enough. *Am Surg* 2015;81(4):395–403.

48. Foks KA, Cnossen MC, Dippel DWJ, Maas A, Menon D, van der Naalt J, Steyerberg EW, Lingsma H, Polinder S. Management of mild traumatic brain injury at the emergency department and hospital admission in Europe: a survey of 71 neurotrauma centers participating in the center-TBI study. *J Neurotrauma* 2017;34.

49. Minor head injury discharge advice - adults. The Brain Injury Association. https://www

.headway.org.uk/media/2767/minor-head-injury-discharge-advice.pdf

50. Gioia GA. Medical-school partnership in guiding return to school following mild traumatic brain injury in youth. *J Child Neurol* 2016;31(1):93–108.

51. McCrory P, Davis G, Makdissi M. Second impact syndrome or cerebral swelling after sporting head injury. *Curr Sports Med Rep* 2012;11(1):21–3.

52. Adult concussion management guidelines (routine). England Rugby 2017. https://www.englandrugby.com//dxdam/86/86c7a5b7-e65a-4f58-ae9c-3c3c1449b519/HEADCASE%20Adult%20Concussion%20Management%20Guidelines.pdf

Early Phase Care of Patients with Moderate and Severe Head Injury

Mark Wilson

Introduction

Worldwide 50 million people have a traumatic brain injury (TBI) each year.[1] It is the leading cause of death in young adults, causes considerable morbidity and has a huge cost to society. Prevention through public health programmes is key; however, once primary injury has occurred, it is our job as clinician/scientists to minimise neuronal loss through secondary brain injury. The time to do this is as early as possible in the pathogenesis of neuronal injury and hence the pre-hospital phase is the most critical of all. The quality of pre-hospital care varies considerably globally – from non-existent through to advanced clinician led, often helicopter-based services that can perform multiple interventions. This chapter will explain the basic processes in the first few hours after TBI and interventions that can be used to minimise secondary injury. Evidence-based guidelines developed by the brain trauma foundation can be found at https://braintrauma.org/guidelines/pre-hospital

Prevention of TBI

Those that practice pre-hospital care are in a unique position to witness directly the mechanisms of injury that cause TBI. The mechanisms range from simple falls from standing through to high-speed mechanisms in road traffic collisions. By recording mechanisms accurately, public health clinicians involved in epidemiology of TBI can make targeted recommendations for legislation (helmet laws, road design, elderly care, etc.). Doctors have a duty to raise awareness and highlight increasing issues such as assaults when they occur in our community.

Impact Brain Apnoea and Airway Obstruction

It is well documented in animal literature that traumatic brain injury often results in a period of apnoea.[2] This applies across all animal species and mechanisms of injury. The greater the force, the longer the period of apnoea, and if artificial ventilation is not initiated during a prolonged period of apnoea, death will occur. The phenomenon is considerably underappreciated in humans because, as health care workers, we usually do not witness the apnoeic period.[3] The hypoxia may well have induced a cardiac arrest and following unsuccessful resuscitation the patient may be labelled as dying from 'traumatic brain injury'. This is not technically correct. They have died of a hypoxic brain injury secondary to trauma. Similarly, if a reduced level of consciousness results in airway obstruction, hypoxia will ensue. Following 'successful' resuscitation, a subsequent CT scan may show the effects of that hypoxia (Figure 8.1) with loss of grey-white differentiation and loss of sulcal spaces. The patient may not have signs of bleeding/significant brain injury and the outcome may well have been different if airway support and

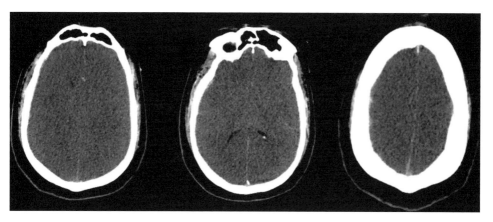

Figure 8.1 Brain CT scan demonstrating hypoxic brain injury – often such patients are labelled with 'traumatic brain injury', but there is minimal contusion and a more correct diagnosis is hypoxic brain injury secondary to trauma-induced apnoea. From M. H. Wilson et al.[3]

ventilation care had been instituted earlier. Addressing this issue is extremely difficult as it requires intervening before the ambulance service arrives. Better training of bystanders, the use of mobile technology to alert nearby first aiders and the use of remote video to guide bystanders are probably the most likely techniques that can impact in this phase.

It is worth noting that Impact Brain Apnoea may also be associated with cardiovascular instability. Although it is often stated that hypotension cannot be caused by an isolated head injury (implying look for other causes of hypovolaemia), recent studies have demonstrated that approximately 15% of 'code red' patients (trauma patients who have a systolic blood pressure of <90 mmHg) have an isolated head injury and this hypotension may be related to a period of impact brain apnoea.[4]

Concussion

Concussion is a poor term[5] that has many definitions. One such definition is '*A clinical syndrome characterised by immediate and transient impairment of neural function, such as alteration of consciousness, disturbance of vision, equilibrium, etc. due to mechanical forces*'. Some definitions relate to a lack of pathology, but this may just reflect the lack of fidelity of our current MRI/imaging techniques (if performed) to demonstrate injury. Other terms such as 'minor brain injury' that recognise the injury within the spectrum of traumatic brain injury are probably better. Concussion is however a term that is in common use, especially in relation to sports injuries.

Assessment of concussion in sporting events is often done using specific tools. For example, the Sport Concussion Assessment Tool (SCAT 5) assesses conscious level and then proceeds to assess orientation, memory, balance and other functions that imply 'concussion' may be present.[6] This chapter will focus more on civilian trauma.

On-Scene Management

Once scene safety is established, it is often possible to infer transfers of energy and mechanisms of injury by 'reading the wreckage': this can predict likely injury patterns.

For example, if a patient has been hit by a vehicle and there is a 'bull's-eyed' windscreen, the patient is likely to have sustained a head injury. If there is blood and hair in the glass, then it is nearly 100% likely to be related to a head injury. Similarly, falls from height, distance of the patient from collision and types of assault weapons can all be used to build a picture.

Whilst establishing and maintaining the airway is the priority, it is often useful to make a concurrent assessment of conscious level (see below) as this will probably guide interventions/decisions.

C-Spine Protection

Cervical spine immobilisation has been the mainstay of Advanced Trauma Life Support (ATLS) teaching for decades. Traditionally this has been triple immobilisation through the application of a collar, sandbags and tape. However, the benefits have been debated for some time, with the value of the cervical collar in addition to blocks and tape being specifically questioned. Recently the complications of spinal immobilisation, in particular the risks of aspiration, pressures sores and raised ICP[7] have resulted in some countries revising their guidelines. Some reviews have been critical of cervical collars,[8] whilst others still recommend their use with blocks and tape.[9] In Norway the use of the lateral position to protect the airways does not appear to be associated with increased spinal injury.[10] The Australian and New Zealand Resuscitation Councils no longer recommend the use of semi-rigid collars.

Agitation

Agitation is common in patients following TBI and can make patient and scene management difficult. There are many reasons a patient may be agitated apart from the actual head injury. Drugs and alcohol, a period of hypoxia, underlying dementia and existing personality can all make control of a situation difficult to attain. Attempts made to verbally calm the patient often fail and sedation (e.g. with midazolam or ketamine) may be required. This in turn will commonly reduce the level of consciousness of the already compromised patient and hence an ability to then control the airway through intubation may be needed. Note, ketamine has previously been contraindicated in TBI; however, it does not appear to raise blood pressure significantly, can possibly act as a neuroprotectant and maintains airway reflexes supporting its utility.[11,12]

Airway Management and Intubation

Patients who have suffered TBI may well have concurrent facial injuries causing blood to well in their airway with the potential for aspiration. With a reduced level of consciousness, they may also obstruct their airway. Simple manoeuvres such as jaw thrust, insertion of nasopharyngeal or oropharyngeal airways can be of critical importance. Nasopharyngeal airways are relatively contraindicated in skull base fractures but can be placed safely with the mouth open watching as the tip passes behind the soft palate into the oropharynx. Torrential facial bleeding may benefit from nasal packing/balloon tamponade, bite blocks ± collar.

Intubation of patients for TBI has previously been controversial. Studies showing increased morbidity and mortality were often poorly conducted, not comparing pre-hospital versus in-hospital but comparing untrained personnel versus trained personnel.[13] The indications for intubation need to be part of a clear and highly governed system and when conducted in a trained, audited and systematic environment, pre-hospital anaesthesia has been demonstrated to be both safe[14] and to improve outcome[15] from severe TBI.

Breathing

In spontaneously breathing patients it can be useful to attach end tidal CO_2 ($EtCO_2$) monitoring during transfer to monitor rate and effectiveness of breathing (TBI patients can both hypo and hyperventilate). In intubated patients, $EtCO_2$ monitoring is essential and a standard part of anaesthesia. Hyperventilation was previously thought to be useful to lower intracranial pressure in TBI; however, it has been demonstrated to reduce cerebral blood flow[16] and hence guidance now is to maintain normal $EtCO_2$ levels (~4.5 kPa).

Circulation

Hypoxia and hypotension are considered the prime secondary brain injuries. Many studies have demonstrated increased mortality with episodes of either.[17,18] A recent study has demonstrated that every 10 mmHg increase in systolic blood pressure was associated with a decrease in the adjusted odds of death of nearly 20%.[19] However, ideal blood pressure may be different for different types of injury (extradural haematoma vs. diffuse axonal injury) and more work is required in this area to define pathology specific targets.

Disability

A rough assessment of conscious level has usually occurred concurrently with the above; however, this should be done formally and documented. This is commonly recorded as the Glasgow Coma Score or using the AVPU (alert, responds to voice, responds to pain, unresponsive) systems. Pupil size, response to light and any lateralising signs (e.g. not moving one side) should also be sought and recorded.

Specific ICP Care

It is usually not possible to assess intracranial pressure (ICP) in the pre-hospital environment. It is therefore best to undertake practices that assume it is raised, or likely to increase. Box 8.1 outlines basic examples of such techniques.

Box 8.1 Techniques to Potentially Lower ICP in the Pre-hospital Environment (Where ICP Is Not Usually Known)

Aim for normoxia, normocarbia and normotension. Treat the cause of raised ICP if it can be established

Loosen collar – improve venous drainage

Position (35° head-up) (tilt the stretcher with a blanket under the head end)

Adequate sedation/analgesia

Paralysis

Normalise $EtCO_2$ if intubated (4.5 kPa) (avoid excessive positive pressure)

Avoid abdominal compression (do not leave oxygen cylinder on abdomen in transfer)

Osmotic diuretics

The benefits of osmotic diuretics have been questioned. Current guidelines vary, but they can be considered in those who have signs of raised ICP (e.g. reduced GCS < 8 and pupil dilatation/fixation). They may be useful to buy a short period of time whilst en route to definitive surgery. Commonly used agents are mannitol (1–2 g/kg) or hypertonic saline (6 ml/kg of 5%). There is some evidence that hypertonic saline results in less acute kidney injury and may be better in those with polytrauma.

Cooling has been thought to be neuroprotectant but recently has fallen out of favour with evidence of harm on intensive care.[20] There are ongoing studies in the prehospital environment, but at the present time, normothermia should be targeted.

TBI and Coagulopathy

Coagulopathy in brain injury can either be pre-existing (e.g. from anticoagulant use or liver failure) or as a result of the brain injury itself.

Pre-existing/Drug-Induced Coagulopathy

Anticoagulant complicated TBI is increasing as the burden of elderly TBI increases. Some anticoagulants are easily reversible, others not.

Warfarin. Warfarin (which mostly reduces prothrombin and factor VII) can be reversed with prothrombin complex concentrates (PCC) or fresh frozen plasma and vitamin K_1.[21] The advent of nearside patient INR testing enables the administration of PCC in the field prior to transfer to hospital and subsequent CT imaging.[22] This can prevent progression of bleeding and haemorrhagic contusion and is likely to be the most significant intervention pre-hospital services can make in the management of traumatic brain injury in the elderly population. Most UK advanced prehospital services will reverse warfarin pre-hospitally.

Novel anticoagulants. Dabigatran is a direct thrombin Factor IIa inhibitor. It can only be reversed with the monoclonal antibody Idarucizumab. *Rivaroxaban* is a factor Xa inhibitor interrupting both the intrinsic and extrinsic pathways. It does not inhibit thrombin or platelets. A potential reversant under investigation is Andexanet alfa (a recombinant derivative of factor Xa). However, prehospital services, and even most in-hospital services, are not able to reverse either of these medications using specific reversal agents yet. The management of patients on such medications is extremely difficult and once in hospital should be undertaken in consultation with haematology.

Anti-platelet agents. Aspirin and Clopidogrel inhibit platelet aggregation, but reducing their effects is difficult to achieve in the pre-hospital phase. dDAVP (0.3 mcg/kg IV in 50 ml NS × 1) and steroids may be of use.[23] Recent evidence of no benefit from supplemental platelets in spontaneous intracerebral haemorrhage implies that there may be little or no benefit from their administration following intracerebral haemorrhage secondary to trauma.[24]

Brain Injury–Induced Coagulopathy

Isolated brain injury is thought to cause coagulopathy in approximately 30% of brain-injured patients resulting in a tenfold increase in death.[25] The pathogenesis of this probably relates to release of tissue factor, activation of protein C pathways, disseminated intravascular coagulopathy and platelet dysfunction.

The use of tranexamic acid (TXA) has been demonstrated to be beneficial in polytrauma.[26] Currently the use of tranexamic acid to reduce clot/contusion progression is being studied in the CRASH 3 trial. This may prove TXA to be the first clinically beneficial neuroprotectant – by stopping bleeding rather than acting on neurons!

Triage and Transfer

It is recognised that patients with TBI managed in a neurotrauma centre have better outcomes than those managed in peripheral units.[27] However, protocols for transfer vary and multiple factors need to be considered. A recent study where potential head injured patients bypassed the local trauma unit (TU) to go directly to a neurosurgical unit found an overtriage rate for neurosurgical intervention of 13:1.[28] With the increasing incidence of elderly TBI, many of whom do not require surgery, long distance transfers from home or a local hospital (Trauma Unit) causes many problems in subsequent social care package development and visiting for relatives. As such, tools that will support diagnosis and decision-making in the pre-hospital environment are much needed. These are under development and can broadly be divided into biomarkers (that will give an indication if brain injury is likely) and imaging (that will indicate the type and location of the pathology).

Biomarkers

There are a number of biomarkers which may be of use in the pre-hospital environment. Their use very much depends on the time course of their concentration rise and the ability to be assessed with patient-side testing. S100 is a biomarker used in emergency departments in Scandinavia to assess if patients who are GCS 14 should proceed to CT scan.[29] Purine levels have been demonstrated to rise rapidly with cerebral ischaemia and may be of use in TBI.[30] MicroRNA can be found in saliva and studies are currently under way looking at its role in concussion assessment.[31]

Imaging

Mobile CT imaging is currently utilised for suspected stroke patients in some European and US cities.[32] It is not yet used for trauma, but as such tools miniaturise, this may be more feasible. Near InfraRed (NIR) tools can be used to detect extra-axial blood clot and may be of use in remote environments where transfer for definitive imaging might be prolonged.[33]

Future Developments

The further development of biomarker and imaging tools over the next 10 years could rapidly change and individualise pre-hospital TBI management. Other advances may include:

Remote Technologies

The development of mobile technologies to both see patients on scene (and provide bystander advice for example to hold an airway open) and crowdsource those with medical training to provide assistance in the first few minutes after injury has the potential to significantly improve outcomes of those patients that otherwise succumb to hypoxia, be that through impact brain apnoea or airway obstruction. These kind of logistical improvements, together with the development of better major trauma pathways, are likely to have the biggest impact.

Neuroprotective Agents

There are many pharmacological agents that have shown benefit in animal studies but have failed to show improved outcome when translated into human studies. This could be because the nature of the injury is different or because time delays in administering the drug in reality mean that damage is already done. Potential agents that have failed to show benefit so far include steroids,[34] progesterone[35] and NMDA antagonists. Current trials of Tranexamic acid and the antimalarial Artesunate, which give the drug in the hyperacute phase of injury (first hour), may demonstrate benefit.

Suspended Animation

A 'Holy Grail' of pre-hospital care is the ability to arrive and 'suspend' pathological processes to enable transfer to hospital and definitive management. With the development of pre-hospital Extracorporeal Membrane Oxygenation (ECMO), the administration of fluids that could potentially slow metabolism and rapidly cool patients may one day become a reality.

Neurosurgical Procedures

The practice of exploratory burr holes has little place in modern TBI care. Timely imaging is available in most parts of the Western world. There may be occasions when a diagnosis is made but transfer is delayed (e.g. distance or weather restriction) in which case burr hole evacuation by a non-neurosurgeon may be indicated.[36] Traditionally, bilateral fixed pupils and GCS 3 has an incredibly poor prognosis[37]; however, if this is due to an extradural, the outcome is often surprisingly good.[38]

Conclusions

Interventions in the first few minutes/hours after injury can have a profound effect on outcome from TBI. Current pre-hospital TBI management is not disease specific. A generic TBI protocol minimising the secondary brain injuries of hypoxia and hypotension and minimising risks of raised ICP is practiced by most advanced pre-hospital services. However, in the future, our ability to diagnose on scene may enable patient- and disease-specific treatments.

Care in this crucial stage of the brain-injured patient pathway is vital in saving lives and keeping the patient the same person they were before the injury.

References

1. Maas PAIR, Menon PDK, Adelson PD, Andelic N, Bell MJ, Belli A, et al. The Lancet Neurology Commission Traumatic brain injury: integrated approaches to improve prevention, clinical care, and research. *Lancet Neurol* 2017;16(12):987–1048. http://doi.org/10.1016/S1474-4422(17)30371-X

2. Atkinson JL, Anderson RE, Murray MJ. The early critical phase of severe head injury: importance of apnea and dysfunctional respiration. *J Trauma* 1998;45(5):941–5.

3. Wilson MH, Hinds J, Grier G, Burns B, Carley S, Davies G. Impact brain apnoea – a forgotten cause of cardiovascular collapse in trauma. *Resuscitation*

2016;105:52–8. http://doi.org/10.1016/j
.resuscitation.2016.05.007

4. Gavrilovski M, El-Zanfaly M, Injury RL.
    Isolated traumatic brain injury results in
    significant pre-hospital derangement of
    cardiovascular physiology. *Injury*
    2018;49:1675–9. http://doi.org/10.1016/j
    .injury.2018.04.019

5. Sharp DJ, Jenkins PO. Concussion is
    confusing us all. *Practical Neurol* 2015;15
    (3):172–86. http://doi.org/10.1136
    /practneurol-2015-001087

6. Sport concussion assessment tool – 5th
    edition. *Br J Sports Med* 2017;51(11):851–8.
    http://doi.org/10.1136/bjsports-2017-
    097506SCAT5

7. Davies G, Deakin C, Wilson A. The effect of
    a rigid collar on intracranial pressure.
    Injury 1996;27(9):647–9. http://doi.org/10
    .1016/S0020-1383(96)00115–5

8. Sundstrøm T, Asbjørnsen H, Habiba S,
    Sunde GA, Wester K. Prehospital use of
    cervical collars in trauma patients: a critical
    review. *J Neurotrauma* 2014;31(6):531–40.
    http://doi.org/10.1089/neu.2013.3094

9. Theodore N, Hadley MN, Aarabi B,
    Dhall SS, Gelb DE, Hurlbert RJ, et al.
    Prehospital cervical spinal immobilization
    after trauma. *Neurosurgery* 2013;72 (Suppl
    2):22–34. http://doi.org/10.1227/NEU
    .0b013e318276edb1

10. Fattah S, Ekås GR, Hyldmo PK, Wisborg T.
    The lateral trauma position: what do we
    know about it and how do we use it? A
    cross-sectional survey of all Norwegian
    emergency medical services. *Scand
    J Trauma Resuscitation Emerg Med* 2011;19
    (1):45. http://doi.org/10.1186
    /1757-7241-19-45

11. Bourgoin A, Bourgoin A, Albanèse J,
    Albanèse J, Wereszczynski N,
    Wereszczynski N, et al. Safety of sedation
    with ketamine in severe head injury
    patients: comparison with sufentanil.
    Critical Care Med 2003;31(3):711–17. htt
    p://doi.org/10.1097/01
    .CCM.0000044505.24727.16

12. Filanovsky Y, Filanovsky Y, Miller P,
    Miller P, Kao J, Kao J. Myth: ketamine
    should not be used as an induction agent

    for intubation in patients with head injury.
    CJEM 2010;12(2):154–7.

13. Davis DP, Davis DP, Hoyt DB, Hoyt DB,
    Ochs M, Ochs M, et al. The effect of
    paramedic rapid sequence intubation on
    outcome in patients with severe traumatic
    brain injury. *J Trauma* 2003;54(3):444–53.
    http://doi.org/10.1097/01
    .TA.0000053396.02126.CD

14. Lockey D, Crewdson K, Weaver A,
    Davies G. Observational study of the
    success rates of intubation and failed
    intubation airway rescue techniques in
    7256 attempted intubations of trauma
    patients by pre-hospital physicians. *Br
    J Anaes* 2014;113(2):220–5. http://doi.org/
    10.1093/bja/aeu227

15. Bernard SA, Nguyen V, Cameron P,
    Masci K, Fitzgerald M, Cooper DJ, et al.
    Prehospital rapid sequence intubation
    improves functional outcome for patients
    with severe traumatic brain injury:
    a randomized controlled trial. *Ann Surg*
    2010;252(6):959–65. http://doi.org/10.1097
    /SLA.0b013e3181efc15f

16. Coles JPJ, Minhas PS, Fryer TD,
    Smielewski P, Aigbirihio F, Donovan T,
    et al. Effect of hyperventilation on cerebral
    blood flow in traumatic head injury:
    clinical relevance and monitoring
    correlates. *Critical Care Med* 2002;30
    (9):1950–9. http://doi.org/10.1097/01
    .CCM.0000026331.91456.9A

17. Chesnut RM, Marshall LF, Klauber MR,
    Blunt BA, Baldwin N, Eisenberg HM,
    et al. The role of secondary brain injury
    in determining outcome from severe
    head injury. *J Trauma* 1993;34
    (2):216–22.

18. Murray GD, Butcher I, McHugh GS, Lu J,
    Mushkudiani NA, Maas AIR, et al.
    Multivariable prognostic analysis in
    traumatic brain injury: results from the
    IMPACT study. *J Neurotrauma* 2007;24
    (2):329–37. http://doi.org/10.1089/neu
    .2006.0035

19. Spaite DW, Hu C, Bobrow BJ, Chikani V,
    Sherrill D, Barnhart B, et al. Mortality and
    prehospital blood pressure in patients with
    major traumatic brain injury: implications
    for the hypotension threshold. *JAMA Surg*

2016. http://doi.org/10.1001/jamasurg
.2016.4686

20. Andrews PJD, Sinclair HL, Rodriguez A,
Harris BA, Battison CG, Rhodes JKJ, et al.
Hypothermia for intracranial hypertension
after traumatic brain injury. *New Engl
J Med* 2015;373(25):2403–12.
http://doi.org/10.1056/NEJMoa1507581

21. Cabral KP, Fraser GL, Duprey J,
Gibbons BA, Hayes T, Florman JE,
Seder DB. Prothrombin complex
concentrates to reverse warfarin-induced
coagulopathy in patients with intracranial
bleeding. *Clin Neurology Neurosurg*
2013;115(6):770–4. http://doi.org/10.1016/
j.clineuro.2012.07.006

22. Lendrum RA, Kotze J-P, Lockey DJ,
Weaver AE. Case studies in prehospital
care from London HEMS: pre-hospital
administration of prothrombin complex
concentrate to the head-injured patient.
Emerg Med J 2003;30(3):247–8.

23. Qureshi A.I, Suri MFK. Acute reversal of
clopidogrel-related platelet inhibition
using methyl prednisolone in a patient with
intracranial hemorrhage. *Am J Neuroradiol*
2008;29(10):e97. http://doi.org/10.3174/aj
nr.A1297

24. Baharoglu MI, Cordonnier C, Al-Shahi
Salman R, de Gans K, Koopman MM,
Brand A, et al. Platelet transfusion versus
standard care after acute stroke due to
spontaneous cerebral haemorrhage
associated with antiplatelet therapy
(PATCH): a randomised, open-label, phase
3 trial. *Lancet* 2015;387(10038):2605–13. h
ttp://doi.org/10.1016/S0140-
6736(16)30392-0

25. Harhangi BS, Kompanje EJO,
Leebeek FWG, Maas AIR. Coagulation
disorders after traumatic brain injury. *Acta
Neurochirurgica* 2008;150(2):165–75;
discussion 175. http://doi.org/10.1007/
s00701-007-1475-8

26. Shakur H, Roberts I, Bautista R,
Caballero J, Coats T, et al. Effects of
tranexamic acid on death, vascular
occlusive events, and blood transfusion in
trauma patients with significant
haemorrhage (CRASH-2): a randomised,
placebo-controlled trial. *Lancet* 2010;376

(9734):23–32. http://doi.org/10.1016/S014
0-6736(10)60835–5

27. Patel HC, Bouamra O, Woodford M,
King AT, Yates DW, Lecky FE, Trauma
Audit and Research Network. Trends in
head injury outcome from 1989 to 2003
and the effect of neurosurgical care: an
observational study. *Lancet* 2005;366
(9496):1538–44. http://doi.org/10.1016/
S0140-6736(05)67626-X

28. Lecky FE, Russell W, McClelland G,
Pennington E, Fuller G, Goodacre S, et al.
Bypassing nearest hospital for more distant
neuroscience care in head-injured adults
with suspected traumatic brain injury:
findings of the head injury transportation
straight to neurosurgery (HITS-NS) pilot
cluster randomised trial. *BMJ Open* 2017;7
(10):e016355–7. http://doi.org/10.1136/
bmjopen-2017–016355

29. Undén L, Calcagnile O, Undén J,
Reinstrup P, Bazarian J. Validation of the
Scandinavian guidelines for initial
management of minimal, mild and
moderate traumatic brain injury in adults.
BMC Med 2015;13 (292):1–9. http://doi.org
/10.1186/s12916-015–0533-y

30. Tian F, Bibi F, Dale N, Imray CHE. Blood
purine measurements as a rapid real-time
indicator of reversible brain ischaemia.
Purinergic Signal 2017;13(4):1–8. http://
doi.org/10.1007/s11302-017-9578-z

31. Zetterberg H, Blennow K. Fluid
biomarkers for mild traumatic brain injury
and related conditions. *Nature Neurol*
2016;12(10):563–74. http://doi.org/10.1038
/nrneurol.2016.127

32. Ebinger M, Winter B, Wendt M, Weber JE,
Waldschmidt C, Rozanski M, et al. Effect of
the use of ambulance-based thrombolysis
on time to thrombolysis in acute ischemic
stroke: a randomized clinical trial. *JAMA*
2014;311(16):1622–31. http://doi.org/10
.1001/jama.2014.2850

33. Leon-Carrion J, Leon-Carrion J,
Dominguez-Roldan JM, Dominguez-
Roldan JM, Leon-Dominguez U, Leon-
Dominguez U, Murillo-Cabezas F. The
Infrascanner, a handheld device for
screening in situ for the presence of brain
haematomas. *Brain Injury* 2010;24

(10):1193–201. http://doi.org/10.3109/026
99052.2010.506636

34. Edwards P, Arango M, Balica L,
Cottingham R, El-Sayed H, Farrell B,
et al. Final results of MRC CRASH,
a randomised placebo-controlled trial of
intravenous corticosteroid in adults
with head injury-outcomes at 6 months.
Lancet 2005;365(9475):1957–9. http://do
i.org/10.1016/S0140-6736(05)66552-X

35. Wei J, Xiao G-M. The neuroprotective
effects of progesteone on traumatic brain
injury: current status and future prospects.
Acta Pharmacol Sin 2013;34:1485–90.

36. Wilson MH, Wise D, Davies G, Lockey D.
Emergency burr holes: 'how to do it'. *Scand*

J Trauma Resuscitation Emerg Med
2012;20:24. http://doi.org/10.1186
/1757–7241-20–24

37. Chaudhuri K, Chaudhuri K, Malham GM,
Malham GM, Rosenfeld JV. Survival of
trauma patients with coma and bilateral
fixed dilated pupils. *Injury* 2009;40
(1):28–32. http://doi.org/10.1016/j
.injury.2008.09.004

38. Scotter J, Hendrickson S, Marcus HJ,
Wilson MH. Prognosis of patients with
bilateral fixed dilated pupils secondary to
traumatic extradural or subdural
haematoma who undergo surgery:
a systematic review and meta-analysis.
Emerg Med J 2014;32:654–9.

Interhospital Transfer of Brain-Injured Patients

Thomas Price, Gareth Allen and Robbie Thorpe

Introduction

Neurosurgical services in the UK are organised regionally into 34 acute neuroscience centres. Brain injury, both traumatic and non-traumatic, is common, and patients often present to local hospitals requiring further treatment in a neuroscience centre. Between April 2014 and June 2015, 15 820 patients suffered a traumatic brain injury in the UK. Of these, 6258 were transferred directly to a neuroscience centre, 5880 were not admitted to a neuroscience centre and 3682 underwent a secondary transfer from the admitting hospital to a neuroscience centre.[1] In addition to traumatic brain injury, indications for non-traumatic causes of brain injury requiring acute transfer to a neuroscience centre continue to increase. Advances in stroke management with intravenous thrombolysis, mechanical thrombectomy, endovascular coiling of aneurysmal haemorrhage and decompressive craniectomy have further increased the demand for rapid transfer of brain-injured patients to neuroscience centres. It has been demonstrated that the process of transfer may have adverse consequences in the general critically ill population, and it is widely accepted that the process of transferring any patient incurs inherent risks.[2] It is important therefore that, during the process of bringing the brain-injured patient to a venue for definitive care, attention should be given to minimising these risks at both individual patient and organisational levels. The need for standards for interhospital transfer was first highlighted in 1994,[3] and since then guidelines have been produced by a number of organisations.[4–6]

Many regions now use centrally based retrieval teams, particularly for the transfer of paediatric patients, reducing the burden on the referring hospital on-call anaesthetic team for prolonged transfers. However mobilisation of retrieval teams takes time, and there is often a need to transfer patients with brain injury urgently. In a situation where neurosurgical intervention is time-critical, such as an expanding intracranial haematoma, transfer by the referring team using the most appropriate members of staff available remains the preferred option.[7] All acute hospitals must retain the ability to resuscitate, stabilise and transfer critically ill patients.[4]

This chapter will discuss the indications for transfer, the conduct of transfer and the training implications.

Indications for Transfer

Accepting that transfer may have risks, it is important to have clear markers to identify patients who stand to benefit from being relocated.

Indications for transfer include

1   patients requiring neurosurgical intervention, for example evacuation of a haematoma, decompressive craniectomy, or drainage of cerebro-spinal fluid (CSF)

2 patients requiring monitoring which cannot be provided at the referring hospital.

3 patients requiring radiological intervention for stroke, for example mechanical thrombectomy or endovascular coiling.

In addition, evidence suggests that the patient with severe brain injury may benefit from care in a specialist neurocritical care centre irrespective of the plans for surgical intervention,[8-12] particularly where this is headed by specialist neurocritical care doctors.[13] However, given that demand may sometimes outstrip supply for these beds, first priority is usually given to patients who require surgery. The Society of British Neurosurgeons (SBNS) advise that admission to a regional neurosurgical unit for life-saving, emergency surgery should never be delayed and lack of critical care beds must not be a reason for refusing admission for patients requiring urgent surgery.[14] The widespread availability of 24 hour computerised tomography (CT) scanning in hospitals receiving trauma has reduced the need for interhospital transfer for neuroimaging, and all patients should be appropriately investigated in a timely manner by secondary care prior to referral to a neuroscience centre.[14]

Conduct of the Transfer

The transfer should be agreed between the doctor in charge at the referring hospital and the receiving neurosurgical team. It is imperative to ensure that the receiving critical care and anaesthesia teams are also aware of the transfer of the patient. The precise destination of the patient, whether operating theatre, intensive care unit (ICU) or emergency department should be ascertained, as well as the urgency of the journey.

Information passed to the neurosurgical team must include the patient's age and medical history, mechanism and time of injury, initial and current neurological status, presence of drugs or alcohol, extracranial injuries, physiological status, details of patient management and findings of imaging. The use of a standardised neurosurgical referral letter has been shown to more consistently provide all relevant information than non-standardised *ad hoc* documents.[5,15]

There should be a referral agreement between all referring hospitals served by a regional neuroscience centre, consistent with national and international guidelines.[6] Such an agreement should include detailed plans on which patients should be referred, which patients require emergency transfer, who is responsible for accepting the patient, clear details of where the patient should be received and the point at which responsibility for the patient is transferred to the receiving team.[6] These referral agreements should be subject to regular review and audit by the neuroscience centre, and governance issues arising should be disseminated to all referring hospitals.[6]

The digital transfer of CT images has greatly improved communication between referring hospitals and neuroscience centres. This has greatly reduced inappropriate patient transfers.[16] It is vital that all hospitals receiving trauma patients have the ability to both obtain and transfer images to the neuroscience centre.

Various problems may occur during transfer, some being unique to the interhospital environment. During movement into and out of the vehicle inadvertent decannulations or extubations may occur. Vehicles used, whether land or air based, often lack space. This coupled with the motion of the vehicle and potential for poor lighting makes patient observation and the performance of procedures more challenging than in the hospital environment. Monitoring alarms and inadvertent disconnections may also take longer to be noticed. The climate within the transport vehicle may be more variable than in a hospital, with patients potentially being exposed to excessive heat or cold depending on the location and the season. The motion of the vehicle may affect the patient's physiology. Hypoxaemia may be precipitated by vibrations loosening secretions and possibly provoking bronchospasm as well as by head-down tilt whilst descending hills. Haemodynamic changes during transport, hypotension and occasionally hypertension, are common and thought to be precipitated by changes in preload and afterload.[17] This is caused by the mass movement of blood volume during acceleration and deceleration as well as by tilt induced by hills. Intracranial pressure (ICP) may be increased by vibration, noise, head down tilt or by worsening of intracranial pathology. Previously undiagnosed conditions may present or treated conditions may deteriorate, all in a location where physical help is usually unavailable. The patient is totally reliant on portable equipment during the transfer. Since 2002 all transfer equipment and vehicles are subject to regulations published by the European Committee for Standardisation (CEN).[18] In addition, although unlikely, road accidents with patient and staff injury have occurred during transfers. It is vital that appropriate medical indemnity and personal injury assurance be provided for the staff undertaking the transfer.

Unsurprisingly therefore problems during transfer have been found to occur in up to 34% of transfers of the critically ill with up to 37% having worse observations after the journey.[19] Audit data obtained by a dedicated critical care transfer team revealed that hypoxaemia was the commonest adverse event (15%), hypotension occurring in 10%, cardiac arrhythmia in 7% and equipment failure in 9%.[17] The need for emergency re-intubation was rare (0.4%). Data from the 1970s and 1980s showed that hypotension and hypoxaemia were very common on arrival at neurosurgical centres – up to 30% of patients in one series.[20] Improvement in these figures has occurred with time, and data from the 1990s shows hypotension occurring in 12% and hypoxaemia in 6% of transfers.[21] More attention to stabilisation of the patient prior to transfer is a key component in this improvement.[22]

Allowing for the fact that time to evacuation of an intracranial haematoma inversely correlates with the chance of a good outcome,[23,24] it is accepted that transfer must be accomplished as rapidly as possible allowing for patient safety. A maximum of 4 hours is taken as the commonly used target between time of injury and starting neurosurgery for life-threatening neurosurgical conditions, although this target is not evidence based.[6] Within stroke management, improved clinical outcomes have been demonstrated with intravenous thrombolysis delivered within 4.5 hours of symptom onset and mechanical thrombectomy delivered up to 6 hours from symptom onset in anterior circulation strokes has been demonstrated to be associated with improved clinical outcomes.[25,26] However this must not occur at the expense of adequate assessment and resuscitation. There is little merit in decreasing the time to surgery at the expense of increasing the degree of systemically originated secondary brain injury. Direct involvement of experienced senior staff in patient management and in the decision-making process is therefore vital. For the reasons outlined above all life-threatening injuries must be attended to at the referring hospital. In one study untreated life-threatening extracranial injuries were present in almost one in ten patients arriving at neurosurgical centres.[27] Scalp injuries are probably the most frequently overlooked injury, and the potential for significant haemorrhage from these must be appreciated.[28] Immobilisation of any fractures should be performed and the cervical spine stabilised appropriately. The use of spinal boards and cervical collars during the secondary transfer of patients does not have a firm evidence base, and the risk of precipitation of severe pressure damage must be appreciated, with the incidence of collar-related pressure ulcers ranging from 6.8 to 38%.[29] These predominantly occur over the occiput, chin, shoulders and back.[29]

Unsurprisingly, formal guidelines are lacking regarding their use in a transfer setting and the decision currently rests with the staff directly involved with each transfer. The Helicopter Emergency Medical Service (HEMS) within the authors region utilises vacuum mattresses with or without a cervical spine collar depending on clinicians preference.

Primary Transfer to Tertiary Referral Centres

Between 2010 and 2014, 27 Major Trauma Networks were developed in England. Using pre-hospital triage tools, the Major Trauma Networks (MTN) aim to transfer triage-positive patients, who are within 45 min transfer time, directly to a Major Trauma Centre (MTC), bypassing all hospitals en route unless life-threatening complications arise such as airway obstruction. During 2012 these Networks treated 16 000 patients and demonstrated a significant improvement in the probability of surviving major trauma.[30]

The benefits of primary transfer to tertiary referral centres are further supported by the fact that as few as 33% of patients undergoing a secondary transfer may arrive within 4 hours of injury at a neurosurgical operating theatre, the median time in one study being over 6 hours.[31]

However a systematic review and meta-analyses of 19 major trauma studies between 1988 and 2012 demonstrated no difference in the outcome for direct transport to a trauma centre versus initial triage in a local hospital.[32] The authors however did acknowledge significant limitations in study design and high levels of heterogeneity in included data.[32]

Primary transfer of the brain-injured patient to the tertiary neuroscience centre requires a number of criteria to be satisfied. Firstly, the patient should be correctly diagnosed as having sustained a traumatic head injury or stroke. To fail in this respect exposes a patient with unconsciousness due to systemic cardiorespiratory insufficiency or drug overdose to risks of a longer transfer whilst unstable, and places further pressure on neurosurgical centre intensive care services. Secondly, there must be effective collaboration between the ambulance service and the regional neuroscience service. Thirdly, facilities must exist to stabilise the patient and then rapidly undertake the longer journey to the neurosurgical centre. These requirements can be met using Helicopter Emergency Medical Services (HEMS), with a suitably experienced, equipped and assisted doctor on board. There are currently more than 20 HEMS operating within the UK.[33] Where systems such as this are in place delays would appear to be consistently less than those cited above; however, several hours may still elapse from injury to surgical intervention.[34] The ability of doctor-led pre-hospital care to perform drug-assisted intubation at the scene of brain injury undoubtedly has its benefits, in particular treating airway obstruction, correcting hypoxia and reducing ICP through appropriate sedation and paralysis. Furthermore, observational data comparing paramedic versus physician staffed emergency medical services attending severe traumatic brain injury patients has demonstrated a reduction in mortality, a reduction in the incidence of hypoxia and an improvement in neurological outcome in patients treated by the physician-led emergency medical service.[35]

It must be borne in mind that helicopter transport presents its own unique set of problems, particularly concerning management of complications occurring *en route*, and the experience and training of the teams involved must be rigorous.[36,37]

Management of 'Non-surgical' Patients in District General Hospitals

Evidence citing improvement in outcome for brain-injured patients by medical management in specialised units has attracted some controversy, large-scale retrospective data suggesting a 26% mortality increment with management in non-neurosurgical centres.[8] Attention must be paid to the content of the care as well as the location. Previously some centres had demonstrated trends towards improved outcome using multi-modal monitoring and protocols for investigation and management of detected abnormalities.[10–12] Available evidence suggests that the average district hospital receiving trauma will care for 15 severe head injuries per year, making hospital volume a potential factor in outcome.[38] District hospitals are less likely to have access to ICP monitoring, and unlikely to have capacity to drain CSF if required. This has led to current National Institute of Clinical Excellence (NICE) guidance recommending that all patients with a severe brain injury (GCS of 8 or less) be transferred to a neuroscience centre irrespective of the need for surgery.[5] However where adequate facilities exist, and in conjunction with general surgical support, some non-neurosurgical centres have shown comparable rsults.[39] Caring for such patients at a distance from full neurosurgical support means that controlled expedient transfer may be needed in the event of a deterioration, for instance if decompressive craniectomy is required, ongoing liaison with the neuroscience unit over clinical management is essential.[5]

Maintaining Standards for Interhospital Transfers

Given the large number of transfers occurring and the associated risks, maintenance of quality is paramount. To this end several guidance documents have been published, most recently by the Association of Anaesthetists in conjunction with the Neuro Anaesthesia & Critical Care Society.[6]

A summary of their recommendations is given in Table 9.1 and several of the points noted bear further examination.

The role of the designated consultants, both in the referring hospital and the neuroscience unit, should be one of quality control and include organisation of audit, incident collation, education and liaison with appropriate staff – medical and non-medical. Previous audit had shown that up to 50% of UK hospitals have not formally identified a staff member for this role.[40]

In addition to those patients with a Glasgow Coma Scale (GCS) of less than or equal to eight, other patients may require pre-emptive intubation in order to preclude the need for this procedure *en route*. They include those with a downward trend in the GCS, those with airway injuries, bilateral mandibular fractures often being cited as an example or those with suboptimal respiratory function.

A 'clinician with appropriate training and experience' is usually taken to mean one capable of performing any necessary procedures during the transfer, and with knowledge of the pathophysiology of brain injury. They should be able to independently initiate,

Table 9.1 Recommendations for the safe transfer of the brain-injured patient: Trauma and stroke, 2019

1 There should be designated consultants in the referring hospitals and the neuroscience units* with overall responsibility for the transfer of patients with brain injuries.

2 Local guidelines should be drawn up between the referring hospital trusts, the neurosciences unit and the local ambulance services; these should be consistent with established national guidelines.

3 Details of the transfer of responsibility for patient care should also be agreed.

4 While transfer is often urgent, thorough resuscitation and stabilisation of the patient must be completed prior to transfer.

5 Patients with a Glasgow Coma Scale (GCS) less than or equal to 8 requiring transfer should undergo tracheal intubation and mechanical lung ventilation.

6 The Working Party has used a consensus technique to devise recommendation on blood pressure targets.

7 Patients with acute ischaemic stroke for thrombectomy should be transferred without delay; those with anterior circulation stroke rarely need airway intervention.

8 Patients with a brain injury should be accompanied by a clinician with appropriate training and experience in the transfer of patients with acute brain injury.

9 Monitoring during transport should adhere to previously published standards.

10 The transfer team must be provided with a mobile phone for urgent communication.

11 Education, training and continuous audit are crucial to maintaining standards of transfer.

Source: Reproduced with permission from the Association of Anaesthetists[6]

administer and modify pharmacology, physiology and lung ventilation to minimise secondary brain injury.[6] If this is a trainee working in an unsupervised role, they should have access to consultant advice by mobile phone.[6] In addition they should be accompanied by a trained assistant, for example an anaesthetic nurse, Operating Department Practitioner (ODP), Advanced Critical Care Practitioner (ACCP) or ICU nurse.[6]

Transfer personnel for brain injury associated with stroke will vary depending on the clinical condition of the patient. Anterior circulation strokes are often not associated with impairment of consciousness and therefore rarely need anaesthetic accompaniment. Posterior circulation, large malignant middle cerebral artery (MCA) stroke and subarachnoid haemorrhages often cause impairment of consciousness and will require anaesthetic input for the transfer.

The standard of monitoring should not be less than that in the hospital from which the patient is leaving, and as a minimum should include ECG, blood pressure (preferably invasive if time permits arterial line insertion), pulse oximetry, capnography and temperature.[4] Although central venous pressure monitoring is usually not essential, the line itself is a reliable port of access and invaluable should the need for vasoactive drugs for maintenance of perfusion pressure be required during transfer. Its placement, however, should not delay transfer, particularly for surgical intervention. The pupillary reflexes must be monitored for signs of neurological deterioration. Airway pressure, inspired oxygen concentration and ventilator settings must be observed. It is essential that all observations and interventions are recorded, an anaesthetic chart is usually well suited to this purpose and specifically designed transfer charts are used in certain regions.

Maintenance and optimisation of cerebral perfusion pressure (CPP) is fundamental to minimising secondary brain injury. Fluid administration should be aimed at correcting hypovolaemia and maintaining cerebral blood flow. Isotonic fluids, such as 0.9% Sodium

Table 9.2 Consensus recommendations for blood pressure targets for brain-injured patient transfer

Brain injury pathology	Blood pressure targets
Traumatic brain injury – uncontrolled haemorrhage or multiple injuries	Aim systolic blood pressure (SBP) 90–100 mmHg Aim mean arterial pressure (MAP) 80 mmHg *N.B. Short term only (<1–2 hours); once haemorrhage controlled, aim for MAP > 90 mmHg*
Traumatic brain injury – controlled haemorrhage or isolated head injury	Aim MAP > 90 mmHg
Acute ischaemic stroke – for intravenous thrombolysis	Aim SBP > 140 mmHg and SBP <180/100 mmHg
Acute ischaemic stroke – for mechanical thrombectomy	Control SBP if > 220 mmHg or MAP > 130 mmHg
Spontaneous intracerebral haemorrhage	Aim SBP <150 mmHg
Aneurysmal subarachnoid haemorrhage	Aim SBP >110 mmHg and <160 mmHg

Source: Adapted from 'Safe transfer of the brain-injured patient: trauma and stroke; 2019', with permission from the Association of Anaesthetists [6]

Chloride, are most commonly used. If fluid resuscitation fails to correct hypovolaemia and the patient remains hypotensive in the absence of ongoing haemorrhage or excess sedation, then vasoactive medication, such as Noradrenaline or Metaraminol, should be considered to maintain cerebral perfusion pressure. The Association of Anaesthetists has produced consensus recommendations on optimal blood pressure targets during transfer of brain-injured patients (Table 9.2).[6]

Checklists

It is recommended that checklists be used when preparing a patient for transfer.[6] As a general rule there should be a suitable doctor, with functioning equipment and a suitable assistant to transfer a suitable patient in a suitable vehicle, to a clear pre-arranged destination. Examples of checklists are shown in Figure 9.1.

Available functioning equipment must include a portable ventilator, adequate oxygen supply, monitors as detailed above, full range of airway management equipment, infusion pumps, equipment for management of pneumothorax, full range of vascular access equipment, equipment for ALS management of cardiac arrest and warming equipment. A supply of sedatives, neuromuscular blocking drugs, analgesics, anticonvulsants, vasoactive drugs and intravenous fluids should be available, as well as osmotic agents for the management of intracranial hypertension. The standard osmotic agent carried for transfer within the authors region is 3% Hypertonic Saline, due to the ease of administration and more favourable side effect profile in comparison to mannitol.

Administration of osmotic agents should be discussed with the neuroscience centre prior to administration, unless impending or actual brain herniation is occurring, in which case emergency administration is the priority to prevent brain stem herniation. Guidelines

Respiratory Checklist

$P_aO_2 > 13.0$ kPa (for AIS aim for $SaO_2 >$ or equal to 95%)
P_aCO_2 4.5–5.0 kPa
Airway protected adequately
Chest drain managed appropriately
Tracheal tube position confirmed (if present)

Circulatory Checklist

Blood pressure target (See Table 9.2)
Two reliable large IV cannulae in situ
Bleeding controlled
Estimated blood loss already replaced
Cross matched blood available (in multiply injured trauma patient)
Arterial line (if time permits)

Brain Checklist

Seizures controlled
Raised ICP appropriately managed
Adequate sedation
GCS and pupils stable
Hypertonic therapy available

Other Injuries

Cervical spine protected
Pneumothorax excluded
Active intrathoracic or intra-abdominal bleeding excluded
Pelvic, long bone fractures

Other Monitoring, Vital Signs

Urinary catheter
Normothermia (and appropriate warming equipment)
Normoglycaemia
Gastric tube position confirmed (if present)

Escort

Transferring team appropriately trained and experienced
Adequate equipment, drugs and oxygen supplies
Case notes
Imaging transferred to the neuroscience centre
Transfer documentation
Destination determined (incl. specific site in receiving unit; e.g. ED, ICU or theatres)
Telephone numbers programmed into mobile phone
Mobile phone battery fully charged
Name and contact details of receiving doctor
Receiving team given estimated time of arrival

Figure 9.1 Transfer checklist. Reproduced with permission from the Association of Anaesthetists.[6]

within the authors HEMS service for administration include the presence of unilateral or bilateral papillary dilatation with a GCS of less than or equal 8 or progressive hypertension (SBP over 160 mmHg) and bradycardia (pulse below 60) in the presence of a GCS less than or equal to 8.[41]

Training

Medical training in general and anaesthesia training in particular have undergone widespread change with the introduction of competency-based training framework.[42] This has provided the opportunity to include transfer skills in a structured training programme.[42] Furthermore, formal assessment by a supervising consultant during an accompanied transfer has been introduced in some areas.[43] Safe Transfer and Retrieval (StaR) courses are organised by the Advanced Life Support Group at venues throughout the UK,[44] and some local hospitals provide 'Training for Transfer'.[45] These courses provide a multidisciplinary 'hands-on' approach promoting best practice and awareness of legislation relating to equipment.

Summary

Interhospital transfer of the brain-injured patient is common and demanding. Hospitals that receive patients with severe brain injuries should retain the capability for their resuscitation, stabilisation and transfer. The goal is the delivery of a patient to the neuroscience unit in a timely fashion, with a safe airway, appropriate blood pressure depending on the underlying pathology, ICP < 22 mmHg, P_aO_2 >13 kPa, P_aCO_2 4.5–5.0 kPa, normothermic and normo-glycaemic, and with no untreated life-threatening extracranial injuries.[46] Extensive high-quality guidelines are available from a number of sources, and checklists should be used during preparation for the transfer. Involvement of senior staff in both administration, clinical decision-making and training is vital in maintaining standards of care.

References

1. Lawrence T, et al. Traumatic brain injury in England and Wales: prospective audit of epidemiology, complications and standardised mortality. *BMJ Open* 2016;6 (11):e012197.

2. Duke G, Green JV. Outcome of critically ill patients undergoing interhospital transfer. *Med J Austr* 2001;174(3): 122–5.

3. Oakley P. The need for standards for interhospital transfer. *Anaesthesia* 1994;49:565–6.

4. Intensive Care Society. Guidelines for the transport of the critically ill adult; 2002. https://www.ficm.ac.uk/sites/default/files/transfer_critically_ill_adult_2019.pdf

5. NICE Guidelines. Head injury: assessment and early management; 2014. www.nice.org.uk/guidance/cg176/chapter/1-recom mendations#transfer-from-hospital-to-a-n euroscience-unit

6. Nathanson MH, et al. Guidelines for the safe transfer of the brain-injured patient: trauma and stroke 2019. Guidelines from the Association of Anaesthetists and Neuro Anaesthesia and Critical Care Society; 2019.

7. Farling P, Smith M. Transfer of brain injured patients – time for a change? *Anaesthesia* 2006;61:1–2.

8. Patel HC, Bouamra O, Woodford M, et al. Trends in head injury outcome from 1989 to 2003 and the effect of neurosurgical care: an observational study. *Lancet* 2005;366 (9496):1538–44.

9. Seeley HM, Hutchinson P, Maimaris C, et al. A decade of change in regional head injury care: a retrospective review. *Br J Neurosurg* 2006;20(1):9–21.

10. Elf K, Nilsson P, Enblad P. Outcome after traumatic brain injury improved by an

organized secondary insult program and standardized neurointensive care. *Critical Care Med* 2002;30(9):2129–34.

11. Clayton TJ, Nelson RJ, Manara AR. Reduction in mortality from severe head injury following introduction of a protocol for intensive care management. *Br J Anaesthesia* 2004;93(6):761–7.

12. Patel HC, Menon DK, Tebbs S, et al. Specialist neurocritical care and outcome from head injury. *Intensive Care Med* 2002;28:547–53.

13. Varelas PN, Conti MM, Spanaki MV, et al. The impact of a neurointensivist-led team on a semiclosed neurosciences intensive care unit. *Critical Care Med* 2004;32 (11):2191–8.

14. Society of British Neurological Surgeons. Care quality statement; October 2015. www .sbns.org.uk/index.php/policies-and-publications/

15. Keaney J, Fitzpatrick MO, Beard D, et al. A standardised neurosurgical referral letter for the interhospital transfer of head injured patients. *J Accident Emerg Med* 2000;17(4):257–60.

16. Eljamel MS, Nixon T. The use of a computer-based image link system to assist interhospital referrals. *Br J Neurosurg* 1992;6(6):559–62.

17. Ridley S, Carter R. The effects of secondary transport on critically ill patients. *Anaesthesia* 1989;44:822–7.

18. Medical vehicles and their equipment – Road ambulances EN 1789; 1999. www .cenorm.be

19. Ligtenberg JJ, Arnold LG, Stienstra Y, et al. Quality of interhospital transport of critically ill patients: a prospective audit. *Critical Care* 2005;9(4):446–51.

20. Gentleman D, Jennett B. Hazards of interhospital transfer of comatose head-injured patients. *Lancet* 1981;2 (8251):853–4.

21. Dunn LT. Secondary insults during the interhospital transfer of head-injured patients: an audit of transfers in the Mersey Region. *Injury* 1997;28 (7):427–31.

22. Andrews PJD, Piper IR, Dearden NM. Secondary insults during intrahospital transport of head-injured patients. *Lancet* 1990;335:327–30.

23. Mendelow AD, Karmi MZ, Paul KS, et al. Extradural haematoma: effect of delayed treatment. *Br Med J* 1979;1(6173):1240–2.

24. Seelig JM, Becker DP, Miller JD, et al. Traumatic acute subdural hematoma: major mortality reduction in comatose patients treated within four hours. *New Engl J Med* 1981;304(25):1511–18.

25. Hacke W, et al. Thrombolysis with Alteplase 3–4.5 hours after Acute Ischemic Stroke. *New Engl J Med* 2008;359 (13):1317–29.

26. Berkhemer OA, et al. A randomised trial of intraarterial treatment for acute ischemic stroke. *New Engl J Med* 2015;372(1):11–20.

27. Henderson A, Coyne T, Wall D, et al. A survey of interhospital transfer of head-injured patients with inadequately treated life-threatening extracranial injuries. *ANZ J Surg* 1992;62(10):759–62.

28. Fitzpatrick MO, Seex K. Scalp lacerations demand careful attention before interhospital transfer of head injured patients. *J Accident Emerg Med* 1996;13 (3):207–8.

29. Ham W, et al. Pressure ulcers from spinal immobilization in trauma patients: a systematic review. *J Trauma Acute Care Surg* 2014;76(4):1131–41.

30. McCullough Al, et al. Major trauma networks in England. *Br J Anaesth* 2014;113:286–94.

31. Lind CR. Transfer of intubated patients with traumatic brain injury to Auckland City Hospital. *ANZ J Surg* 2005;75 (10):858–62.

32. Pickering, A, et al. Impact of prehospital transfer strategies in major trauma and head injury: systematic review, meta-analysis, and recommendations for study design. *J Trauma Acute Care Surg* 2015;78(1):164–77.

33. Association of Air Ambulances. Framework for High Performing Air Ambulance Service; 2013. www.associatio nofairambulances.co.uk/resources/events/

AOAAFramework%19202013-OCT13-%2
0Final%20Document.pdf

34. Wright KD, Knowles CH, Coats TJ, et al. 'Efficient' timely evacuation of intracranial haematoma – the effect of transport direct to a specialist centre. *Injury* 1996;27 (10):719–21.

35. Pakkanen T, et al. Pre-hospital severe traumatic brain injury – comparison of outcome in paramedic versus physician staffed emergency medical services. *Scand J Trauma Resuscitation Emerg Med* 2016;24:62.

36. Bernard SA. Paramedic intubation of patients with severe head injury: a review of current Australian practice and recommendations for change. *Emerg Med Austr* 2006;18(3):221–8.

37. Davis DP, Stern J, Sise MJ, et al. A follow-up analysis of factors associated with head-injury mortality after paramedic rapid sequence intubation. *J Trauma Injury Infection Critical Care* 2005;59 (2):486–90.

38. McKeating EG, Andrews PJ, Tocher JI, et al. The intensive care of severe head injury: a survey of non-neurosurgical centres in the United Kingdom. *British Journal of Neurosurgery* 1998;12 (1):7–14.

39. Havill JH, Sleigh J. Management and outcomes of patients with brain trauma in a tertiary referral trauma hospital without neurosurgeons on site. *Anaesthesia Intensive Care* 1998;26(6):642–7.

40. Allen G, Farling P, Mullan B. Designated consultants for the interhospital transfer of patients with brain injury. *J Intensive Care Soc* 2006;7(2):13–15.

41. C Brown, D Monaghan. NIHEMS: Head Injury Standard Operating Procedure; 2017.

42. Anaesthetic CCT Curriculum 2020. See https://www.rcoa.ac.uk/training-careers/training-anaesthesia/anaesthetic-cct-curriculum-2020

43. Spencer C, Watkinson P, McCluskey A. Training and assessment of competency of trainees in the transfer of critically ill patients. *Anaesthesia* 2004;59:1242–55.

44. Advance Life Support Group Course Dates and venues. https://www.alsg.org/home/mod/url/view.php?id=1127

45. Mark J. Transfer of the critically ill patient. *Anaesthesia News*, July 2004;2–4.

46. Carney N, et al. Guidelines for the management of severe traumatic brain injury, fourth edition. *Neurosurgery* 2017;80(1):6–15.

Principles of Head Injury Intensive Care Management

Martin Smith

Introduction

Traumatic brain injury (TBI) encompasses a continuum of primary and secondary injurious processes. Primary injury describes the irreversible structural damage sustained at the time of impact. It initiates a host response which results in a cascade of biochemical, cellular and molecular events that lead to further (secondary) brain injury.[1] Advances in neuromonitoring and neuroimaging techniques, in association with improved understanding of the pathophysiology of TBI, have led to the introduction of more effective critical care treatment strategies aimed at preventing or minimising secondary injury that have translated into improved outcomes for patients.

All patients with severe TBI should be managed in an intensive care unit (ICU) offering immediate access to multidisciplinary clinical neuroscience teams and other relevant specialties, supported by appropriate imaging and investigational facilities. Those with mild or moderate TBI may also require admission to an ICU for a variety of indications (Table 10.1).

Monitoring

As well as the close monitoring and assessment of systemic physiological variables relevant to all critically ill patients, neuromonitoring provides information about cerebral (patho)physiology and its response to treatment. Fundamental to neuromonitoring is serial clinical assessment of neurological status, and the Glasgow coma scale remains the mainstay of clinical assessment more than 40 years since its first description.[2] Clinical monitoring is limited in sedated patients or

Table 10.1 Indications for intensive care unit admission of head-injured patients

- Severe traumatic brain injury (post-resuscitation Glasgow Coma Scale score ≤8)
- Clinical or radiological evidence of raised intracranial pressure
- Requirement for mechanical ventilation
  - Decreased conscious level
  - Bulbar dysfunction
  - Acute respiratory failure
- Cardiovascular instability requiring intensive haemodynamic monitoring and management
- Invasive neurological and systemic monitoring
- Systemic organ support
- Post-operatively following neurosurgical interventions
- Multiple trauma
- Status epilepticus

those with decreased conscious level; in such circumstances, neuromonitoring can be used to identify brain insults and guide therapeutic interventions after TBI. Several techniques are available for global and regional brain monitoring, providing assessment of cerebral perfusion, oxygenation and metabolic status, and early warning of impending brain hypoxia/ischaemia and metabolic disturbance.[3,4]

The 2017 Brain Trauma Foundation guidelines recommend that intracranial pressure (ICP) should be monitored in all salvageable patients with severe TBI and an abnormal CT scan (haematomas, contusions, swelling, herniation or compressed basal cisterns), or a normal CT and two of the following: age >40, motor posturing, or hypotension (systolic blood pressure <90 mmHg).[5] Alternative guidelines from a group of mainly European clinical experts (the Milan consensus) provide pragmatic and specific recommendations for ICP monitoring in different TBI scenarios and computed tomography findings.[6] Unlike the Brain Trauma Foundation, the Milan consensus does not recommend routine ICP monitoring in comatose TBI patients with a normal computed tomography scan, but, instead, advises a second scan and institution of monitoring only if there is radiological worsening (Table 10.2).

Table 10.2 Indications for intracranial pressure monitoring in traumatic brain injury

Brain Trauma Foundation Guidelines[5]

- Salvageable patients with severe TBI (GCS ≤ 8) and an abnormal cranial CT scan
- Salvageable patients with severe TBI and a normal scan and two or more of the following:
  - Age > 40 years
  - Unilateral or bilateral motor posturing
  - Systolic blood pressure < 90 mmHg

Milan Consensus Recommendations[6]

- Comatose TBI patients with an initial CT scan showing minimal signs of injury that subsequently worsen
- Comatose TBI patients with cerebral contusions when interruption of sedation to check neurological status is contra-indicated, or when the clinical examination is unreliable
- Comatose TBI patients with large bifrontal contusions and/or haemorrhagic mass lesions close to the brain stem irrespective of initial GCS
- Following secondary decompressive craniectomy
- Following evacuation of an acute supratentorial intracranial haematoma in salvageable patients at high risk of intracranial hypertension, including those with:
  - GCS motor score ≤5
  - Pupillary abnormalities
  - Prolonged/severe hypoxia and/or hypotension
  - Compressed or obliterated basal cisterns
  - Midline shift >5 mm
  - Additional extra-axial haematomas, contusions or intraoperative brain swelling
- ICP monitoring should also be considered in the context of TBI and multiple trauma
- ICP monitoring should not be implemented in comatose TBI patients with a normal initial CT
  - A second interval CT scan is recommended, urgently if the patient deteriorates neurologically

Note: ICP = intracranial pressure; CPP = cerebral perfusion pressure; CT = computed tomography; GCS = Glasgow Coma Scale; TBI = traumatic brain injury.

Intracranial and cerebral perfusion pressures are routinely monitored in most centres, but they provide limited assessment of the adequacy of cerebral perfusion. Cerebral ischaemia can occur in the presence of normal values of ICP and cerebral perfusion pressure (CPP).[7] Cerebral oxygenation monitoring provides information about the balance between cerebral oxygen delivery and utilisation, and therefore of the adequacy of cerebral perfusion.[8] A Phase II randomised clinical trial demonstrated that management of severe TBI guided by brain tissue oxygenation monitoring in addition to ICP reduced the incidence of tissue hypoxia with a trend towards lower mortality and more favourable outcome compared to ICP monitoring-guided treatment.[9] Multimodality neuromonitoring allows individualised treatment decisions to be guided by monitored changes in cerebral physiology rather than pre-determined and generic targets.[10] In current clinical practice this most commonly involves the simultaneous measurement of ICP/CPP and brain tissue oxygen tension, although assessment of autoregulatory state is increasingly being adopted into clinical practice. Any impact of monitor-guided therapy on outcomes is dependent on the thresholds chosen to initiate intervention and subsequent management in response to changes in monitored variables, these remain undefined in many circumstances.[4] Furthermore, which variables are modifiable targets for treatment rather than surrogates of injury severity is also unclear.

Neuromonitoring techniques are reviewed in detail elsewhere[4] and discussed in Chapters 11 and 12.

General Intensive Care Management

The critical care management of TBI requires a coordinated approach providing meticulous general intensive care support as well as interventions targeted to the injured brain.[11] Treatment focuses on prevention of intracranial complications, optimisation of systemic physiology, and management of non-neurological complications (Table 10.3).[12] Continuous monitoring and rigorous management by a multidisciplinary neurocritical care team is associated with improved outcomes after TBI.[13]

Cardiorespiratory Support

Secondary systemic physiological insults, particularly hypotension and hypoxaemia, have adverse effects on outcome. A single episode of hypoxaemia ($PaO_2 < 8$ kPa or $SpO_2 < 90\%$) or hypotension (systolic BP < 90 mmHg) is strongly associated with worse outcomes after severe TBI, and the combination of the two is more deleterious than either insult alone.[14] To decrease mortality and improve neurological outcomes in survivors, the Brain Trauma Foundation recommends that systolic BP should be maintained ≥ 100 mmHg in patients aged 50 to 69 years and ≥ 110 mm Hg in those aged 15 to 49 years or older than 70 years.[5]

Fluid management is a key component of TBI management, and maintenance of euvolaemia with intravenous isotonic crystalloids is the primary cardiovascular goal.[15] Albumin is associated with increased mortality and should be avoided, as should hypotonic fluids because of the risk of worsened cerebral oedema.[16] Continuous infusion of hypertonic saline has been associated with survival benefits in TBI-related intracranial hypertension.[17] A vasopressor is indicated if adequate intravascular filling is insufficient to maintain arterial blood pressure and CPP targets. There is no evidence to support the use of one agent over another, but norepinephrine has a predictable and consistent effect on blood pressure and cerebral haemodynamics, and is widely used.

Table 10.3 General aspects of the critical care management of severe head injury

Ventilation	• PaO$_2$ > 10 kPa
	• PaCO$_2$ 4.5–5.0 kPa
	• Lung protective ventilation strategies (tidal volume 6 ml/kg ideal body weight, PEEP 6–12 mmHg and recruitment manoeuvres) as brain-directed therapy permits
	• Ventilator 'care bundle' to minimise risk of pneumonia
	– Head-up positioning
	– Oral hygiene
	– Peptic ulcer prophylaxis
	– Daily sedation holds if ICP permits
Cardiovascular	• SBP ≥ 100 mmHg in patients 50 to 69 years of age
	• SBP ≥ 110 mm Hg in patients aged 15 to 49 years or older than 70 years
	• Euvolaemia with isotonic crystalloids
	• Vasopressors/inotropes if insufficient response to fluid
ICP and CPP targets	• CPP 60–70 mmHg
	• ICP < 22 mmHg
Other	• Blood glucose < 10 mmol/L
	• Normothermia
	• Seizure control
	• Enteral nutrition
	• Thromboembolic prophylaxis

Note: CPP = cerebral perfusion pressure; ICP = intracranial pressure; SBP = systolic blood pressure; PEEP = positive end-expiratory pressure.

Endotracheal intubation and mechanical ventilation are mandatory after severe TBI. There is a high risk of loss of airway control, respiratory compromise, pulmonary aspiration and pneumonia. PaO$_2$ should be maintained > 10 kPa, but increasing FiO$_2$ beyond that which is necessary to maintain oxygenation targets is not recommended because of the potential risk of harm from hyperoxia. High tidal volume ventilation is a major risk factor for the development of acute lung injury after TBI, and a protective ventilation strategy (tidal volume < 6 ml/kg) should be used if brain-directed therapy permits.[18] Moderate levels of PEEP (≤15 cmH$_2$O) do not have clinically significant effects on ICP or CPP and can be applied safely to optimise PaO$_2$ as part of a protective ventilation strategy.[19] Maintenance of normocapnoea minimises the risk of hyperventilation-associated cerebral ischaemia, and routine hyperventilation is no longer recommended. Short-term moderate hyperventilation may be considered as a temporising measure to reduce critically elevated ICP, but should be avoided during the first 24 hours after injury when cerebral blood flow is often critically reduced.

Many TBI patients require tracheostomy because of a prolonged requirement for mechanical ventilation and/or airway protection. A meta-analysis of eight studies including almost 1700 patients suggested that early tracheostomy (<10 days after injury) may reduce infection rates and accelerate ventilator weaning and ICU discharge after TBI.[20]

Glycaemic Control

Hyperglycaemia (blood glucose >10 mmol/L) exacerbates secondary neuronal injury after TBI and is associated with worse outcomes compared to normoglycaemia.[21] A systematic review and meta-analysis of 10 randomised controlled trials including 1066 TBI patients found that intensive glycaemic control with intravenous insulin was not associated with reduced mortality, although a (non-significant) trend towards lower rates of poor neurological outcomes was identified despite a greatly increased incidence of hypoglycaemia.[22] The apparent contradiction between the high rates of hypoglycaemia and signal of lower rates of poor outcomes requires further investigation. In the meantime, moderate level glucose control is recommended, maintaining serum glucose concentration < 10 mmol/L while avoiding hypoglycaemia (serum glucose < 3.5 mol/L) and large swings in glucose concentration.[23]

Temperature Management

Pyrexia develops in more than half of critically ill TBI patients from multiple causes including infection and hypothalamic dysfunction. Although high temperature is independently associated with worse outcomes, there is no prospective evidence that fever reduction to normothermia leads to improved outcome.[24]

In preclinical studies, therapeutic hypothermia (TH) has established neuroprotective actions through stabilisation of the blood-brain barrier, ICP reduction and inhibition of inflammation and intracellular calcium overload. Several single-centre clinical studies have demonstrated benefit of TH after TBI, but this has not been confirmed by large-scale randomised trials.[25] Moderate TH (34°–35°C) is an effective means of reducing raised ICP and is often incorporated into ICP management protocols despite lack of evidence of improved outcomes. The Eurotherm3235 study, which investigated TH as part of a tiered approach to ICP management, was suspended early because of worse functional outcomes and higher mortality in the hypothermia group.[26] While this study provides evidence against the early use of hypothermia to control ICP, it does not address its role in the management of refractory intracranial hypertension for which it is most commonly used in clinical practice.

Seizures

Early post-traumatic seizures occur in more than 20% of TBI patients, and guidelines recommend 7 days of antiepileptic drug therapy to reduce the incidence of early post-traumatic seizures.[5] However, prophylaxis is controversial because early seizures have not been clearly associated with worse outcomes, and it does not prevent late onset seizures. If prophylaxis is used, treatment should be continued for no more than 7 days in patients who remain seizure free. Levetiracetam may be superior to phenytoin because of its more favourable safety profile.[27]

Other Supportive Measures

Acute traumatic coagulopathy develops in over one-third of patients with isolated TBI, and is associated with worse outcome.[28] Management relies on standard interventions including combinations of fresh frozen plasma and prothrombin complex concentrate according to local protocols. The optimal haemoglobin concentration to trigger red cell transfusion after TBI has not been established.[29] A randomised controlled trial demonstrated no statistically significant difference in outcome between haemoglobin concentration of 70 versus 100 g/L, but the higher transfusion threshold was associated a higher rate of thromboembolic events.[30]

TBI leads to a hypermetabolic state, and enteral feeding initiated within 48 hours is associated with reduced rates of mortality, poor outcomes, and infectious complications.[31] Physical methods to minimise the risk of venous thromboembolism must be provided from admission to the ICU, but the timing of pharmacological prophylaxis is more controversial. Based on evidence from more than 5000 TBI patients, initiation of chemoprophylaxis after 48 hours appears to be safe in those at low risk of haematoma expansion and after 72 hours in patients at medium or high risk.[32]

Brain-Directed Therapies

In addition to general supportive measures and optimisation of systemic physiology as outlined above, brain-directed therapies are a key component of the critical care management of TBI. The sole goal of identifying and treating intracranial hypertension has been superseded by a focus on the prevention of secondary brain injury by a multi-faceted neuroprotective strategy incorporating a systematic, stepwise approach to maintenance of cerebral perfusion and oxygen/substrate delivery.[33]

Management of Intracranial and Cerebral Perfusion Pressures

Intracranial hypertension has been associated with increased mortality in large cohort studies of TBI,[34,35] and the Brain Trauma Foundation recommends treatment of ICP $\geq$ 22 mmHg based on evidence that this may reduce in-hospital and 2 week post-injury mortality.[5] The neurocritical care management of intracranial hypertension incorporates tiered strategies administered in a stepwise manner, starting with safer, first-line, interventions while reserving higher-risk options for patients with intractable intracranial hypertension or multimodal neuromonitoring evidence of resistant brain hypoxia/ischaemia.[36] The relative risk of death is increased by 60% if escalation from first to second tier ICP-lowering interventions is necessary.[37] The management of intracranial hypertension is discussed in Chapter 13 and has been reviewed in detail elsewhere.[36]

All clinical guidelines advocate early treatment of intracranial hypertension [5;6], but there is little evidence that monitoring and managing ICP improves clinical outcomes.[38] The only randomised controlled trial investigating the impact of ICP monitoring (BEST-TRIP) found no difference in outcomes when treatment was guided by ICP monitoring compared to treatment guided by imaging and clinical examination in the absence of ICP monitoring.[39] Since both treatment approaches provided satisfactory outcomes despite the absence of ICP monitoring in one, this study challenges the established practice of maintaining ICP below a universal and arbitrary threshold.[40] It is increasingly recognised that treatment interventions can be best optimised by individualised interpretation of ICP values in association with other neuromonitoring variables, patient characteristics, and after assessment of the potential benefits and risks of treatment.[4]

Guidelines recommend that CPP should be maintained between 60 and 70 mmHg through manipulation of arterial blood pressure and ICP,[5] with evidence of adverse outcomes if CPP is lower or higher.[35] An alternative approach, the Lund concept, targets a lower CPP (50 mmHg) to minimise increases in intra-capillary hydrostatic pressure and intracerebral water content in an attempt to avoid secondary increases in ICP.[41] The Lund concept does not have a strong evidence base and is not universally accepted. In any case it is likely that the CPP threshold resulting in cerebral hypoperfusion and ischemia exists on an individual basis. Targeting an individualised 'optimal' CPP range, identified by continuous monitoring of cerebral autoregulatory state, might be associated with improved outcomes.[42]

Whichever approach is taken to its management, the accurate measurement of CPP (calculated as mean arterial pressure – ICP) requires the same zero reference point for arterial pressure and ICP, that is at the level of the brain using the tragus of the ear as the external landmark.[43] Because of hydrostatic effects, actual CPP may be up to 11 mmHg lower than calculated CPP in a patient with 30° head elevation if ICP is referenced to the level of brain and mean arterial pressure to the level of the heart. Despite the importance of this issue, a narrative literature review was unable to determine how mean arterial pressure was measured in the calculation of CPP in 50% of 32 widely cited studies of CPP-guided management.[44]

Neurosurgical Intervention

Evacuation of an expanding intracranial haematoma is the primary goal of neurosurgical treatment, and life-saving surgery should be available within 4 hours of injury.[45] Not replacing the bone flap – primary decompressive craniectomy – is an option to minimise the adverse impact of further brain swelling on ICP.[46] Secondary decompressive craniectomy, which involves removal of the skull and opening of the underlying dura, is most commonly undertaken after TBI as a last-tier intervention in a patient with severe, refractory intracranial hypertension. In the RESCUEicp trial, secondary decompressive craniectomy was associated with lower mortality but higher rates of vegetative state and severe disability in survivors compared to maximal medical therapy in patients with ICP >25 mmHg for >1 hour refractory to other interventions.[47]

Other Neuroprotective Interventions

Several therapies have shown promise as neuroprotective agents in pre-clinical and early clinical studies, but these benefits have not been confirmed in prospective clinical trials.[48] Progesterone reduces inflammation, promotes cell proliferation and is antiapoptotic, but large phase 3 clinical trials have not demonstrated improved survival or neurological outcome in moderate or severe TBI.[49] Erythropoietin has non-haemopoietic beneficial effects on endothelial cells, neurons and glia in pre-clinical studies, and a meta-analysis of randomised controlled clinical trials found that it was associated with a significant reduction in mortality after TBI.[50] However, a potential benefit on neurological outcome did not reach statistical significance in this analysis.

Systemic Complications

Non-neurological organ system dysfunction and failure are common after TBI. They are independently associated with increased morbidity but, with the exception of hypotension and acute kidney injury, not with increased mortality.[51] Systemic complications may be related to neurogenic causes such as brain injury-related catecholamine and neuroinflammatory responses, or occur as a complication of brain-directed therapies.[52]

Cardiac Complications

TBI-induced catecholamine release from cardiac sympathetic nerves results in myocyte dysfunction and the neurogenic stunned myocardium syndrome.[53] This reversible neurologically mediated cardiac injury is characterised by ECG changes, elevated cardiac troponin and a spectrum of ventricular dysfunction in the absence of coronary ischaemia. Systemic catecholamine release can cause neurogenic pulmonary oedema and other organ damage. Neurones and glial cells produce pro-inflammatory cytokines in response to injury and intense local and systemic inflammatory responses.[54] Disruption of autonomic and neuroendocrine pathways can also cause immunosuppression and high rates of infective complications after TBI.

Pulmonary Complications

Up to 80% of TBI patients develop respiratory complications; those with the severest injury are most at risk.[55] Ventilator acquired pneumonia is a particular concern and develops in 45%–60% of patients.[56] While the application of ventilator 'care bundles' and protective ventilation strategies reduce the incidence of acute lung injury after TBI, there can be conflict between ventilation and brain-directed strategies and therapy may be a compromise on a case-by-case basis.[57]

Electrolyte and Endocrine Dysfunction

TBI can result in alterations in hypothalamic–pituitary–adrenal axis function, disruption of the anterior hypothalamus and related hormones, and alteration of regulation of sodium and fluid balance. Risk factors for electrolyte and endocrine dysfunction include older age, diffuse axonal injury, severe cerebral oedema, traumatic vasospasm and skull base fractures. Both hyponatraemia and hypernatraemia have adverse effects on the injured brain, and a systematic approach to diagnosis and treatment is essential.[58] Hypothalamic-pituitary axis dysfunction leading to adrenal insufficiency occurs in up to 50% of patients with severe TBI, and the effects can be long lasting and affect recovery into the chronic phases of rehabilitation.[59] Hormone replacement is not well studied, but hydrocortisone should be considered in the presence of refractory hypotension.

For a detailed review of the aetiology and management of non-neurological complications the reader is referred elsewhere[52,60] and to Chapter 14.

Benefits of Neurocritical Care

Neurocritical care encompasses the management of all critically ill patients with neurological disease, including those with TBI, but different models of care delivery exist. Neurocritical care can be provided by neurointensivists in specialised neurocritical care units, or by neurointensivists in a mixed ICU. Alternatively, in some centres, critically ill neurological patients are managed in a mixed ICU without specialty-specific arrangements. While there is some evidence that outcomes are improved when head injured patients are managed in a specialist neurocritical care unit compared to a general ICU, the reasons for this are likely to be multifactorial and not only (or at all) related to the location of care delivery. Implementation of management protocols, improved management of systemic physiological variables and multi-disciplinary neurocritical care teams have all been shown to contribute to improved outcomes after TBI.[13]

Management Protocols

The complex pathophysiology of TBI makes it unlikely that any intervention in isolation will modulate outcome. However, the combination of multiple interventions into a management protocol designed to avoid or minimise secondary brain injury has been associated with mortality reductions and improved neurological outcomes after severe TBI.[61] Increased compliance with protocols leads to greater outcome improvements.[62]

The Neurocritical Care Team

A multi-professional neurocritical care team comprising medical, nursing and other health care professionals supervised by a neurointensivist and with involvement of senior neuro-surgeons has a positive impact on patient management and outcomes after TBI. Experienced neurocritical care staff ensure that individualised therapies aimed at preventing secondary brain injury are applied in a timely and consistent fashion, and within the context of the complex interactions between systemic physiology and the injured brain.[12]

Length of Stay and Cost-Effectiveness

Some early single centre studies suggested that management of TBI patients in a neurocritical care unit was associated with shorter length of stay and lower resource usage compared to management in a general ICU, but more recent data indicate the contrary.[13] A population-based study found that neurocritical care unit length of stay increased as patient outcomes improved over time, possibly because of more aggressive and longer duration therapy and lower rates of early treatment withdrawal.[63] In a UK study, management of patients with severe TBI in specialised neurocritical care units was associated with a higher 6 month cost but also with higher quality of life and lower long-term health can social care costs compared to management in general ICUs, suggesting that specialist units may be cost-effective.[64]

Therapeutic Nihilism

Accurate early prognostication after severe TBI is notoriously difficult. There is limited evidence from controlled studies to guide decision-making, and risk prediction models are insufficiently precise for use in individual patients.[65] A period of physiological stabilisation and observation is strongly recommended to improve the quality of decision-making and to avoid the 'self-fulfilling prophecy' of early withdrawal of life sustaining therapies leading to death.[66] In one study, up to 15% of severe TBI patients who ultimately had a favourable outcome did not begin to follow commands until beyond 2 weeks after injury.[67] Despite early and aggressive support some patients will not achieve a degree of neurological recovery which is acceptable to them, and there should be a timely switch to compassionate and individualised end-of-life care as soon as this is recognised.[68]

Summary

The critical care management of TBI is complex and requires a coordinated and stepwise approach including meticulous general intensive care support as well as interventions targeted to the injured brain. Treatment focuses on prevention and management of intra-cranial complications, optimisation of systemic physiological variables, and management of non-neurological complications. Advances in neuromonitoring and neuroimaging techniques, in association with improved understanding of the pathophysiology of TBI, have led to the introduction of more effective critical care treatment strategies that have translated into improved outcomes for patients. While clinical guidelines have developed with international consensus, advances in multimodality neuromonitoring have allowed individualised treatment decisions to be guided by monitored changes in cerebral physiology rather than pre-determined and generic targets. Implementation of ICU management protocols, improved management of systemic physiology and care delivery by multi-disciplinary neurocritical care teams have all contributed to improved outcomes after TBI.

References

1. McGinn MJ, Povlishock JT. Pathophysiology of traumatic brain injury. *Neurosurg Clin N Am* 2016;27:397–407.

2. Teasdale G, Maas A, Lecky F, Manley G, Stocchetti N, Murray G. The Glasgow Coma Scale at 40 years: standing the test of time. *Lancet Neurol* 2014;13:844–54.

3. Oddo M, Villa F, Citerio G. Brain multimodality monitoring: an update. *Curr Opin Crit Care* 2012;18:111–18.

4. Smith M. Multimodality neuromonitoring in adult traumatic brain injury: a narrative review. *Anesthesiology* 2018;128:401–15.

5. Carney N, Totten AM, O'Reilly C, et al. Guidelines for the management of severe traumatic brain injury, fourth edition. *Neurosurgery* 2017;80:6–15.

6. Stocchetti N, Picetti E, Berardino M, et al. Clinical applications of intracranial pressure monitoring in traumatic brain injury: report of the Milan consensus conference. *Acta Neurochir (Wien)* 2014;156:1615–22.

7. Oddo M, Levine JM, Mackenzie L, et al. Brain hypoxia is associated with short-term outcome after severe traumatic brain injury independently of intracranial hypertension and low cerebral perfusion pressure. *Neurosurgery* 2011;69:1037–45.

8. Kirkman MA, Smith MB. Oxygenation monitoring. *Anesthesiol Clin* 2016;34:537–56.

9. Okonkwo DO, Shutter LA, Moore C, et al. Brain oxygen optimization in severe traumatic brain injury phase-II: a phase II randomized trial. *Crit Care Med* 2017;45:1907–14.

10. Makarenko S, Griesdale DE, Gooderham P, Sekhon MS. Multimodal neuromonitoring for traumatic brain injury: a shift towards individualized therapy. *J Clin Neurosci* 2016;26:8–13.

11. Kinoshita K. Traumatic brain injury: pathophysiology for neurocritical care. *J Intensive Care* 2016;4:29.

12. Wijdicks EF, Menon DK, Smith M. Ten things you need to know to practice neurological critical care. *Intensive Care Med* 2015;41:318–21.

13. Kramer AH, Zygun DA. Neurocritical care: why does it make a difference? *Curr Opin Crit Care* 2014;20:174–81.

14. McHugh GS, Engel DC, Butcher I, et al. Prognostic value of secondary insults in traumatic brain injury: results from the IMPACT study. *J Neurotrauma* 2007;24:287–93.

15. van der Jagt M. Fluid management of the neurological patient: a concise review. *Crit Care* 2016;20:126.

16. Gantner D, Moore EM, Cooper DJ. Intravenous fluids in traumatic brain injury: what's the solution? *Curr Opin Crit Care* 2014;20:385–9.

17. Asehnoune K, Lasocki S, Seguin P, et al. Association between continuous hyperosmolar therapy and survival in patients with traumatic brain injury – a multicentre prospective cohort study and systematic review. *Crit Care* 2017;21:328.

18. Mascia L, Zavala E, Bosma K, et al. High tidal volume is associated with the development of acute lung injury after severe brain injury: an international observational study. *Crit Care Med* 2007;35:1815–20.

19. Boone MD, Jinadasa SP, Mueller A, et al. The effect of positive end-expiratory pressure on intracranial pressure and

cerebral hemodynamics. *Neurocrit Care* 2017;26:174–81.

20. Lu Q, Xie Y, Qi X, Li X, Yang S, Wang Y. Is early tracheostomy better for severe traumatic brain injury? A meta-analysis. *World Neurosurg* 2018;Jan 11 Epub ahead of print.

21. Jauch-Chara K, Oltmanns KM. Glycemic control after brain injury: boon and bane for the brain. *Neuroscience* 2014;283:202–9.

22. Hermanides J, Plummer MP, Finnis M, Deane AM, Coles JP, Menon DK. Glycaemic control targets after traumatic brain injury: a systematic review and meta-analysis. *Crit Care* 2018;22:11.

23. Godoy DA, Behrouz R, Di Napoli M. Glucose control in acute brain injury: does it matter? *Curr Opin Crit Care* 2016;22:120–7.

24. Bohman LE, Levine JM. Fever and therapeutic normothermia in severe brain injury: an update. *Curr Opin Crit Care* 2014;20:182–8.

25. Lewis SR, Evans DJ, Butler AR, Schofield-Robinson OJ, Alderson P. Hypothermia for traumatic brain injury. *Cochrane Database Syst Rev* 2017;9: CD001048.

26. Andrews PJ, Sinclair HL, Rodriguez A, et al. Hypothermia for intracranial hypertension after traumatic brain injury. *N Engl J Med* 2015;373:2403–12.

27. Xu JC, Shen J, Shao WZ, et al. The safety and efficacy of levetiracetam versus phenytoin for seizure prophylaxis after traumatic brain injury: a systematic review and meta-analysis. *Brain Inj* 2016;30:1054–61.

28. Epstein DS, Mitra B, O'Reilly G, Rosenfeld JV, Cameron PA. Acute traumatic coagulopathy in the setting of isolated traumatic brain injury: a systematic review and meta-analysis. *Injury* 2014;45:819–24.

29. Lelubre C, Bouzat P, Crippa IA, Taccone FS. Anemia management after acute brain injury. *Crit Care* 2016;20:152.

30. Robertson CS, Hannay HJ, Yamal JM, et al. Effect of erythropoietin and transfusion threshold on neurological recovery after traumatic brain injury: a randomized clinical trial. *JAMA* 2014;312:36–47.

31. Wang X, Dong Y, Han X, Qi XQ, Huang CG, Hou LJ. Nutritional support for patients sustaining traumatic brain injury: a systematic review and meta-analysis of prospective studies. *PLoS One* 2013;8: e58838.

32. Abdel-Aziz H, Dunham CM, Malik RJ, Hileman BM. Timing for deep vein thrombosis chemoprophylaxis in traumatic brain injury: an evidence-based review. *Crit Care* 2015;19:96.

33. Kirkman MA, Smith M. Intracranial pressure monitoring, cerebral perfusion pressure estimation, and ICP/CPP-guided therapy: a standard of care or optional extra after brain injury? *Br J Anaesth* 2014;112:35–46.

34. Badri S, Chen J, Barber J, et al. Mortality and long-term functional outcome associated with intracranial pressure after traumatic brain injury. *Intensive Care Med* 2012;38:1800–9.

35. Balestreri M, Czosnyka M, Hutchinson P, et al. Impact of intracranial pressure and cerebral perfusion pressure on severe disability and mortality after head injury. *Neurocrit Care* 2006;4:8–13.

36. Stocchetti N, Maas AI. Traumatic intracranial hypertension. *N Engl J Med* 2014;370:2121–30.

37. Stocchetti N, Zanaboni C, Colombo A, et al. Refractory intracranial hypertension and 'second-tier' therapies in traumatic brain injury. *Intensive Care Med* 2008;34:461–7.

38. Yuan Q, Wu X, Sun Y, et al. Impact of intracranial pressure monitoring on mortality in patients with traumatic brain injury: a systematic review and meta-analysis. *J Neurosurg* 2015;122:574–87.

39. Chesnut RM, Temkin N, Carney N, et al. A trial of intracranial-pressure monitoring

in traumatic brain injury. *N Engl J Med* 2012;367:2471–81.

40. Chesnut RM. Intracranial pressure monitoring: headstone or a new head start: the BEST TRIP trial in perspective. *Intensive Care Med* 2013;39:771–4.

41. Koskinen LO, Olivecrona M, Grande PO. Severe traumatic brain injury management and clinical outcome using the Lund concept. *Neuroscience* 2014;283:245–55.

42. Needham E, McFadyen C, Newcombe V, Synnot AJ, Czosnyka M, Menon D. Cerebral perfusion pressure targets individualized to pressure-reactivity index in moderate to severe traumatic brain injury: a systematic review. *J Neurotrauma* 2017;34:963–70.

43. Smith M. Cerebral perfusion pressure. *Br J Anaesth* 2015;115:488–90.

44. Kosty JA, LeRoux PD, Levine J, et al. Brief report: a comparison of clinical and research practices in measuring cerebral perfusion pressure: a literature review and practitioner survey. *Anesth Analg* 2013;117:694–8.

45. Leach P, Childs C, Evans J, Johnston N, Protheroe R, King A. Transfer times for patients with extradural and subdural haematomas to neurosurgery in Greater Manchester. *Br J Neurosurg* 2007;21:11–15.

46. Kolias AG, Kirkpatrick PJ, Hutchinson PJ. Decompressive craniectomy: past, present and future. *Nat Rev Neurol* 2013;9:405–15.

47. Hutchinson PJ, Kolias AG, Timofeev IS, et al. Trial of decompressive craniectomy for traumatic intracranial hypertension. *N Engl J Med* 2016;375:1119–30.

48. Stocchetti N, Taccone FS, Citerio G, et al. Neuroprotection in acute brain injury: an up-to-date review. *Crit Care* 2015;19:186.

49. Lu XY, Sun H, Li QY, Lu PS. Progesterone for traumatic brain injury: a meta-analysis review of randomized controlled trials. *World Neurosurg* 2016;90:199–210.

50. Liu WC, Wen L, Xie T, Wang H, Gong JB, Yang XF. Therapeutic effect of erythropoietin in patients with traumatic brain injury: a meta-analysis of randomized controlled trials. *J Neurosurg* 2016;127(1):8-15.

51. Corral L, Javierre CF, Ventura JL, Marcos P, Herrero JI, Manez R. Impact of non-neurological complications in severe traumatic brain injury outcome. *Crit Care* 2012;16:R44.

52. Gaddam SS, Buell T, Robertson CS. Systemic manifestations of traumatic brain injury. *Handb Clin Neurol* 2015;127:205–18.

53. Krishnamoorthy V, Mackensen GB, Gibbons EF, Vavilala MS. Cardiac dysfunction after neurologic injury: what do we know and where are we going? *Chest* 2016;149:1325–31.

54. Anthony DC, Couch Y. The systemic response to CNS injury. *Exp Neurol* 2014;258:105–11.

55. Zygun DA, Kortbeek JB, Fick GH, Laupland KB, Doig CJ. Non-neurologic organ dysfunction in severe traumatic brain injury. *Crit Care Med* 2005;33:654–60.

56. Zygun DA, Zuege DJ, Boiteau PJ, Laupland KB, Henderson EA, Kortbeek JB, Doig CJ. Ventilator-associated pneumonia in severe traumatic brain injury. *Neurocrit Care* 2006;5:108–14.

57. Young N, Rhodes JK, Mascia L, Andrews PJ. Ventilatory strategies for patients with acute brain injury. *Curr Opin Crit Care* 2010;16:45–52.

58. Tisdall M, Crocker M, Watkiss J, Smith M. Disturbances of sodium in critically ill adult neurologic patients: a clinical review. *J Neurosurg Anesthesiol* 2006;18:57–63.

59. Vespa PM. Hormonal dysfunction in neurocritical patients. *Curr Opin Crit Care* 2013;19:107–12.

60. Lim HB, Smith M. Systemic complications after head injury: a clinical review. *Anaesthesia* 2007;62:474–82.

61. English SW, Turgeon AF, Owen E, Doucette S, Pagliarello G, McIntyre L. Protocol management of severe traumatic brain injury in intensive care units: a systematic review. *Neurocrit Care* 2013;18:131–42.

62. Gerber LM, Chiu YL, Carney N, Hartl R, Ghajar J. Marked reduction in mortality in patients with severe traumatic brain injury. *J Neurosurg* 2013;119:1583–90.

63. Kramer AH, Zygun DA. Declining mortality in neurocritical care patients: a cohort study in Southern Alberta over eleven years. *Can J Anaesth* 2013;60:966–75.

64. Harrison DA, Prabhu G, Grieve R, et al. Risk Adjustment In Neurocritical care (RAIN) – prospective validation of risk prediction models for adult patients with acute traumatic brain injury to use to evaluate the optimum location and comparative costs of neurocritical care: a cohort study. *Health Technol Assess* 2013;17:vii–viii.

65. Stevens RD, Sutter R. Prognosis in severe brain injury. *Crit Care Med* 2013;41:1104–23.

66. Harvey D, Butler J, Groves J, et al. Management of perceived devastating brain injury after hospital admission: a consensus statement from stakeholder professional organizations. *Br J Anaesth* 2018;120:138–45.

67. Vedantam A, Robertson CS, Gopinath SP. Clinical characteristics and temporal profile of recovery in patients with favorable outcomes at 6 months after severe traumatic brain injury. *J Neurosurg* 2018;129(1): 234-40.

68. Smith M. Treatment withdrawal and acute brain injury: an integral part of care. *Anaesthesia* 2012;67:941–5.

Intracranial Pressure Monitoring in Head Injury

Adam J. Wells, Peter Smielewski, Rikin A. Trivedi
and Peter J. Hutchinson

Introduction

Intracranial pressure (ICP) is well recognised as a critical parameter to both measure and influence in the management of the head injured patient. Since Lundberg's seminal studies, ICP has arguably become the major focus of monitoring in head injury, as well as a number of other neurosurgical scenarios.[1] Mean ICP and the features that make up the ICP waveform provide insight into the state of elastance and compliance of the injured brain, impending trends and events related to changes in intracranial pathophysiology, and also end-prognosis in traumatic brain injury (TBI).

Definitions and Pathophysiology

ICP can be interpreted as the environmental pressure acting within the cranial vault. Three different pressures contribute to ICP: atmospheric, hydrostatic and filling pressure. Atmospheric pressure is transmitted via the cerebral vasculature and is relative to altitude; however, ICP is described clinically relative to atmospheric pressure and therefore this contribution is generally ignored.[2] Hydrostatic pressure depends on the weight of the fluid of the contents of the skull above the point of measurement,[3,4] and filling pressure is determined by the volume of the intracranial contents and their elastance.

There are three main volumetric elements that contribute to ICP: the brain parenchyma, intracranial blood volume, and cerebrospinal fluid (CSF). These three elements are contained within the fixed volume of the rigid bony skull, and the relationship between the volume of the intracranial components and ICP is described by the Monro-Kellie doctrine.[5] For two centuries it has been understood that any increase in volume of one of the intracranial components must result in a decrease in volume of one or both of the other two components in order to maintain a constant ICP. As compensatory reserve diminishes ICP begins to rise in an exponential manner (Figure 11.1).

The effects of an increased ICP are twofold: raised ICP can result in herniation of the brain substance beyond normal anatomical compartments, and ICP directly influences cerebral blood flow (CBF) via its effect on cerebral perfusion pressure (CPP) (Figure 11.2). ICP acts as an opposing influence to the intrinsic driving force of mean arterial pressure (MAP) as defined by the equation CPP=MAP-ICP. In normal physiologic states CBF is maintained across a wide range of CPP by the process of autoregulation (Figure 11.3); however, following TBI, autoregulation is frequently impaired, putting the brain at risk of ischaemia or hyperaemia. One of the main management strategies in TBI is preventing secondary brain injury, and one of the biggest secondary insults is cerebral hypoxia, hence

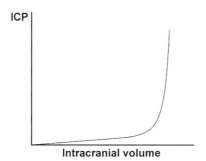

Figure 11.1 Relationship between intracranial pressure (ICP) and increasing volume of intracranial contents, including exponential rise in ICP as compensatory reserve exhausts.

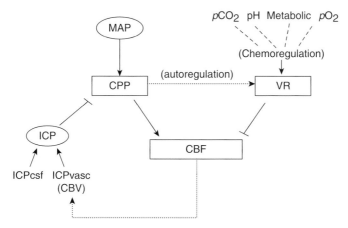

Figure 11.2 Relationship between intracranial pressure and cerebral blood flow. CBF, cerebral blood flow; CBV, cerebral blood volume; CPP, cerebral perfusion pressure; ICP, intracranial pressure (composed of distinct contributions from cerebrospinal fluid (ICPcsf) and the vascular compartment (ICPvasc)); MAP, mean arterial pressure; VR, cerebral vascular resistance; →, excitatory; –|, inhibitory; –>, variable influences.

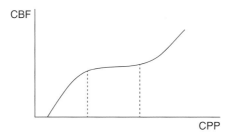

Figure 11.3 Autoregulation of cerebral blood flow (CBF). A relatively constant CBF is maintained over a range of cerebral perfusion pressure (CPP) (dotted lines).

ICP and MAP measurements are vital to calculate CPP and to focus therapy on ICP and CPP targets.

Technology of ICP Monitoring

There are several methods of measuring ICP; however, all techniques currently used employ one or two general modalities, being fluid-filled catheters or pressure micro-transducers. The 'gold standard' for measuring ICP remains an intraventricular catheter connected to an external pressure transducer, which measures ICP at the level of the interventricular foramen of Monro where there is relatively unobstructed flow of CSF, and this is generally accepted as the physiological reference point for ICP.[6,7] In addition to accurately measuring ICP, ventricular catheters have the added advantage of being able to withdraw CSF as a therapeutic measure for intracranial hypertension. The disadvantages of ventricular catheters include increased technical skill in insertion, particularly following TBI where the ventricular target is small, and higher infection rates compared with parenchymal micro-transducers. Ventricular catheter infection generally increases with time since insertion, with acceptable rates reported ranging from 6% to 8%.[8,9]

Technological advances in microsensor design and reliability have allowed evolution of Millar-type peizoresistive strain-gauge and fibre-optic microsensors, which have an excellent frequency response suitable for investigating high-frequency components, and can be placed anywhere within the cranial cavity.[10] One of the most commonly used devices is the Codman ICP microsensor (Codman & Shurtleff Inc., MA), with the most common location of insertion being intraparenchymal via a frontal burr hole. In addition to the technical ease of insertion they have the added advantage of a lower infection rate when compared to ventricular catheters. Although they cannot be re-zeroed after insertion, they tend to have negligible zero-drift over days and even weeks following insertion.[11,12] The main disadvantages with microsensors include increased expense and the focal nature of the ICP reading. Although ICP should equilibrate there may often be pressure gradients within the cranial cavity, particularly in the presence of space occupying lesions, and as such parenchymal ICP could be under- or over-reported relative to the laterality of insertion.[13]

Other locations for measuring ICP via a microsensor include the epidural, subdural and subarachnoid spaces, and although they are slightly less invasive than intraparenchymal devices they are also less likely to provide an accurate measure of true ICP. Lumbar CSF can be coupled to a fluid filled catheter and an external pressure transducer much like an intraventricular catheter, but in the context of TBI lumbar pressures are not a reliable reflection of ICP and may even be dangerous in the presence of intracranial hypertension or a space occupying lesion, as lumbar CSF drainage may promote tonsillar herniation.[6,7] Non-invasive methods of ICP measurement currently in development are based on either morphology (magnetic resonance, computed tomography, ultrasound, fundoscopy) or physiology (transcranial Doppler, tympanometry, near-infrared spectroscopy), and although they do not have the infective and haemorrhagic risks associated with invasive devices, they are not yet reliable enough to employ clinically.[14,15] The advantages and disadvantages for the different methods and locations for measuring ICP are summarised in Table 11.1.

Normal ICP Values and Treatment Thresholds

Although ICP is frequently taught to have a normal range of 5–15 mmHg, in reality there is no universal 'normal' ICP value. ICP varies between and within individuals, and depends on

Table 11.1 Different methods of measuring intracranial pressure, advantages and disadvantages

Monitor type	Advantages	Disadvantages
Intraventricular catheter	Measures 'true' ICP Ability to remove CSF Able to be re-zeroed	Most invasive Highest infection risks Difficulty with insertion
Intraparenchymal probe	Lower infection rates Easier insertion Most accurate of the microtransducer probes	Not as accurate as ventricular catheter Possible zero-drift
Subarachnoid probe	Lower infection rates Less invasive	Limited accuracy High failure rate
Epidural probe	Lower infection rates Less invasive Easy insertion	Limited accuracy
Lumbar CSF manometer	Extracranial percutaneous insertion Ability to remove CSF	Unreliable measure of ICP Dangerous and contraindicated in intracranial mass lesions
Non-invasive methods	Non-invasive No haemorrhagic or infection complications	Not reliable enough for clinical use

Note: CSF = cerebrospinal fluid; ICP = intracranial pressure.

age, body posture and clinical condition. Pressure may not be evenly distributed within the cranial cavity, particularly in the presence of space occupying mass lesions.[13] In healthy male adults in the horizontal position, it ranges from 7 to 15 mmHg[16]; however, in the vertical position, it can be slightly negative (but not lower than −15 mmHg).[17]

Any underlying clinical context also influences ICP significantly; idiopathic intracranial hypertension for example has diagnostic criteria of lumbar puncture opening pressure >25 cmH_2O (18.4 mmHg), with pressures often ranging from 30 to 40 cmH_2O (22.1–29.4 mmHg).[18] In TBI ICP > 20 mmHg is considered abnormal, and aggressive therapy is frequently initiated with ICP > 25 mmHg. Recommended treatment thresholds vary between institutions; however, the current official upper threshold for ICP in TBI as reported by the Brain Trauma Foundation is 22 mmHg, based on a single centre class 2 study that demonstrated improved rates of mortality and favourable outcome.[19,20]

Common ICP Patterns after Head Injury

ICP varies with time, taking the form of a wave. In acute states, continuous monitoring of ICP reveals a few patterns,[6] which may be classified as follows (Figure 11.4):

1   Low and stable ICP (<20 mmHg), typically seen following uncomplicated head injury or in the early stages post-trauma.
2   High and stable ICP (>20 mmHg), the most common following head trauma.

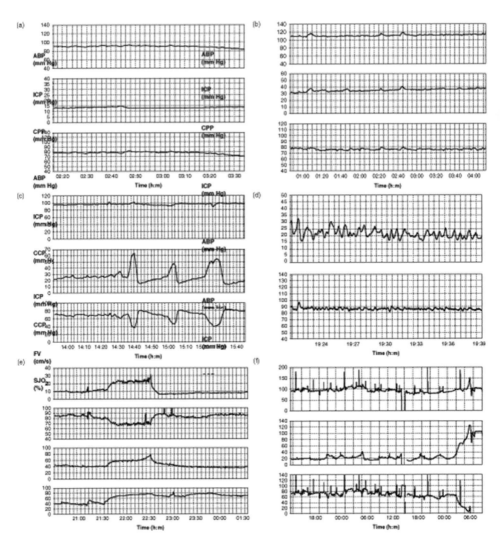

Figure 11.4 ICP patterns. (a) Low and stable ICP; (b) high and stable ICP; (c) plateau waves; (d) B waves; (e) hyperaemia; (f) development of refractory intracranial hypertension.

3 Vasogenic waves: Plateau 'A' waves (steep increases in ICP remaining at a high level for 5–20 min) and 'B' waves (oscillations at 0.5–2 Hz).
4 ICP waves related to changes in cerebral blood flow (transient hyperaemic events).
5 Refractory intracranial hypertension – refers to a large and rapid rise in ICP that is often fatal unless drastic aggressive measures such as decompressive craniectomy are instigated.

Analysis of ICP Waveforms

ICP is a modality of a highly rich content. Commonly only instantaneous (at the bed side), hourly mean values or (worse still) end-of-hour point values are available to clinicians and saved in electronic record systems. This is largely the case even today in most critical care units, despite so much having been published on the subject of ICP waveforms and the additional information carried by them. In fact, one relatively recent clinical trial of ICP orientated therapy failed to show outcome benefits from using ICP measured in this basic way,[21] and it was subsequently argued that only through analysis of ICP waveforms that added benefit could be seen.[22] Minute-by-minute records of ICP monitoring is becoming more commonplace now, and with that measures such as dose of ICP, including total or hourly dose, have become possible. Several authors have shown benefits of using such a measure over simple ICP mean, and of course end-hour point value.[23,24] But even that is only touching the tip of the iceberg. The truly remarkable thing about ICP modality is that it provides us with a reliable and stable window into intracranial dynamics from which many properties of cerebrovascular and cerebrospinal circulation can be derived. There is no other neuromonitoring modality that would offer such high temporal (up to 100 Hz) insights into mechanical properties of the cranium over such long time periods of days or even weeks. But in order to take advantage of this information one must rely on computer supported analysis, ideally performed in real time at the bedside, such as offered by software solutions like ICM+ (http://icmplus.neurosurg.cam.ac.uk)

ICP Waveform Components

The ICP waveform appears to exhibit complex patterns that do not get simpler when examined at different time scales, but merely seem to change the apparent features (Figure 11.5). In order to appreciate the composition of ICP of different (and to a large extent independent) components, one can reach out for a mathematical tool that allows separating those time scales via the frequency decomposition, most commonly using Fourier spectral analysis.[6] If several hours long segments of ICP waveforms are examined, this way one can distinguish several components (Figure 11.6). The most well defined are the arterial pulse derived components (period of 50–180 beats/min) and respiratory cycle derived components (period of 8–20 cycles/min). In addition there are what is now collectively termed slow waves (waves or duration of about 10 s and longer). These include M-waves (cyclic waves related to baroreceptors and chemoreceptors, with frequency of about 6/min),[25] B-waves (related to modulation of cerebral blood volume via arterial vasodilatation and constriction),[26] and A-waves (also known as plateau waves), which are large in magnitude (reaching 40 mmHg and more) and lasting for at least 5 min, attributed to the so-called vasodilatatory cascade in conditions of exhausted brain compliance.[27] Each of these wave types require a different analytical strategy.

Pulse waveform analysis can be approached either in time domain, by examining morphology of a single, representative, pulse pressure wave, or in frequency domain, by investigating the frequency decomposition of the pulse. These two broad types of approaches, despite their quantitative differences, are qualitatively equivalent. They both allow easier access to different metrics of the pulse, with some of them having more physiological relevance than others. For example, the most intuitive metric of the pulse wave is its amplitude, which in time domain is defined as peak-to-peak pressure difference (Figure 11.7). This metric has been shown to be associated with clinical outcome in TBI,[28] as well as in patients treated for hydrocephalus.[29] In both cases increased pulse amplitude provides evidence of either reduced cerebral compliance or increased cerebral arterial blood load, which in the case of TBI is usually associated with increased ICP and/or decreased

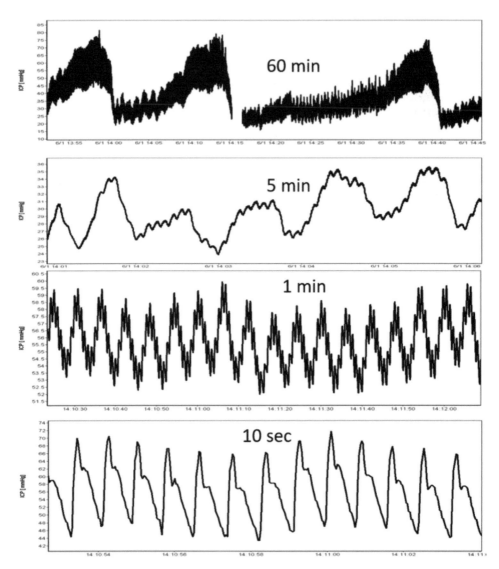

Figure 11.5 An ICP recording from a single TBI patient, with the four separate panels representing different timescales of the same recording. Note how each timescale reveals distinct waveform patterns.

CPP. However, it has also been shown that other metrics derived from the pulse wave are equally interesting indicators of cerebral compliance and have stronger clinical associations. These are mainly derived from the relationship between three distinctive peaks that could be observed in the shape of the pulse, P1 (percussion), P2 (tidal) and P3 (dicrotic), with P1 to P2 ratio believed to reflect brain compliance (Figure 11.7).[30] But perhaps the most thorough analysis of the morphology of ICP pulse has been conducted by Hu and colleagues,[31] who have identified 28 basic metrics using their MOCAIP algorithm, including individual peaks amplitude, location, curvatures and slope/decay-related indices. Using this large number of

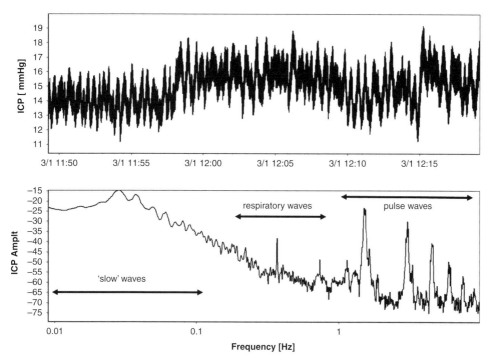

Figure 11.6 An example of a 30-min-long recording of ICP, shown as a time series trace demonstrating a complex pattern of waves (top panel) and as a Fourier frequency spectrum decomposing the waveforms into the three main components (bottom).

derived measures however does not by itself offer any benefits over interpretation of individual samples of the pulse. ICP pulse can be sufficiently represented by the first 10 harmonics, which corresponds to 20 samples per pulse. However, this approach offers a non-linear transformation of the original data which allows amplification of certain features making the final, combined, index or indices more robust. For example, they have shown that by using machine learning derived classifier derived from their basic metrics they could predict ICP elevation 5 min prior to its onset with high specificity and sensitivity.[32]

In frequency domain we can examine a pulse pressure segment after digital Fourier transformation (Figure 11.8). This mathematical tool produces representation of the pulse as a superposition of a number (equal to half of the number of samples contained in the pulse) of scaled and phase shifted sinusoids. Here too, one has to define a small subset of features of this decomposition for the technique to offer any dimensionality reduction benefits. Two such features that have been studied in the context of clinical associations are the amplitude of the fundamental harmonic (the amplitude of the main sinusoidal element of the decomposition, with period equal to the pulse period) and the centre of gravity of the frequency decomposition (high-frequency centroid, HFC). The former, often denoted 'AMP' in the literature, has been shown to be useful as a pulse amplitude metric, offering similar interpretation and clinical correlations as peak-to-peak amplitude, with good direct correlation between the two measures.[33] This spectral measure of amplitude is a lot more robust in the

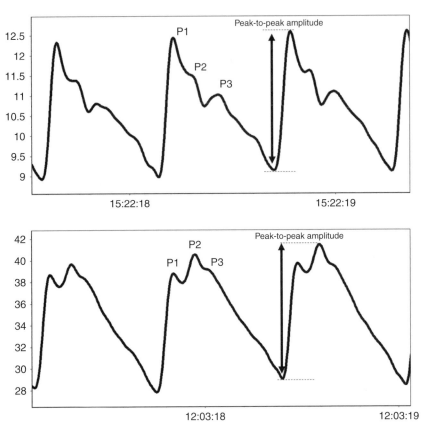

Figure 11.7 ICP pulse waves from the same patient at two separate intervals, at a normal ICP (top panel) and at hypertensive levels (bottom panel), demonstrating three distinctive peaks: P1 (percussion wave related), P2 (tidal wave related) and P3 (dicrotic wave related). Note that the peak-to-peak amplitude metric at normal ICP reflects P1 and at hypertensive levels P2.

presence of noise and other high-amplitude waves (e.g. respiratory component), but is more sensitive to pronounced cardiac arrhythmias. HFC, on the other hand, provides an index of 'complexity' of the pulse shape (Figure 11.8). HFC has been originally defined as the power-weighted average frequency within the 4 to 15 Hz band of the ICP spectrum,[34] and it has been demonstrated that it inversely correlates with ICP volume index (PVI) with high values indicating exhaustion of intracranial volume-buffering capacity. This is usually associated with high ICP, but it is likely a reflection of low cerebral compliance.[33,34] These findings are consistent with current interpretations of the components of the ICP waveform.

Which approach produces more robust metrics is debatable. What it comes down to in reality is how robust are the techniques to noise and cardiac arrhythmias and how much this can be controlled by appropriate signal conditioning and other pre-processing steps. This of course depends on the software available at the bed-side, as none of these pulse shape descriptor indices are routinely available on most critical care monitors, not even pulse amplitude of ICP.

The respiratory component of the ICP waveform has not so far been found to be particularly useful, as its frequency is normally too high to probe cerebral autoregulatory

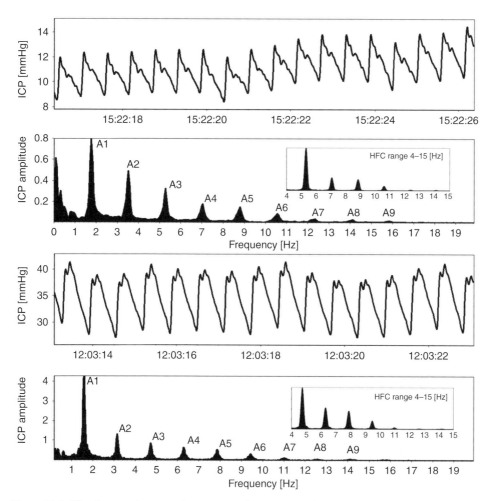

Figure 11.8 ICP pulse wave frequency decomposition for a patient with normal ICP (top two panels, time series and spectrum respectively) and a patient with intracranial hypertension (bottom two panels, time series and spectrum respectively). The pulse wave is composed of sinusoidal components of amplitudes A1–A9, the so-called harmonics of the fundamental component A1. Frequency range 4–15 Hz originally used for calculating the centre of gravity of the decomposition (HFC, High Frequency Centroid) is demonstrated inset to the spectrum charts. The centre of gravity (HFC) shifts to the right with intracranial hypertension.

capacity, and its almost sinusoidal shape does not offer any interesting features to exploit. One application that can be mentioned here involves comparison of a pulse shape feature, the pulse slope, at inspiration and expiration (I:E) (Figure 11.9); the I:E pulse slope ratio has been found to reflect the degree of venous volume buffering available. Values approaching unity seem to be associated with the loss of intracranial volume buffering and are indicative of a critical change in intracranial volume prior to the point at which ICP starts to rise steeply with further increases in volume (Figure 11.10).[35,36]

Things get more interesting again when one considers frequencies below 0.1 Hz. These waves are highly irregular and have been shown to have non-stationary

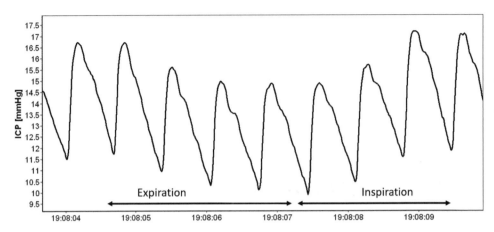

Figure 11.9 ICP pulse waveforms over one respiratory cycle. The ratio of the upstroke slopes of the pulse wave at inspiration and expiration phase is expressed as the I:E index and reflects intracranial volume buffering.

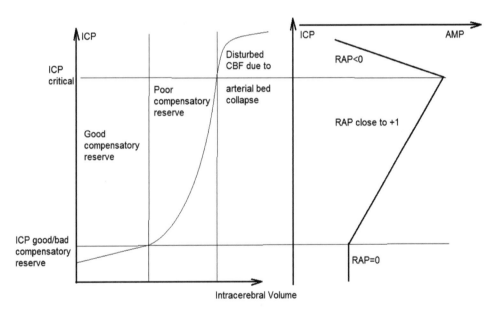

Figure 11.10 The cerebral pressure volume characteristic and derived pulse amplitude to mean ICP relationship. The chart on the left depicts a conceptual drawing of the pressure-volume curve with two distinct breakpoints: the first one separates good from exhausted compensatory reserve (where small changes in volume result in large changes in pressure) and the second one marking the point where cerebral vessels begin collapsing due to insufficient filling pressure. The chart on the right depicts the corresponding relationship between the pressure pulse amplitude and mean ICP, again differentiating the three states.

properties. Analytical approaches include estimation of the total power within a particular range of frequencies (e.g. 0.33–3 cycles/min), examination of duration and incidence of longer lasting waves, and assessment of their 'chaotic' properties. The latter approach is particularly attractive as it does not require assumption of stationarity nor linearity of the underlying processes, and allows an assessment of the overall 'health' of the network of interconnected dynamic components (intracranial and systemic) which collectively form the homeostatic system.[37] Methods like fractal analysis, looking at fractal dimensionality (i.e. self-similarity) of the slow waves and Entropy analysis,[38,39] looking at the overall complexity of the slow waves features, reveal a strong association between these global measures of 'health' of the homeostatic system with the patient outcome after severe brain trauma.[40] These do not point to a single particular aspect of physiology and thus do not offer any basis for selection of treatment, but may provide an early warning system, as an indicator of a general homeostatic deterioration.

Slow Wave–Derived Indices

Probably the most clinically useful benefit of analysis of slow waves comes from the fact that they can be treated as spontaneous, and thus non-interventional, probes modulating mean value of ICP, and thus CPP, allowing assessment of such properties as cerebral autoregulation and cerebrospinal compensatory reserve.

Cerebral Autoregulation Assessment Using Pressure Reactivity Index (PRx)

By its definition cerebral autoregulation should technically be assessed by quantifying response in cerebral blood flow to slow changes in mean cerebral perfusion pressure (slow, because of the inherent inertia of this mechanism, with time constant of several seconds). However, if one notes that stabilisation of cerebral flow is achieved through active cerebral arterial vasoconstriction and vasodilation, then intuitively one can visualise changes in cerebral blood volume brought about by these effects (Figure 11.11). Cerebral blood volume changes in turn will produce changes in ICP, of magnitude dependent on the brain compliance.[41] Thus, if analysis of mean ICP responses to slow changes (waves) of mean arterial blood pressure by means of phase shift is performed, it can be seen that with impaired autoregulation there is a passive response in ICP (passive distension of arterial bed), giving it a phase shift of 0, while with active autoregulation there is positive phase shift of about 150° (which would have been 180° if the autoregulation acted instantaneously) (Figure 11.12).[42] When the ABP to ICP relationship is expressed as a correlation coefficient, termed PRx,[41] it gives values of +1 for impaired vascular reactivity, and highly negative (but higher than −1) for fully functioning reactivity. In practical terms it is calculated as Pearson correlation between 30 consecutive 10 s averages of ICP and ABP. The index has been validated in experimental work, against a direct measure of cerebral autoregulation based on Laser Doppler flowmetry as well as in TBI patients against outcome (see later in this chapter).[43] Because of its conceptual and technical simplicity, a large volume of evidence in TBI, and the fact that it does not require any additional measurements than the ones already available in patients undergoing neuromonitoring, its popularity has soared over the last decade and it has found its way into recent TBI management guidelines. However there is still more work to be done to improve its robustness, in particular in circumstances of high brain compliance such as that seen in TBI patients after decompressive craniectomy.[44]

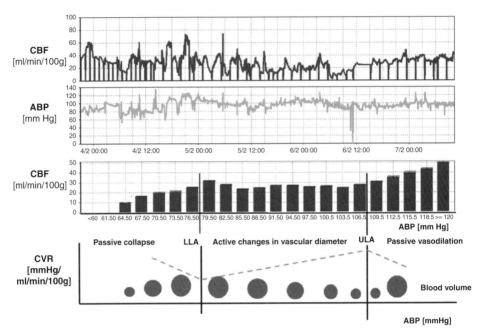

Figure 11.11 Example of a recording from a TBI patient using Hemedex thermodilution measure of cerebral blood flow. The classically described autoregulatory curve obtained from those measurements is demonstrated in the third panel. Conceptual behaviour of the cerebral arterial vasculature is depicted in the bottom panel, with changes in luminal diameter to counteract changes in arterial blood pressure (more accurately cerebral perfusion pressure) or passively expanding or collapsing with pressure outside of the autoregulatory range.

Cerebrospinal Compensatory Reserve (RAP)

This index reflects the relationship between mean ICP and its pulse amplitude, in the form of a correlation coefficient between the two. In order to interpret this index one must picture the cerebrospinal pressure/volume characteristic (Figure 11.10). At the lower end (low volume) it assumes flat, approximately linear relationship. In this part changes in volume (brain swelling or cerebral vasodilatation) will produce small and approximately linear increases in pressure. As more volume is added (e.g. due to continued post-traumatic cerebral oedema) the characteristic becomes steeply exponential. It turns out that with some simplifying assumptions the current location on the pressure/volume curve can be derived, the so-called compensatory reserve, by examining the correlation between mean ICP and its pulse amplitude.[45] This can be done as a running correlation between the two, and the resulting index termed RAP. As was the case with PRx, RAP is calculated as a Pearson correlation coefficient between 30 consecutive 10 s averages of mean ICP and its pulse amplitude (calculated using the spectral method). With good compensatory reserve (the flat part of pressure volume curve) RAP is around 0, while in conditions of a tight brain (the steep, exponential part) RAP becomes close to +1.[46] But there is yet another part to it, perhaps more relevant to TBI patients. With continued volume expansion the cerebral vasculature eventually starts to shut down, causing the pulse propagation to decrease despite steady increase in mean ICP, resulting in negative RAP (Figure 11.13). This effect is only

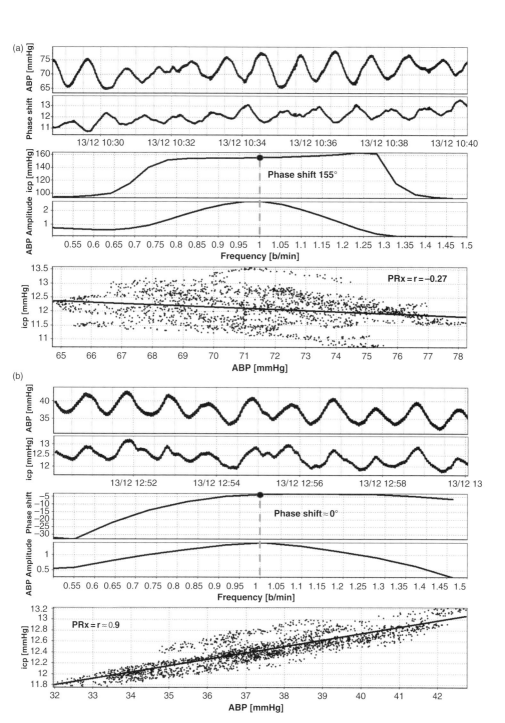

Figure 11.12 The relationship between arterial blood pressure (ABP) and ICP waveforms reflects cerebral autoregulation. This figure shows an example of a low-pass filtered (10 s moving average) ICP recording taken during experimental arterial hypotension in piglets.[74] The relationship at normal ABP values and fully functioning autoregulation is depicted in (a), whereas (b) demonstrates the relationship at the end of the experiment at severe arterial hypotension. In this study a steady oscillation of ABP was induced by modulating positive end expiratory pressure at a frequency of 1/min. The two middle panels in each figure show a section of the Fourier amplitude spectrum of ABP demonstrating well-defined peaks at frequency 1/min, and the ABP -> ICP transfer function phase shift at that point.

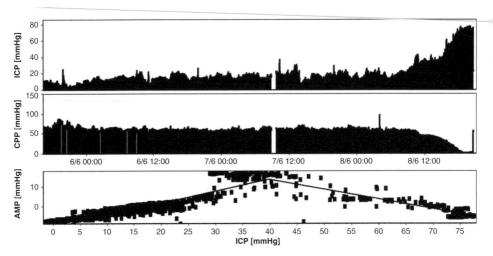

Figure 11.13 Three day ICP recording from a patient with refractory intracranial hypertension. The bottom panel shows the linear relationship between ICP and pulse amplitude (AMP) for lower ICP values (with correlation coefficient RAP close to +1), and for critically high ICP values (>45 mmHg) when the relationship becomes negative (correlation coefficient RAP highly negative).

observed in conditions of refractory intracranial hypertension and signals highly critical levels of ICP.

Other ICP Waveform-Based Indices

Over the years there have emerged other (related) moving correlation principle-based indices that use a combination of pulse amplitude and mean values of ICP, ABP, and CPP signals. In particular indices PAx (the pulse amplitude version of PRx),[47] wPRx (wavelet-based PRx)[48] and RAC (pulse amplitude and CPP correlation)[49] have potential to overcome some of the shortcomings of PRx related to its dependence on brain compliance, or as is the case of RAC, attempt to combine information of cerebral autoregulation with compliance. An informative review of the various autoregulatory indices derived from multi-modality monitoring and their relation to each other is presented by Zeiler et al.[50]

ICP Related to Clinical Outcomes in TBI

One of the main objectives in TBI monitoring and research is to develop a method of predicting imminent decompensation. So far, four of these measures have proven useful as predictors of clinical outcome: mean ICP, RAP, PRx and slow wave content.

Elevated mean ICP correlates with mortality rate following head injury. Remarkably however, no difference in mean ICP is seen between TBI survivors with severe disability and favourable outcome (Figure 11.14).[51] Data such as this has prompted the investigation of decompressive craniectomy as a life-saving procedure for patients with medically refractory intracranial hypertension following TBI, as surgical decompression has shown to be a powerful method to control elevated ICP following TBI.[52] Two independent multi-centre randomised controlled trials have now demonstrated that although decompressive craniectomy achieves its goal of reducing mean ICP and mortality following severe TBI, it

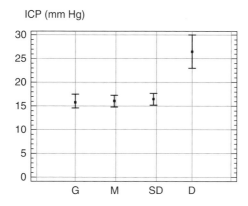

ICP (mm Hg)

Figure 11.14 ICP related to clinical outcome. Mean and 95% confidence intervals of ICP in different outcome groups. G, good outcome; M, moderate outcome; SD, severe disability; D, death.

does so at the expense of increased survivors with a spectrum of outcome categories, whether it is performed as an early intervention[53] or as a rescue procedure.[54]

CPP on the other hand is not always predictive of outcome except at very high values, where the incidence of favourable outcome decreases, and as a predictor of mortality carries less significance than ICP.[51] Whether or not CPP can influence clinical outcome as an independent parameter separate from ICP and MAP, where CPP-orientated protocols are in place, is yet to be determined.[19]

RAP has been a useful tool in indicating the patient's position on the pressure–volume curve as a measure or cerebral compliance. Low average RAP has been shown to be associated with worse outcome when it is detected along with raised ICP.[55] More specific predictions have also been made using RAP; these include prediction of ICP response to hyperventilation (in a preliminary study)[56] and recovery of good compensatory reserve after decompressive craniectomy.[57] Furthermore, a significant correlation between RAP and CBF (as assessed by positron emission tomography) and the width of ventricles and contusion size in closed head injury have been observed.[58,59]

PRx as a measure of pressure-reactivity in the cerebrovascular bed has shown a number of useful clinical correlates. PRx has been shown to be predictive of outcome in head injury, independently of mean ICP, age or severity of injury.[60] It has been shown that PRx correlates with CBF (as predicted by PET and $CMRO_2$);[61] PRx has also been demonstrated as an indicator of loss of autoregulatory reserve in ICP-plateau waves and in refractory intracranial hypertension.[62]

Plotting PRx against CPP reveals a U-shaped curve, suggesting a defined range of CPP over which PRx is optimal (CPPopt; Figure 11.15). Based on early evidence that an optimum range of CPP in terms of brain tissue oxygenation does indeed exist, it has been suggested that PRx might be used as an indicator of the optimum CPP to target in CPP-orientated therapy.[58,63] Real-time CPPopt can be determined in the majority of TBI patients monitored in modern critical care centres, and 6 month clinical outcomes are more likely to be favourable in patients with median CPP close to CPPopt compared to patients in which CPP was not individualised.[64] Further work on the subject of PRx and CPPopt may lead to personalised thresholds and targets with minute-by-minute adjustments to facilitate critical care monitoring and management and to optimise intracranial homeostasis post-TBI.[65–67]

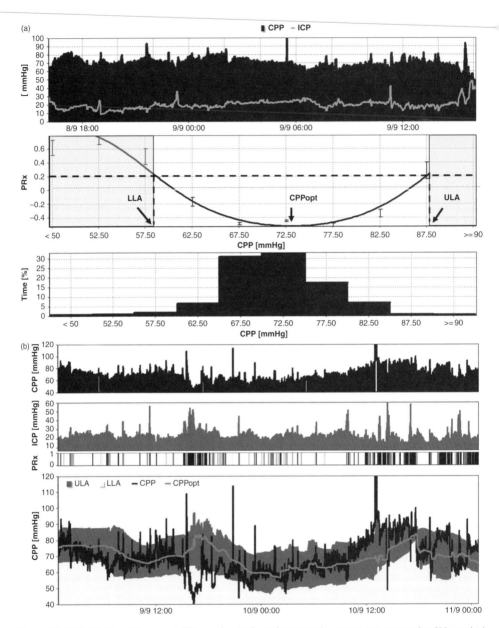

Figure 11.15 (a) Plotting PRx against CPP reveals a U-shaped curve with a vertex pointing to the CPP at which autoregulation works best. This point has been termed optimal CPP (CPPopt). If a horizontal line is drawn at a borderline PRx value of 0.2 (between impaired and intact autoregulation), CPP levels corresponding to lower limit of autoregulation (LLA) and upper limit of autoregulation (ULA) can be determined. Keeping the patient's CPP within this range (LLA-ULA), and possibly close to CPPopt, has been proposed to be associated with better outcome after TBI. (b) Demonstration of ICM+ software, which enables tracking of CPPopt and limits of regulation in real time.

Clinical Use of ICP Monitoring in TBI

ICP monitoring is so fundamental to the modern management of TBI that it has been included in every guideline for TBI published by the Brain Trauma Foundation since its inception. The current Guidelines for the Management of Severe Traumatic Brain Injury recommend the use of ICP monitoring in severe TBI patients to reduce both in-hospital and 2 week post-injury mortality based on level 2 evidence.[19] The previous edition was somewhat more specific in its recommendations for ICP monitor use in patients at risk of intracranial hypertension: salvageable TBI patients who present in coma (Glasgow Coma Scale score of ≤8 after resuscitation) and who have an abnormal CT scan were recommended to have an ICP monitor inserted, and ICP and CPP targeted therapy initiated. Furthermore, TBI patients in coma with normal CT were also recommended to have an ICP monitor inserted if they meet two of three further criteria, being age >40 years, uni- or bilateral motor posturing or systolic blood pressure <90 mmHg.[68] The choice of monitoring device should be driven by unit protocol; however, it should also be influenced by patient's intracranial pathology and the advantages and disadvantages of the different monitor types as illustrated in Table 11.1. Particular consideration for the type of monitor used should be given to the need for CSF diversion or the addition of multimodality monitoring devices, such as microdialysis or brain tissue oxygen probes.

Because of the relatively routine use of ICP monitoring in the developed world there still remains an apparent lack of equipoise regarding its benefits. As such, the evidence for using ICP monitoring in TBI is largely secondary to observational studies that have demonstrated worse clinical outcomes associated with intracranial hypertension.[51] In fact, the only study that has directly compared ICP-driven therapy against imaging and clinical examination without ICP monitoring, performed in central America where ICP monitoring is not currently considered the standard of care, demonstrated that treatment focused on maintaining ICP <20 mmHg was no superior to non-ICP driven management strategies, only that ICP monitored patients had improved efficiency of care.[21] This of course does not mean that ICP monitoring should be abandoned in the management of TBI; in countries and regions without readily available ICP technology, protocols based on radiology and clinical examination can be sophisticated and can act as a surrogate for monitoring ICP, and management strategies are still based on the assumption of intracranial hypertension. Where ICP technology exists however its widespread use promotes real-time feedback on not only mean intracranial pressure and evolving intracranial events, but other useful pathophysiological data regarding intracranial compliance and homeostasis that can be used to guide clinical decision-making, and continued study in the extra information that ICP monitoring allows will increase our knowledge in this still burgeoning area. Despite some lingering doubt regarding superiority of ICP monitor driven treatment protocols,[69] the bulk of the literature is consistent in its conclusion that the use of ICP monitoring in conjunction with clinical examination, data from other monitoring devices and investigation results is associated with lower mortality and improved clinical outcomes.[70–73]

Central to the approach of ICP targeted therapy is an upper threshold for which mean ICP should be kept below, but in reality this concept remains simplistic in nature. Although current ICP-driven protocols rely on a single universal value to target therapy, in reality TBI is a hugely heterogenous population for which a one-size-fits-all approach to ICP is unrealistic at best. In future, management of TBI must become more individualised for each patient, with the acceptance that ICP is 'more than a number'.[58] At present, good neurocritical care relies not only on ICP targeted therapy, but also clinical examination and the results of radiology and other investigations. ICP monitoring must evolve to include other measures of intracranial compliance, autoregulatory reserve, oxygenation and substrate supply, such that treatment becomes targeted towards providing the injured brain the environment it needs to avoid secondary injury and aid maximal recovery. ICP-derived parameters such as RAP and PRx, together with multimodality monitoring, imaging and clinical examination, may be the future of individualised TBI management, to predict response to surgical decompression and prognosticate clinical outcomes.

References

1. Lundberg N. Continuous recording and control of ventricular fluid pressure in neurosurgical practice. *Acta Psychiatr Scand Suppl* 1960;36(149):1–193.

2. Pollock LJ, Boshes B. Cerebrospinal fluid pressure. *Arch Neurol Psychiatr* 1936;36(5):931–74.

3. Magnaes B. Body position and cerebrospinal fluid pressure. Part 2: clinical studies on orthostatic pressure and the hydrostatic indifferent point. *J Neurosurg* 1976;44(6):698–705.

4. Magnaes B. Body position and cerebrospinal fluid pressure. Part 1: clinical studies on the effect of rapid postural changes. *J Neurosurg* 1976;44(6):687–97.

5. Wilkins R, Wilkins G. *Neurosurgical Classics II*: Thieme, 2000.

6. Czosnyka M, Pickard JD. Monitoring and interpretation of intracranial pressure. *J Neurol Neurosurg Psychiatr* 2004;75(6):813–21.

7. Steiner LA, Andrews PJ. Monitoring the injured brain: ICP and CBF. *Br J Anaesth* 2006;97(1):26–38.

8. Aucoin PJ, Kotilainen HR, Gantz NM, et al. Intracranial pressure monitors: epidemiologic study of risk factors and infections. *Am J Med* 1986;80(3):369–76.

9. Mayhall CG, Archer NH, Lamb VA, et al. Ventriculostomy-related infections. A prospective epidemiologic study. *New Engl J Med* 1984;310(9):553–9.

10. de Jong W. Blood pressure variability in neonates [PhD thesis]. Technical University of Eindhoven; 2000.

11. Citerio G, Piper I, Cormio M, et al. Bench test assessment of the new Raumedic Neurovent-P ICP sensor: a technical report by the BrainIT group. *Acta Neurochir* 2004;146(11):1221–6.

12. Fernandes HM, Bingham K, Chambers IR, et al. Clinical evaluation of the Codman microsensor intracranial pressure monitoring system. *Acta Neurochir Suppl* 1998;71:44–6.

13. Wolfla CE, Luerssen TG, Bowman RM, et al. Brain tissue pressure gradients created by expanding frontal epidural mass lesion. *J Neurosurg* 1996;84(4):642–7.

14. Padayachy LC. Non-invasive intracranial pressure assessment. *Child's Nervous Syst* 2016;32(9):1587–97.

15. Robba C, Bacigaluppi S, Cardim D, et al. Non-invasive assessment of intracranial pressure. *Acta Neurol Scand* 2016;134(1):4–21.

16. Albeck MJ, Borgesen SE, Gjerris F, et al. Intracranial pressure and cerebrospinal fluid outflow conductance in healthy subjects. *J Neurosurg* 1991;74(4):597–600.

17. Chapman PH, Cosman ER, Arnold MA. The relationship between ventricular fluid pressure and body position in normal subjects and subjects with shunts: a telemetric study. *Neurosurgery* 1990;26(2):181–9.

18. Chan JW. Current concepts and strategies in the diagnosis and management of

idiopathic intracranial hypertension in adults. *J Neurol* 2017;264(8):1622–33.

19. Carney N, Totten AM, O'Reilly C, et al. Guidelines for the management of severe traumatic brain injury, fourth edition. *Neurosurgery* 2017;80(1):6–15.

20. Sorrentino E, Diedler J, Kasprowicz M, et al. Critical thresholds for cerebrovascular reactivity after traumatic brain injury. *Neurocrit Care* 2012;16 (2):258–66.

21. Chesnut RM, Temkin N, Carney N, et al. A trial of intracranial-pressure monitoring in traumatic brain injury. *New Engl J Med* 2012;367(26):2471–81.

22. Chesnut RM. Intracranial pressure monitoring: headstone or a new head start. The BEST TRIP trial in perspective. *Intensive Care Med* 2013;39(4):771–4.

23. Sheth KN, Stein DM, Aarabi B, et al. Intracranial pressure dose and outcome in traumatic brain injury. *Neurocrit Care* 2013;18(1):26–32.

24. Vik A, Nag T, Fredriksli OA, et al. Relationship of 'dose' of intracranial hypertension to outcome in severe traumatic brain injury. *J Neurosurg* 2008;109(4):678–84.

25. Julien C. The enigma of Mayer waves: Facts and models. *Cardiovascul Res* 2006;70 (1):12–21.

26. Spiegelberg A, Preuß M, Kurtcuoglu V. B-waves revisited. *Interdiscip Neurosurg* 2016;6:13–17.

27. Castellani G, Zweifel C, Kim DJ, et al. Plateau waves in head injured patients requiring neurocritical care. *Neurocrit Care* 2009;11(2):143–50.

28. Radolovich DK, Aries MJ, Castellani G, et al. Pulsatile intracranial pressure and cerebral autoregulation after traumatic brain injury. *Neurocrit Care* 2011;15 (3):379–86.

29. Eide PK, Sorteberg W. Diagnostic intracranial pressure monitoring and surgical management in idiopathic normal pressure hydrocephalus: a 6-year review of 214 patients. *Neurosurgery* 2010;66(1):80–91.

30. Kirkness CJ, Mitchell PH, Burr RL, et al. Intracranial pressure waveform analysis: clinical and research implications. *J Neurosci Nurs* 2000;32(5):271–7.

31. Hu X, Xu P, Scalzo F, et al. Morphological clustering and analysis of continuous intracranial pressure. *IEEE Trans Bio-med Eng* 2009;56(3):696–705.

32. Hu X, Xu P, Asgari S, et al. Forecasting ICP elevation based on prescient changes of intracranial pressure waveform morphology. *IEEE Trans Bio-med Eng* 2010;57(5):1070–8.

33. Czosnyka Z, Keong N, Kim DJ, et al. Pulse amplitude of intracranial pressure waveform in hydrocephalus. *Acta Neurochir Suppl* 2008;102:137–40.

34. Robertson CS, Narayan RK, Contant CF, et al. Clinical experience with a continuous monitor of intracranial compliance. *J Neurosurg* 1989;71(5 Pt 1):673–80.

35. Foltz EL, Blanks JP, Yonemura K. CSF pulsatility in hydrocephalus: respiratory effect on pulse wave slope as an indicator of intracranial compliance. *Neurol Res* 1990;12(2):67–74.

36. Westhout FD, Pare LS, Delfino RJ, et al. Slope of the intracranial pressure waveform after traumatic brain injury. *Surg Neurol* 2008;70(1):70–4; discussion 74.

37. Gao L, Smielewski P, Czosnyka M, et al. Cerebrovascular Signal Complexity Six Hours after Intensive Care Unit Admission Correlates with Outcome after Severe Traumatic Brain Injury. *J Neurotrauma* 2016;33(22):2011–18.

38. Burr RL, Kirkness CJ, Mitchell PH. Detrended fluctuation analysis of intracranial pressure predicts outcome following traumatic brain injury. *IEEE Trans Bio-med Eng* 2008;55(11):2509–18.

39. Sourina O, Ang B, Nguyen MK. Fractal-based approach in analysis of intracranial pressure (ICP) in severe head injury. In *Proceedings of the 10th IEEE International Conference on Information Technology and Applications in Biomedicine*; 2010.

40. Lu CW, Czosnyka M, Shieh JS, et al. Complexity of intracranial pressure correlates with outcome after traumatic brain injury. *Brain* 2012;135(Pt 8): 2399–408.

41. Czosnyka M, Smielewski P, Kirkpatrick P, et al. Continuous assessment of the cerebral vasomotor reactivity in head injury. *Neurosurgery* 1997;41(1):11–17; discussion 17–19.

42. Fraser CD, 3rd, Brady KM, Rhee CJ, et al. The frequency response of cerebral autoregulation. *J Appl Physiol* 2013;115 (1):52–6.

43. Brady KM, Lee JK, Kibler KK, et al. Continuous measurement of autoregulation by spontaneous fluctuations in cerebral perfusion pressure: comparison of 3 methods. *Stroke* 2008;39 (9):2531–7.

44. Wang EC, Ang BT, Wong J, et al. Characterization of cerebrovascular reactivity after craniectomy for acute brain injury. *Br J Neurosurg* 2006;20(1):24–30.

45. Avezaat CJ, van Eijndhoven JH, Wyper DJ. Cerebrospinal fluid pulse pressure and intracranial volume-pressure relationships. *J Neurol Neurosurg Psychiatr* 1979;42 (8):687–700.

46. Liu X, Donnelly J, Czosnyka M, Aries M, Brady K, Cardim D, Robba C, Cabeleira M, Kim D-J, Haubrich C, Hutchinson P, Smielewski P. Cerebrovascular pressure reactivity monitoring using wavelet analysis in traumatic brain injury patients: A retrospective study. *PLoS Med* 2017;14. doi:10.1371/journal. pmed.1002348.

47. Aries MJ, Czosnyka M, Budohoski KP, et al. Continuous monitoring of cerebrovascular reactivity using pulse waveform of intracranial pressure. *PLoS Med* 2012;17(1):67–76.

48. Liu X, Donnelly J. Cerebrovascular pressure reactivity monitoring using wavelet analysis in traumatic brain injury patients: a retrospective study. *PLoS Med* 2017;14(7):e1002348.

49. Zeiler FA, Donnelly J, Menon D, et al. A description of a new continuous physiologic index in TBI using the correlation between pulse amplitude of icp and cerebral perfusion pressure. *J Neurotrauma* 2018 Feb 9. doi:10.1089/ neu.2017.5241. [Epub ahead of print]

50. Zeiler FA, Donnelly J, Menon DK, et al. Continuous autoregulatory indices derived from multi-modal monitoring: each one is not like the other. *J Neurotrauma* 2017;34 (22):3070–80.

51. Balestreri M, Czosnyka M, Hutchinson P, et al. Impact of intracranial pressure and cerebral perfusion pressure on severe disability and mortality after head injury. *Neurocrit Care* 2006;4(1):8–13.

52. Hutchinson P, Timofeev I, Kirkpatrick P. Surgery for brain edema. *Neurosurg Focus* 2007;22(5):E14.

53. Cooper DJ, Rosenfeld JV, Murray L, et al. Decompressive craniectomy in diffuse traumatic brain injury. *New Engl J Med* 2011;364(16):1493–502.

54. Hutchinson PJ, Kolias AG, Timofeev IS, et al. Trial of Decompressive Craniectomy for Traumatic Intracranial Hypertension. *New Engl J Med* 2016;375(12):1119–30.

55. Czosnyka M, Guazzo E, Whitehouse M, et al. Significance of intracranial pressure waveform analysis after head injury. *Acta Neurochir* 1996;138(5):531–41; discussion 41–2.

56. Steiner LA, Balestreri M, Johnston AJ, et al. Predicting the response of intracranial pressure to moderate hyperventilation. *Acta Neurochir* 2005;147(5):477–83; discussion 83.

57. Whitfield PC, Patel H, Hutchinson PJ, et al. Bifrontal decompressive craniectomy in the management of posttraumatic intracranial hypertension. *Br J Neurosurg* 2001;15(6):500–7.

58. Czosnyka M, Smielewski P, Timofeev I, et al. Intracranial pressure: more than a number. *Neurosurg Focus* 2007;22(5):E10.

59. Hiler M, Czosnyka M, Hutchinson P, et al. Predictive value of initial computerized

tomography scan, intracranial pressure, and state of autoregulation in patients with traumatic brain injury. *J Neurosurg* 2006;104(5):731–7.

60. Balestreri M, Czosnyka M, Steiner LA, et al. Association between outcome, cerebral pressure reactivity and slow ICP waves following head injury. *Acta Neurochir Suppl* 2005;95:25–8.

61. Steiner LA, Coles JP, Johnston AJ, et al. Assessment of cerebrovascular autoregulation in head-injured patients: a validation study. *Stroke* 2003;34 (10):2404–9.

62. Balestreri M, Czosnyka M, Steiner LA, et al. Intracranial hypertension: what additional information can be derived from ICP waveform after head injury? *Acta Neurochir* 2004;146(2):131–41.

63. Steiner LA, Czosnyka M, Piechnik SK, et al. Continuous monitoring of cerebrovascular pressure reactivity allows determination of optimal cerebral perfusion pressure in patients with traumatic brain injury. *Crit Care Med* 2002;30(4):733–8.

64. Aries MJ, Czosnyka M, Budohoski KP, et al. Continuous determination of optimal cerebral perfusion pressure in traumatic brain injury. *Crit Care Med* 2012;40 (8):2456–63.

65. Aries MJ, Wesselink R, Elting JW, et al. Enhanced visualization of optimal cerebral perfusion pressure over time to support clinical decision making. *Crit Care Med* 2016;44(10):e996-9.

66. Depreitere B, Guiza F, Van den Berghe G, et al. Pressure autoregulation monitoring and cerebral perfusion pressure target recommendation in patients with severe traumatic brain injury based on minute-by-minute monitoring data. *J Neurosurg* 2014;120(6):1451–7.

67. Donnelly J, Czosnyka M, Adams H, et al. Individualizing thresholds of cerebral perfusion pressure using estimated limits of autoregulation. *Crit Care Med* 2017;45 (9):1464–71.

68. Bratton SL, Chestnut RM, Ghajar J, et al. Guidelines for the management of severe traumatic brain injury. VI. Indications for intracranial pressure monitoring. *J Neurotrauma* 2007;24 (Suppl 1):S37-44.

69. Yuan Q, Wu X, Sun Y, et al. Impact of intracranial pressure monitoring on mortality in patients with traumatic brain injury: a systematic review and meta-analysis. *J Neurosurg* 2015;122 (3):574–87.

70. Chesnut R, Videtta W, Vespa P, et al. Intracranial pressure monitoring: fundamental considerations and rationale for monitoring. *Neurocrit Care* 2014;21 (Suppl 2):S64–84.

71. Farahvar A, Gerber LM, Chiu YL, et al. Increased mortality in patients with severe traumatic brain injury treated without intracranial pressure monitoring. J Neurosurg 2012;117(4):729–34.

72. Gerber LM, Chiu YL, Carney N, et al. Marked reduction in mortality in patients with severe traumatic brain injury. *J Neurosurg* 2013;119(6):1583–90.

73. Talving P, Karamanos E, Teixeira PG, et al. Intracranial pressure monitoring in severe head injury: compliance with Brain Trauma Foundation guidelines and effect on outcomes: a prospective study. *J Neurosurg* 2013;119(5):1248–54.

74. Brady KM, Easley RB, Kibler K, et al. Positive end-expiratory pressure oscillation facilitates brain vascular reactivity monitoring. *J Appl Physiol* 2012;113(9):1362–8.

Chapter 12

Multimodality Monitoring in Head Injury

Tamara Tajsic, Andrew Gvozdanovic, Ivan Timofeev and Peter J. Hutchinson

Introduction

The major determinant of outcome from TBI is the severity of the primary injury; however, not all brain damage happens at that time point. Invariably, primary injury activates cellular and molecular cascades which mediate potentially reversible, secondary injury in the ensuing hours and days. These events can lead to progressive brain swelling and increased intracranial pressure (ICP) thus compromising cerebral perfusion pressure (CPP) and cerebral blood flow (CBF) resulting in tissue ischaemia, hypoxia and cellular energy failure. Further cell damage exacerbates the brain swelling, forming part of a vicious circle that can lead to life-threatening brain herniation. A large body of evidence links post-traumatic intracranial hypertension at levels above 20 to 25 mmHg with excess mortality and worse functional outcomes. Similar findings have been shown for reduced CPP at levels below 50 to 55 mmHg.[2,3,4,7] The control of ICP and preservation of CPP has therefore been the mainstay of neuro-intensive care management of TBI for several decades. Tier-based protocols employing neuroprotective measures such as sedation, controlled hyperventilation, therapeutic hypothermia, hyperosmolar therapies, barbiturate coma and ventricular drainage have been recommended and are widely used in intensive care units to control intracranial hypertension and facilitate cerebral perfusion and oxygenation.[4]

The International Multidisciplinary Consensus Conference on Multimodality Monitoring in Neurocritical Care in 2014[15] performed a systematic review of the published literature to help develop evidence-based practice recommendations on bedside physiological monitoring. It has been recognised that ICP elevations may be an insensitive and late indicator of secondary brain injury, and that monitoring and treating other physiological parameters may improve patient care.[6,19,21] Most commonly used neuromonitoring methods can provide real-time bedside information about cerebral metabolism (cerebral microdialysis), cerebral oxygenation (measurement of jugular venous oxygenation, brain tissue oxygen, near infrared spectroscopy) and cerebral blood flow (extrapolated from cerebral blood velocity measurements from Transcranial Doppler, laser Doppler and thermal diffusion). This chapter describes the principles of these monitoring techniques and their application following head injury.

The Utility of Microdialysis in the Management of Traumatic Brain Injury

Introduction

In the context of monitoring following TBI, cerebral microdialysis continues to establish its role as a unique and powerful tool. It allows dynamic sampling of the brain extracellular fluid *in vivo* for a range of molecules from neuronal metabolites, to drugs and cytokines, providing a wealth of information on the underlying physiological and pathological processes that follow neuronal injury. Initially envisaged as a research tool, it is now used clinically in an increasing number of centres across the world, primarily for monitoring of energy metabolism at the bedside. Microdialysis has also been used in other neurosurgical conditions such as subarachnoid haemorrhage and in the monitoring of ischaemia during temporary clip placement in cerebral aneurysm surgery.[5,12,13,14]

Prevention of secondary injury in TBI focuses primarily on intracranial pressure monitoring and maintenance of cerebral perfusion pressure. The ideal cerebral perfusion pressure that maintains aerobic metabolism without exacerbating cerebral oedema remains contentious. Furthermore, this value may vary between patients and may vary in the same patient over time. CPP values reflect substrate and oxygen provision, but microdialysis allows a more direct, quantitative measure of cerebral metabolism: the substrate delivery and its utilisation at the cellular level. Used together with ICP and CPP, it has provided us with a better understanding of how brain metabolism following acute injury relates to clinical outcome. Additionally, microdialysis allows sampling of a large number of inflammatory cytokines and chemokines which has provided insight into the neuroinflammatory processes following brain injury. As it matures as a clinical monitoring tool, its combined use with other modalities, such as cerebral oximetry and ICP monitoring, could lead the way to a more individualised management of patients with severe TBI.[14]

Principles of Microdialysis

Microdialysis sampling is based on the free diffusion of molecules (analytes) across the semi-permeable ('dialysis') membrane. The microdialysis catheter is a flexible plastic probe inserted into the brain parenchyma through a twist drill hole, transcranial bolt or craniotomy. It consists of two concentric lumina ending in a semi-permeable ('dialysis') membrane at the tip. A physiological fluid (the 'perfusate') is pumped down one lumen to the dialysis membrane using a small, battery operated pump. This fluid then travels back up the other lumen where it is collected and termed the microdialysate (Figure 12.1). Typical flow rates for this process are 0.3–2 μl/min, allowing time for molecules in the extracellular space to diffuse from the extracellular space into the fluid within the catheter. Thus, the constitution of the microdialysate closely reflects that of the extracellular space.[12–14]

Molecules recovered by the microdialysis catheter are limited to those that can diffuse across the microdialysis membrane. The most important practical considerations are the molecular weight of the molecule of interest and its hydrophobicity. The efficiency of recovery of a molecule of interest by microdialysis is termed the 'relative recovery' for that molecule. It is defined as the concentration of a molecule in the microdialysate divided by the concentration in the external solution multiplied by 100 and expressed in percentages. Relative recovery can be calculated *in vitro* or *in vivo* and can allow direct quantification of the concentration in the extracellular fluid from microdialysis data. As one would expect small molecular weight hydrophilic molecules such as lactate and pyruvate have high relative recoveries of the order of 95% whilst larger molecules such as cytokines have relative recoveries around only 40% with the same catheter.[12,13]

Several other factors impact on relative recovery such as the size of the dialysis membrane pores, the perfusion fluid content and the flow rate of the perfusate. These factors can be manipulated to allow a range of molecules to be recovered at sufficient concentration for assay. Different pore size catheters can be used depending on the

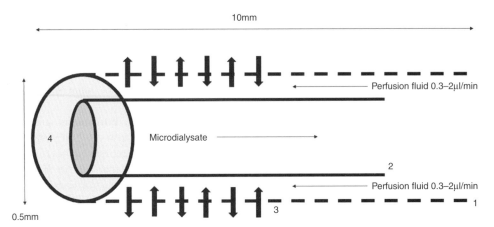

Figure 12.1 Microdialysis catheter. The catheter is made up of outer (1) and inner (2) concentric tubes with a semi-permeable dialysis membrane (20–100 kDa) at the distal end (3). The golden tip (4) facilitates visualisation on CT imaging. Perfusion fluid circulation via the catheter can be seen with extracellular molecules entering the perfusate by a process of diffusion across the dialysis membrane.

molecular weights of the molecules of interest. The standard 20 kDa molecular weight cut-off membrane recovers metabolites such as glucose, pyruvate, lactate, glycerol, glutamate and other small hydrophilic molecules. Larger-pore membranes such as the 100 kDa weight cut-off membrane can be used to also recover larger molecules such as cytokines and chemokines in addition to the small hydrophilic metabolites. Relative recovery of larger molecules can be significantly improved by supplementing the crystalloid perfusion fluid with colloid solutions such as albumin or dextran. Concerns have been expressed with regard to leakage of perfusate which could alter the catheter microenvironment. Supplementation with higher molecular weight colloids (500 kDa) has been shown to avoid such problems.[12–14]

Microdialysis catheters are of small diameter, very flexible and safe to use. The rare adverse events associated with microdialysis use are related to the insertion of catheter and the technique used rather than the catheter itself.[14]

Microdialysis Markers of Cerebral Metabolism and Injury

The pathophysiology of traumatic brain injury and development of secondary injury is a complex dynamic interplay of tissue ischaemia, hypoxia, inflammation, metabolic derangements, cell wall and mitochondrial dysfunction, excitotoxicity and cellular death. Microdialysis enables recovery of some of the key molecular markers of these pathological processes.[14]

Glucose is believed to be the main source of energy in the brain. Measurement of glucose concentration in the extracellular space allows assessment of substrate availability in the first place. Although serum glucose concentration and glycaemic control influence brain glucose concentrations, the relationship may be perturbed in the injured brain. Brain glucose levels can be reduced as a consequence of ischaemia but also by other pathological processes such as seizures or spreading depolarisation. The optimal glucose concentration range in TBI remains to be established. Low glucose (less than 0.8 mM/L and certainly less than 0.2 mM/L) has been linked to poor outcomes. The same has been suggested for brain tissue hyperglycaemia but there is insufficient data to define the absolute cut off.[5,14]

Cerebral metabolism is altered following brain injury, but the full extent and nature of the changes are not yet completely understood. Cells metabolise glucose to pyruvate (a process termed glycolysis) which, during aerobic metabolism, enters the tricarboxylic acid (TCA) cycle and is ultimately metabolised to carbon dioxide and water (Figure 12.2). Reducing equivalents generated within the TCA cycle are used to generate ATP molecules from ADP via the electron chain on the mitochondrial membrane. Alternatively, in pathological conditions where pyruvate cannot be metabolised through the TCA cycle, it is converted to lactate by the action of lactate dehydrogenase and exported into the extracellular space. This is believed to happen in the context of brain injury as brain tissue ischaemia and hypoxia develop, restricting the availability of oxygen for metabolic consumption in the TCA cycle which results in pyruvate being diverted away from being used for energy production in the TCA cycle and towards lactate production and accumulation (Figure 12.2). Mitochondrial dysfunction is a less well understood mechanism which results in disrupted glucose metabolism in TBI. Mitochondria are the powerhouse of cells, and the depressed activity of several mitochondrial dehydrogenases as well as the disruption of the delicate electron transport chains in TBI leads to suboptimal utilisation of pyruvate and accumulation of lactate even in the context of normal tissue oxygenation. Further sources of lactate in the injured brain are believed to arise from the alternative glucose metabolic pathway (the pentose phosphate pathway aka the 'hexose monophosphate shunt') which does not require oxygen and/or through 'aerobic glycolysis' (Warburg Effect) in which there

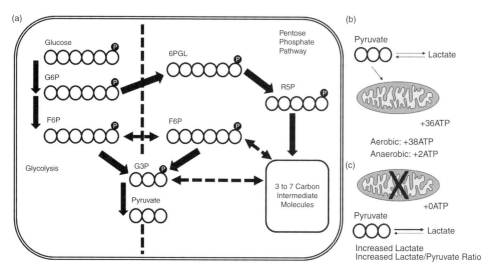

Figure 12.2 Intra-cellular production of energy under aerobic and anaerobic conditions. (a) A simplified diagram representing the glycolysis and pentose phosphate pathways as routes of pyruvate production. Abbreviations: G6P, glucose-6-phosphate; F6P, fructose-6-phosphate; 6PGL, 6-phosphogluconolactone; R5P, ribulose-5-phosphate; G3P, glyceraldehyde-3-phosphate. (b) Aerobic metabolism: glycolysis/pentose phosphate pathway produces pyruvate which enters into the tricarboxylic acid (TCA) cycle. This requires an adequate oxygen supply and normal mitochondrial function. (c) Anaerobic metabolism: Ischaemia or hypoxia leads to reduced availability of tissue oxygen and/or impaired mitochondrial function. Pyruvate is therefore metabolised to lactate with a subsequent rise in the lactate/pyruvate ratio (LPR). Cellular damage will release glycerol from the cell membrane (which may be measured using microdialysis).

are high cellular glycolytic levels in the absence of ischaemia (i.e. there is an adequate supply of oxygen). This phenomenon, where cells show a predilection for using the less energy efficient glycolysis despite ready oxygen supply, has been traditionally linked to cancer cells but is now also recognised to happen in the injured brain. Furthermore, recent evidence suggested that neurons in the injured brain can metabolise lactate *via* the TCA cycle. If the TCA cycle is disturbed due to restricted oxygen supply or mitochondrial disruption, the lactate will remain unutilised and accumulate in the extracellular space.[5]

Both lactate and pyruvate are small molecules that can be readily taken up from the extracellular fluid using microdialysis. The absolute amounts of pyruvate and lactate are not the most accurate reflection of the metabolic state of the injured brain given the multitude of metabolic derangements and alternative pathways employed. Rather, the lactate/pyruvate ratio (LPR) has been the most commonly used marker of disturbed glucose metabolism in clinical studies. It is believed that a raised LPR in the presence of low pyruvate is typically associated with ischaemia, whilst a raised LPR in the presence of normal/high pyruvate indicates mitochondrial dysfunction (Figure 12.2).[5,14] An LPR greater than 25 is associated with unfavourable tissue and clinical outcomes.[14]

Other commonly assayed molecules following TBI include glutamate and glycerol.

The cell membrane is largely made up of a bi-layer of phospholipids which, as well as acting as a hydrophobic barrier for the cell, also suspends a range of membrane bound proteins within it which act as signalling molecules. Following cellular death, the phospholipids within the membrane are enzymatically digested into their constituent components, fatty acid and glycerol. Thus, glycerol levels are thought to reflect cell death. Glycerol monitoring in microdialysis is of limited specificity and limited clinical importance as it is influenced by systemic concentrations; its levels reflect stress response and/or the systemic administration of glycerol containing substances.[14]

Glutamate is an excitatory neurotransmitter and excess levels have been thought to be an additional injurious insult which may exacerbate damage from TBI/SAH. Glutamate release is associated with ischaemia and seizures. There is some evidence to suggest that measuring cerebral glutamate may be useful in estimating prognosis.

The inflammatory component of the complex injury cascade following brain injury may also be monitored using microdialysis. Targeted, focal recovery of inflammatory cytokines and chemokines has contributed greatly to the understanding of neuroinflammatory processes following TBI and its impact on secondary injury progression and functional outcomes.[6,14]

Microdialysis Catheter Placement

Microdialysis is a focal technique. The probe can only sample of small volume of surrounding brain tissue limited by the diffusion distance of the molecule of interest. The heterogeneity of brain injury means that brain chemistry varies in different regions of the brain. It is therefore paramount that any clinical decisions based on microdialysis derived data take into account the exact positioning of the catheter.

The microdialysis catheter can be inserted through a burr hole or a cranial access device ('bolt') or can be placed at the time of craniotomy or craniectomy. In terms of catheter location, the 2014 Microdialysis Consensus statement recommends that for diffuse injury the microdialysis catheter should be inserted into the non-dominant frontal cortex, and for focal injury, in peri-contusional/haematoma tissue with the option of a second catheter to monitor 'normal' brain as determined by CT scan. The microdialysis catheter has a radiopaque tip which allows easy identification on CT imaging (Figure 12.3).

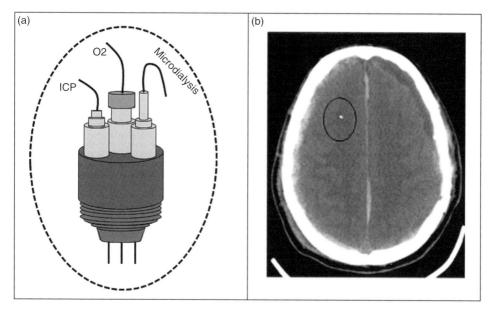

Figure 12.3 (a) Triple bolt allows easy insertion of an intracerebral pressure monitor, brain tissues oxygen sensor and microdialysis catheter. (b) Tip of the microdialysis catheter visible in the right frontal lobe white mater on unenhanced computer tomography imaging of the brain (circled).

The Future of Microdialysis in TBI

The International Consensus Statement from the 2014 International Microdialysis Forum summarises data on the utility and prognostic power of microdialysis derived parameters and strongly supports its use in TBI treatment, although no universally accepted microdialysis parameter guided clinical protocols exist to date. New emerging microdialysis techniques which provide continuous measurements may have the potential to increase the granularity of collected data in response to different clinical events and treatment strategies. As part of a multi-modality monitoring approach, it is likely that microdialysis will be able to help guide management of patients in an individualised and targeted fashion.

As increasing numbers of molecules are being recovered by microdialysis from the human brain after TBI there are ever more innovative uses for this technique. For example, microdialysis can be used to determine pharmacokinetic data for centrally acting drugs and antibiotic. Endogenous molecules such as cytokines are also being increasingly investigated as potential biomarkers of injury severity and secondary injury propagation as well as changes in cytokine profile and concentrations in response to TBI therapies. As well as a monitoring tool, we are beginning to see the benefits of microdialysis in helping to produce new targeted therapies such as recombinant interleukin antagonists and biochemical adjuncts such as infusions of sodium lactate and sodium pyruvate for the treatment of TBI.[14]

Assessment of Cerebral Blood Flow and Oxygenation

Brain tissues rely on an uninterrupted supply of oxygen and energy substrates (primarily glucose, but also ketones and lactate) to maintain cellular metabolism and viability. Multimodality monitoring of a TBI patient in the intensive care setting involves continuous measurements of mean arterial pressure and its derivative cerebral perfusion pressure (CPP) as well as repeated measurements of peripheral blood oxygenation and correction of these parameters according to now well-established guidelines for the treatment of TBI. However, despite optimal systemic perfusion and oxygenation, cerebral ischaemia and hypoxia can develop independently and are major contributors to secondary injury. Additionally, observational studies demonstrate that brain tissue hypoxia may occur even when ICP and CPP are adequate, resulting from microvascular ischaemia and tissue level barriers to oxygen diffusion. These pathological changes are more often regional, and this makes monitoring even more challenging. Yet, early detection of these changes may help both diagnose and treat evolving secondary injury.[15,16]

Assessment of Cerebral Blood Flow (CBF)

CBF is defined as the blood volume that flows per unit mass per unit time in brain tissue and is typically expressed in units of ml blood/100 g tissue/min. The normal average cerebral blood flow (CBF) in adult humans is about 50 ml/100 g/min, with lower values in the white matter [~20 ml/100 g/min] and greater values in the grey matter [~80 ml/100 g/min]. CBF is a function of the driving pressure (CPP), cerebral vascular resistance (CVR) and blood viscosity. Regulation of CBF in healthy and even more so in the injured brain is a complicated and complex phenomenon and relies greatly on the ability of the brain to 'autoregulate', that is adjust the vessels' radius in response to changes in CPP, calcium concentration, changing concentrations of vasoactive metabolites and direct stimulation from perivascular neurones to ultimately match the changing perfusion requirements of brain tissue.

Numerous imaging approaches can be employed to assess CBF and perfusion including nuclear medicine techniques (single photon emission computer tomography and positron emission tomography), perfusion CT or MRI (dynamic susceptibility contrast magnetic resonance imaging and arterial spin labelling magnetic resonance imaging); however, they only provide a 'snapshot' rather than continuous monitoring which limits their clinical utility in managing acute brain injury.

Other techniques such as transcranial Doppler (TCD), thermodilution methods and optical techniques which can provide continuous monitoring at the bedside may have more usability in the intensive care setting.[15,16,18,19,21–24]

Transcranial Doppler (TCD) is a non-invasive simple bedside procedure that does not measure cerebral blood flow directly but provides extrapolated data based on the velocity of blood in large arteries. The technique requires a cranial window allowing ultrasound to penetrate thin bone without being excessively damped. Different segments of the arterial system at the base of the skull give signals which are then identified. The transtemporal acoustic window which is found above the zygomatic arch provides view of the branching of the supraclinoid ICA (internal carotid artery) into the ACA (anterior cerebral artery) and MCA (middle cerebral artery). TCD sonography measures the flow velocity in cerebral arteries which changes with the phases of the cardiac cycle. The Doppler signals are used to derive systolic, average mean flow and end-diastolic flow velocities. The mean carries the highest physiological significance as it correlates with perfusion better than the peak and trough values. The basic principle is that an ultrasound wave at a given frequency (f) experiences a Doppler frequency shift (Δf) as it gets reflected by the red blood cells that are moving at a certain speed. That speed (i.e. flow velocity) can then be calculated if using the known variables (the frequency of the ultrasound wave and the speed of ultrasound in tissues), the angle between the direction of propagation of ultrasound and the direction of the blood vessel. The relationship between vB and Δf is as follows:

$$vB = cs2f \quad \cos(\theta)\Delta f,$$

where cs is the speed of ultrasound in tissue, and θ is the angle between the direction of propagation of ultrasound and the direction of the blood vessel. The uncertainty in the angle θ complicates accurate measurements of vB. Furthermore, the variability in blood vessel diameter introduces an additional uncertainty in translating the speed of BF (in units of cm/s) into a measure of volumetric BF (in units of ml/s) in the blood vessel. Even a good estimate of volumetric BF would still require knowledge of the brain mass perfused by the artery in order to estimate an absolute CBF. For these reasons, TCD provides only a relative index of CBF.

TCD is operator dependent and requires training and experience to perform and interpret results. Although it can provide indirect information on cerebral blood flow and state of autoregulation after head injury, technical difficulties of continuous reliable TCD monitoring limit its practical applications in patients with TBI. The introduction of the automated TCD monitors of CBF through the MCA (such as Presto 1000 TCD system, PhysioSonics, Bellevue, WA) may be able to remedy some of the issues such as continuity and the reliability of the collected data.[1,15,16,23]

Thermodilution methods rely on injection of a known quantity of a cold fluid miscible with blood (typically saline) that introduces a thermal perturbation. This allows direct measurement of blood flow velocity by assessing sequential changes in blood temperature within a large blood vessel that drains the brain, such as the internal jugular vein. Temperature is measured by a thermistor in the distal catheter tip in the vein of interest and allows for continuous or repeated measurements (in the cases of continuous infusion or cold bolus input, respectively). It is typically referred to as jugular thermodilution.[9,11,15,24]

More recently, the similar principle of *thermal diffusion flowmetry* (TDF) has been employed in intracerebral CBF measurement devices. The ability of brain tissue to dissipate heat is directly related to local cerebral blood flow. This technique can measure a spherical volume of about 20 to 30 mm^3 surrounding the probe (sensor), which is placed within brain tissue, providing continuous and invasive bedside monitoring of local CBF. Thermal diffusion sensors contain two thermistors: a passive one that measures brain temperature and is maintained at this temperature (neutral plate) and an active one held at a slightly higher temperature (heated plate). The heat dissipation in the tissue between thermistors reflects local blood flow and the later can be estimated quantitatively in conventional units (ml/100 g/min) assuming that the conduction properties of the surrounding brain are constant.[11,19,21,22]

Laser Doppler flowmetry (LDF) is an invasive technique for the continuous monitoring of cerebral blood flow using optical methodology. LDF samples a superficial volume of 1–2 mm^3 in tissue and requires removal of scalp and skull for access to the human brain. The LDF instrument consists of a fibre-optic probe and uses monochromatic light in the range of 670 to 810 nm. The movement of red blood cells induces a Doppler shift in the light that is proportional to the velocity and number of red blood cells. A photodetector measures the scattered light that has been Doppler shifted and these measurements are translated to a time-varying voltage that is proportional to changes in CBF.[11,19,21,22]

Ideally, the technology to measure CBF should be inexpensive, easy to use, non-invasive, safe, reliable and continuous, allowing real-time dynamic assessment of change and response to treatment, but none of the technologies available so far meets the criteria and most of these methods are still predominantly used in a research-related setting.

Assessment of Cerebral Oxygenation

Systemic monitoring of oxygen (PaO_2, SaO_2, SpO_2) and CO_2 ($PaCO_2$, end-tidal CO_2) is recommended in patients who require neurocritical care and is in routine use in intensive care settings, worldwide. In the past two decades, numerous studies showed a correlation between low brain oxygen levels and higher mortality rate and unfavourable outcome. In 2007, brain oxygen monitoring was added into the Brain Trauma Foundation guidelines suggesting that brain tissue oxygen tension thresholds below 15 mmHg may require treatment.[15–18]

Brain tissue oximetry, the invasive monitoring of cerebral oxygen levels, plays an increasingly important role in managing patients with severe head injury. Cerebral oxygenation also plays a key part in our interpretation of other systemic parameters and more specifically cerebral blood flow, cerebrovascular reactivity and microdialysate as well as evaluation of cerebral autoregulation. Combined monitoring of ICP and brain tissue oxygen tension has shown to be superior to ICP alone. Most importantly, the BOOST-II trial,[17] a recently published Phase II trial designed to assess whether a neurocritical care management protocol could improve $P_{bt}O_2$ levels in patients with severe TBI, found that multi-modal ICP and $P_{bt}O_2$ monitoring reduced brain tissue hypoxia with a trend towards lower mortality and more favourable outcomes compared to ICP-only treatment. A follow-on Phase III efficacy study is now under way.

Measuring devices currently available for clinical use employ two different techniques to monitor the partial oxygen pressure in the surrounding brain tissue and some offer simultaneous monitoring of partial carbon dioxide pressure, temperature and ICP. The most commonly used sensors, such as the Licox® Brain Oxygen Monitoring System (Integra) and Neurovent® catheters (Raumedic) are based on Clark's principle and consist of two electrodes and an outer polyethylene membrane, permeable to oxygen. Following insertion of the catheter, oxygen, driven by its partial pressure, diffuses from the tissue into internal compartment of the sensor via its wall and is reduced at the internal cathode, thus generating a voltage difference with the second reference electrode. This difference is proportional to the partial tissue oxygen tension ($P_{bt}O_2$). These catheters are pre-calibrated. The second technique used for brain tissue oxygen measurement is based on fluorescence quenching in which a marker changes colour according to the ambient amount of gas. This type of oxygen sensor requires bedside calibration and the accuracy and clinical stability seem to be less than with the Clark principle-based catheters. Both methods require direct placement of the sensor into cerebral tissue either via cranial access (bolt) device or following craniotomy with tunnelling under skin. Once inserted, the monitors provide continuous measurement of $P_{bt}O_2$ with an output at a bedside screen and require minimum further maintenance.[11,15–18]

Brain tissue oximetry provides information only about several mm^3 of cerebral tissue. This is the single most important fact that needs to be taken into account for accurate interpretation of the recorded values. Most sensors can be easily identified on conventional cerebral computed tomography scans, and location of the probe and its relation to cerebral parenchymal or extra-axial lesions need to be recorded in all cases following insertion. In most cases it can be assumed that a sensor located in the macroscopically, radiologically 'normal' brain, with predominantly diffuse injury, provides values, which correlate well with regional and global oxygenation values measured by other monitoring and imaging modalities and can therefore be used as an equivalent of 'global' monitoring technique. Although at present it is virtually impossible to accurately define an area of 'penumbra' around traumatic parenchymal lesions, sensors placed in the immediate vicinity of such lesions are more likely to provide very 'focal' information on oxygen levels, albeit from the most vulnerable tissue. There are pros and cons for targeting 'normal' and 'perilesional' brain tissue during the placement of the catheters, and in certain cases there may be a need for more than one catheter. However, interpretation of the values and their integration with other monitoring modalities for optimisation of the therapy needs to be based on clear acknowledgement of probe position and sampled tissue.[15-18]

Interpretation of the reduced $P_{bt}O_2$ values follows the pattern of other cerebral oxygen monitoring techniques, with reduction representing reduced delivery or increased consumption. Currently recommended clinical thresholds are by and large based on observational evidence and assume the 'safe' cerebral oxygenation levels above 20–25 mmHg, with levels below 10 mmHg generally considered pathological. Theoretically higher values of $P_{bt}O_2$ can be due to a number of reasons; however, much less is known about their practical significance. Current clinical use of $P_{bt}O_2$ includes detection of cerebral ischaemia, optimisation of CPP and protection from deleterious effects of hyperventilation.[15-18]

Although invasive, brain tissue oxygen probes have a very good safety profile: the level of haemorrhagic and infectious complications is very low. Focal artefacts (microhaematomas during insertion, proximity to a large vessel, local inflammatory response, etc.) and probe displacement during prolonged use may also affect accuracy of recordings.[15-17]

Further prospective evidence/randomised control trials into the effect of invasive monitoring of cerebral oxygenation and 'oxygen-driven' therapy on functional outcome after traumatic brain injury is still required to support wider use of these monitoring modalities. At present, these techniques provide unique information that may optimise an individual patients' therapy; they are therefore gaining acceptance as a clinical tool in an increasing number of neurocritical care units.[15-17]

NIRS (near-infrared spectroscopy) provides a non-invasive way to assess real-time regional cortical oxygenation using scalp probes. NIRS employs light with wavelength of 600–1000 nm and relies on the principles that each chromophore has unique absorption characteristics which then allows deconvolution of the detected light spectrum to quantify relative amounts of specific chromophores in target tissue. Specifically, deoxygenated and oxygenated haemoglobin have different absorption spectra. This allows quantification of oxyhaemoglobin and deoxyhaemoglobin and calculation of the total haemoglobin concentration and oxygen saturation of haemoglobin in cerebral tissues. The near infrared light is partially absorbed as it passes through the tissue which results in a change in the intensity (concentration of the light beam). Because of the highly scattering nature of NIR light in tissue, light does not travel on a linear path. Therefore, variability in the detected signal cannot simply be attributed to changes in chromophore concentration. Consequently, some form of computational reconstruction is required. Newer NIRS technologies use atlas-based anatomical tissue registration and computational models to predict absorption and scatter through tissues, demonstrating whether the observed parameters are reflective of target brain tissue rather than superficial tissues, scalp or cranium. Signal contamination from superficial tissues has limited the use of NIRS in TBI patients. Furthermore, the signal is confounded by the presence of extracranial and intracranial haematomas.[8,11,15]

NIRS has found clinical applications in cerebral oxygenation monitoring in neonates and, in adult patients, in the context of cardiac and vascular surgery, in which close monitoring of cerebral perfusion is required during periods of cardiopulmonary bypass. These situations most frequently involve normal cerebral anatomy and autoregulation. The fact that both of these are disrupted by TBI makes interpretation of the observed parameters following trauma much more complicated. It is currently accepted that the intervention threshold for a drop in Hb saturation as observed by cerebral NIRS is between 13% and 17% to avoid damage to brain tissue. These thresholds are derived from non-TBI applications but in the context of TBI, the utility of this threshold is less clear.[8,15,19,21]

In a small number of investigations, NIRS-based parameters have been demonstrated to have a reasonably robust temporal relationship with ICP. However, the data regarding the sensitivity of NIRS to detect or predict changes in ICP is lacking.[8,15]

Although NIRS is an attractive monitor since it is non-invasive, with its limitations and no proven benefit for patient outcomes it has limited if any role in the monitoring and management of patient with TBI. Current guidelines do not recommend its routine use in the context of TBI.[15]

The profound effect that the presence of haematomas or intracranial mass lesions can have on the cerebral NIRS parameters yielded within the context of TBI has led to this modality being examined as a screening tool for the presence of these lesions in situations where computer tomography imaging may not be readily available.[19,21]

Jugular venous oximetry (SjvO$_2$) is performed by inserting a catheter into the internal jugular vein with its tip positioned in the jugular bulb. For best results, the catheter should be inserted into the dominant IJV (the right in most cases) and the tip should be proximal to the first extra-cranial tributary. Blood can be sampled intermittently or continuously (using fibre-optic catheters) to derive jugular bulb oxygen saturation (SjvO$_2$) and the difference on the arterial and jugular bulb oxygenation and lactate concentration to help assess cerebral perfusion. Normal SjvO$_2$ is between 55% and 75%. Although various definitions have been used, SjvO$_2$ values <55% are consistent with cerebral ischemia.

Catheters need frequent calibration usually every 8–12 h. Complications from clot formation/venous thrombosis, inaccurate placement and inadequate calibration reduce the accuracy of monitored data to 40%–80% of monitored time. Resulting diluted signal, together with its low sensitivity for focal and regional ischaemia and inferiority to invasive tissue oxygen monitoring, has significantly reduced the routing use of SjvO$_2$ monitoring in TBI patients.[15,16]

Electrophysiological Monitoring

Electrophysiology is a well-established diagnostic method for neurological monitoring. In animal models the monitoring of sensory evoked potentials was shown to be useful in detecting the course of brain injury and early phases of injury.

Continuous EEG (cEEG) monitoring provides early detection of seizures, particularly in the context of the high incidence of subclinical seizures in moderate to severe TBI patients. EEG-based studies in TBI patients showed a direct correlation between ICP elevations and durations of EEG burst and suppression intervals. Short periods of electrical activity in EEG of burst-suppressed patients were followed by transient ICP elevations. Prolonged seizures can result in increased ICP, increased metabolic demand and excitotoxicity. Cortical spreading depolarisation (CSD) is the generic term for pathologic waves of abrupt, sustained mass depolarisation that propagate at velocities of 1.7–9.2 mm/min throughout the grey matter. CSDs are increasingly recorded during multimodal neuromonitoring in neurocritical care as a causal biomarker providing a diagnostic summary measure of metabolic failure and excitotoxic injury. Focal ischaemia causes spreading depolarisation within minutes and further spreading depolarisations arise for hours to days due to energy supply–demand mismatch in viable tissue. Spreading depolarisations exacerbate neuronal injury through prolonged ionic breakdown and spreading depolarisation-related hypoperfusion, that is 'spreading ischemia'. Therefore, indications for cEEG monitoring after TBI are unexplained or prolonged altered consciousness.[10,11,15,19,21]

Continuous EEG monitoring can be achieved using scalp, subdural or cortical electrodes. With its non-invasive nature, scalp electrodes are favoured for continuous monitoring in the neurointensive care setting.[10]

Non-invasive Intracranial Pressure Monitoring

The role of ultrasound in TBI has seen a substantial shift to its use in the non-invasive estimation of intracranial pressure by measuring the optic nerve sheath diameter (ONSD). The optic nerve sheath is continuous with the meninges of the central nervous system and is surrounded by the subarachnoid membrane, which contains cerebrospinal fluid (CSF). When the pressure in the subarachnoid space increases, CSF accumulates in the optic nerve sheath thereby widening its diameter. Ultrasound examination of the ONSD using a linear ultrasound probe placed on the closed upper eyelid without exerting pressure on the eye, with the patient in the supine position. In the two-dimensional mode, ONSD is measured 3 mm behind the globe in the sagittal and transverse plane and the final ONSD is taken as the mean. Several studies have demonstrated a linear correlation between ONSD and ICP, and in human studies ONSD changes occur in minutes. ONSD of 5 mm roughly translates to an ICP of 20 mmHg. Inter-/intra-observer variability does not appear to be a limiting factor in this technology. However, ONSD variation is dependent on individual factors such as age and underlying pathology; this has made it difficult to create an absolute ONSD cut-off value for ICP crises.[20]

Another ophthalmologic approach that is being studied to indirectly assess ICP has been the pupillometer. The automated Neurological Pupil index (NPi) reflects pupillary reactivity. Values range from 0 to 5 with values <3 being associated with poor outcome and trend with elevated ICP.[20]

There is considerable interest and research concentrated on the use of TCD and pulsatility index (PI). By examining the systolic and diastolic velocities within each cardiac cycle, these velocity changes provide the PI value and can allow for ICP trends to be tracked. PI > 1.6 has been associated with higher ICP values and worse outcomes. A combination of PI and ONSD may increase the correlation between the non-invasive and invasive ICP measurements further. Although these non-invasive bedside technologies can provide a quick and easy method of ICP assessment in the pre-hospital and emergency departments setting, there is still a lack of evidence on how they can be used as real-time continuous ICP monitoring at a standard comparable to invasive techniques.[20]

References

1. Alexandrov AV, Joseph M. Transcranial Doppler: an overview of its clinical applications. *Internet J Emerg Intensive Care Med* 2000;4(1).

2. Badri S, Chen J, Barber J, Temkin MR, Dikmen SS, Chestnut RM, et al. Mortality and long-term functional outcome associated with intracranial pressure after traumatic brain injury. *Intensive Care Med* 2012;38(11):1800–9.

3. Balestreri M, Czosnyka M, Hutchinson P, Steiner LA, Hiller M, Smilevski P, et al. Impact of intracranial pressure and cerebral perfusion pressure on severe disability and mortality after head injury. *Neurocrit Care* 2006;4(1):8–13.

4. Carney N, Totten AM, O'Reilly C, Ullman JS, Hawryluk GWJ, Bell MJ, et al. Guidelines for the management of severe traumatic brain injury, fourth edition. *Neurosurgery* 2017;80:6–15.

5. Carpenter KLH, Jalloh I, Hutchinson PJ. Glycolysis and the significance of lactate in traumatic brain injury. *Front Neurosci* 2015;9:112.

6. Carteron L, Bouzat P, Oddo M. Cerebral microdialysis monitoring to improve individualised neurointensive care therapy: an update on recent clinical data. *Front Neurol* 2017;8:601.

7. Chambers IR, Treadwell L, Mendelow AD. Determination of threshold levels of cerebral perfusion pressure and intracranial pressure in severe head injury by using receiver-operating characteristic curves: an observational study in 291 patients. *J Neurosurg* 2001;94(3):412–16.

8. Davies DJ, Zhangije S, Clancy MT, Lucas SJE, Dehghani H, Logan A, Belli A. Near-infrared spectroscopy in the monitoring of adult traumatic brain injury: a review. *J Neurotrauma* 2015;32 (13):933–41.

9. Donnelly J, Budohoski KP, Smielewski P, Czosnyka M. Regulation of the cerebral circulation: bedside assessment and clinical implications. *Crit Care* 2016;20:129.

10. Dreier JP, Fabricius M, Ayata C, Sakowitz OW, Shuttleworth CW, Dohmen C, et al. Recording, analysis, and interpretation of spreading depolarizations in neurointensive care: review and recommendations of the COSBID research group. *J Cereb Blood Flow Metab* 2017;37 (5):1595–625.

11. Fantini S, Sassaroli A, Tgavalekos KT, Kornbluth J. Cerebral blood flow and autoregulation: current measurement techniques and prospects for non-invasive optical methods. *Neurophotonics* 2016;3 (3):031411.

12. Helmy A, Carpenter KL, Skepper JN, Kirkpatrick PJ, Pickard JD, Hutchinson, PJ. Microdialysis of cytokines: methodological considerations, scanning electron microscopy, and determination of relative recovery. *J Neurotrauma* 2009;26:549–61.

13. Hillered L, Dahlin AP, Clausen F, Chu J, Bergquist J, Hjort K, Enblad P, Lewen A. Cerebral microdialysis for protein biomarker monitoring in the neurointensive care setting – a technical approach. *Front Neurol* 2014;5:245.

14. Hutchinson PJ, Jalloh I, Helmy AE, et al. Consensus statement from the 2014 International Microdialysis Forum. *Intensive Care Med* 2015;41(9):1517–28.

15. Le Roux P, Menon DK, Citerio G, Vespa P, Bader MK, Brophy G, et al. The International Multidisciplinary Consensus Conference on Multimodality Monitoring in Neurocritical Care: evidentiary tables: a statement for healthcare professionals from the Neurocritical Care Society and the European Society of Intensive Care Medicine. *Neurocrit Care* 2014;21 (Suppl 2):S297–361.

16. Oddo M, Bösel J. Participants in the International Multidisciplinary Consensus Conference on Multimodality Monitoring: monitoring of brain and systemic oxygenation in neurocritical care patients. *Neurocrit Care* 2014;21(Suppl 2):S103–20.

17. Okonkwo DO, Shutter LA, Moore C, Temkin NR, Puccio AM, Madden CJ, et al. Brain Tissue Oxygen Monitoring and

Management in Severe Traumatic Brain Injury (BOOST-II): a phase II randomized trial. *Crit Care Med* 2017;45(11):1907–14.

18. Purins K, Lewén A, Hillered L, Howells T, Enblad P. Brain tissue oxygenation and cerebral metabolic patterns in focal and diffuse traumatic brain injury. *Front Neurol* 2014:1(5):64.

19. Reis C, Wang Y, Akyol O, Ho WM, Applegate R, Stier G, et al. What's new in traumatic brain injury: update on tracking, monitoring and treatment. *Int J Mol Sci* 2015;16(6):11903–65.

20. Robba C, Bacigaluppi S, Cardim D, Donnelly J, Bertuccio A, Czosnyka M. Non-invasive assessment of intracranial pressure. *Acta Neurol Scand* 2016;134(1):4–21.

21. Roh D, Park S. Brain multimodality monitoring: updated perspective. *Curr Neurol Neurosci Rep.* 2016;16(6):56.

22. Schutt S, Horn P, Roth H, et al. Bedside monitoring of cerebral blood flow by transcranial thermo-dye dilution technique in patients suffering from severe traumatic brain injury or subarachnoid haemorrhage. *J Neurotrauma* 2001;18(6): 595–605.

23. Sloan MA, Alexandrov AV, Tegeler CH, et al. Assessment: transcranial Doppler ultrasonography: report of the Therapeutics and Technology Assessment Subcommittee of the American Academy of Neurology. *Neurology* 2004;62:1468–81.

24. Zeiler FA, Donnelly J, Cardim D, Menon DK, Smielewski P, Czosnyka M. ICP versus laser Doppler cerebrovascular reactivity indices to assess brain autoregulatory capacity. *Neurocrit Care* 2018;28(2):194–202.

Chapter 13

Therapeutic Options in Neurocritical Care
Optimising Brain Physiology

Chiara Robba and Rowan Burnstein

Traumatic Brain Injury (TBI) is a major cause of mortality and morbidity. The severity of primary injury is the major determinant of outcome and occurs during the initial insult, as result of displacement of the physical structures of the brain. However, several factors can occur in the post-injury phase and have also been independently demonstrated to contribute to 'secondary brain injury' and to worsen patients' outcome. These include intracranial hypertension, systemic hypotension, hypoxemia, hyperpyrexia, hypocapnoea and hyper- and hypoglycaemia; many of these factors are amenable to clinical manipulation. It is not well understood how much primary and secondary injuries respectively contribute towards the clinical manifestations of TBI. The exact mechanisms leading to secondary brain injury are not fully elucidated, but exacerbation of cerebral ischaemia and cerebral hypoperfusion are thought to be crucial factors. The integrated management of these factors forms the basis for specialist neurocritical care.

Protocol-Driven Therapy

The development of clinical protocols based on both laboratory and clinical data have underpinned the success of neurocritical care in the management of severe TBI. There is good evidence that such protocol-based treatments lead to improved outcomes after TBI. The evidence for the superiority of any one protocol over other regimes remains controversial.[1,2] Further improvement in outcomes may also be associated with treatment in a specialist neurocritical care unit.[3,4] Most protocols developed for the critical care management of TBI incorporated both surgical and non-surgical components. All rely on the provision of good basic intensive care. They are essentially divided into two schools: maintenance of cerebral perfusion pressure (CPP) as central management of TBI,[5] and the 'Lund protocol'.[6,7]

However, in the last few years, the distinction between such approaches has become increasingly blurred. Improvements in neuromonitoring and imaging of brain tissue and its interpretation are leading to a more individualised approach to TBI management.

Lund Protocol

The 'Lund concept' for the management of TBI was developed in Sweden in 1990.[7,8] This theory focuses on brain volume regulation with the aim to prevent secondary brain injury. The pathophysiological hypothesis is based on reduction in the capillary hydrostatic pressure, avoidance of cerebral oedema and maintenance of plasma oncotic pressure to support brain volume regulatory mechanisms, primarily targeting intracranial pressure (ICP). The Lund protocol accepts levels of CPP between 50 and 60 mmHg, generally lower compared with the CPP-based theory, and aims to target an ICP < 20 mmHg utilising a variety of surgical and non-surgical treatments.[9]

Surgical options include early evacuation of mass lesions, but generally, cerebrospinal fluid drainage is avoided. Decompressive craniectomy can be considered after failed medical therapy to attempt the reduction of ICP. The non-surgical element of Lund therapy includes maintenance of normocapnoea, normal oxygenation and normothermia. Euvolaemia is mandatory and red cell and albumin transfusions are used to achieve haemoglobin levels of 12–14 g/dL and sustain plasma oncotic pressure, respectively. The overall aim is for a negative fluid balance. Effective sedation and stress reduction is achieved by a combination of sedatives, α_2 agonists and β_1 blockade. Sedation is achieved with propofol, midazolam and thiopentone either alone or in combination; the latter is used in 'low doses' of 2–3 mg/kg as boluses to avoid barbiturate side effects. ICP is modulated by optimising plasma oncotic pressure and by maintaining blood pressure using antihypertensive or catecholamine agents. Prostacyclin may also be used to improve the microcirculation in pericontusional areas.[10]

Sustained ICP rises can be also treated with dihydroergotamine, which is a last option before craniectomy. Outcome studies for Lund therapy have suggested favourable results. The incidence of cardiorespiratory complications appears to be lower than that seen with CPP-targeted therapy.[11–13]

CPP Target Therapy

Cerebral ischaemia is the single most important factor to influence outcome from severe TBI, and it is the basis from which Cerebral Perfusion Pressure (CPP)-driven protocols have been developed.[14,15] CPP is defined as the difference between mean arterial pressure (MAP) and ICP, and it is the driving force responsible for brain perfusion and oxygenation. When ICP increases, CPP decreases resulting in inadequate brain perfusion. Therefore, an ICP increase is followed by an impairment of cerebral blood flow (CBF), which is responsible for subsequent metabolic and functional alterations.[15] Low CPP has been associated with a poor outcome after TBI.[16,17]

Rosner et al. in a retrospective study first demonstrated an improvement of outcome from TBI with maintenance of CPP> 70 mmHg.[5] The most recent Brain Trauma Foundation guidelines[18] published in 2016 recommend the management of severe TBI patients using guideline-based recommendations for CPP monitoring to decrease mortality at 2 weeks. The recommended target CPP value for survival and favourable outcomes is between 60 and 70 mm Hg. CPP maintenance is initially focused on ensuring an appropriate MAP by using intravascular fluids targeting a central venous pressure of 5–10 mmHg: vasopressors are used if necessary.

However, the ideal target for post-traumatic CPP continues to be a source of contention, and it is not clear whether 60 or 70 mmHg is the minimum optimal CPP threshold. This is because demonstrating the lower limit of the ischaemic threshold in any individual patient has been elusive and hence the degree to which CPP augmentation might be beneficial is not well established. It is likely that the ischaemic threshold is between 50 and 60 mmHg (BTF guidelines). However, the significant metabolic heterogeneity within the injured brain may render some areas ischaemic at a CPP value that appears to be globally sufficient.[19–21] Moreover, if autoregulation is impaired, increasing CPP will result in increased cerebral blood volume and hence ICP. Furthermore, increasing hydrostatic pressure across the capillary bed may exacerbate vasogenic oedema particularly in regions with poor autoregulation. Therefore, it is becoming increasingly accepted over the last few years that the concept of an individualised CPP should be based on the autoregulatory status of the patient,[17] coupled with bedside monitoring.

The relationship between ICP and MAP can be defined and calculated as the Pressure Reactivity Index (PRx), which is considered as a marker of autoregulatory reserve. Negative PRx values indicate an inverse correlation between ICP and MAP and hence preservation of cerebral autoregulation. Values approaching 1.0 indicate a strong positive association between the two parameters, consistent with poor autoregulation.[22]

The CPP at which the PRx is most negative is used as a surrogate for the point at which autoregulation is best for that individual over the measured time frame. Hence an 'optimum CPP' is identified for an individual patient, with a stronger indication of autoregulation when 'CPPopt' is based on a PRx of less than −0.2. However, prospective evidence to support targeting this opt CPP is yet to be demonstrated prospectively.[17]

CPP-based therapy is not without its hazards; in particular it has been associated with an increased risk of cardiorespiratory complications, such as pulmonary oedema and myocardial ischaemia. For patients at risk of respiratory failure, the current guidelines suggest avoidance of aggressive attempts to maintain CPP >70 mmHg with fluids and vasopressors. However, data suggest that, if autoregulation is intact, CPP-driven therapy may be associated with better outcome compared to the Lund protocol.[23]

General Criteria and Initial Management Goals

Initial management and first-line therapies are directed towards the maintenance of physiological homeostasis and prompt correction of underlying causes associated with intracranial hypertension. Mass lesions amenable to surgical treatment should be evacuated and dilated ventricles should be drained. Baseline laboratory and radiological investigations are shown in Table 13.1.

Airway protection and ventilatory support is crucial. Often patients with TBI require prompt tracheal intubation and mechanical ventilation to protect the airway and optimise oxygen (O_2) and carbon dioxide (CO_2) levels. Hypoxia (oxygen partial pressure (PaO_2) <60 mmHg (8 kPa), or oxygen saturation (SpO_2) <90%) and hypercapnoea (carbon dioxide partial pressure ($PaCO_2$) >45 mmHg/6 kPa) are well-known causes of secondary brain insult and should be avoided.[24] On the other hand, hyperoxia may be detrimental after brain injury and is associated with poor outcome. In addition, hypocapnoea leads to vasoconstriction and cerebral hypoperfusion:[25] there is a narrow optimal window for optimal O_2 and CO_2 levels in TBI.

Haemodynamic stability is crucial in order to avoid hypotension and cerebral hypoperfusion; moreover, in patients with preserved cerebrovascular reactivity and decreased intracranial compliance, hypotension can induce compensatory cerebral vasodilation, increased ICP and further reduction of CPP. The reduction of CPP leads to a vicious circle by further compensatory vasodilation and sustained plateau waves (vasodilatory cascade).[24]

Hypertension can cause intracranial haemorrhage and cerebral oedema, especially in patients with evidence of haemorrhagic contusions and active intracranial bleeding.[26] Fluid resuscitation should aim to maintain euvolaemia and prevention of drops in plasma osmolality, which can cause or worsen cerebral oedema. Hence hypo-osmotic solutions should be avoided.[27]

Table 13.1 Baseline investigations and monitoring used at Addenbrookes Hospital, Cambridge, UK

Baseline investigations	Full blood count
Troponin (if ECG done) crossmatch blood	Clotting screen
	Arterial blood gases
	Glucose
	LFTs
	CRP
	CXR (+ other X-rays/CT as indicated)
	ECG
Basic and advanced monitoring	Capnography
	Pulse oximetry
	Invasive arterial pressure monitoring
	Urinary catheter: hourly urine output and fluid balance recording
	Core and peripheral temperature
	Triple lumen line for CVP measurement
	Cranial access device: ICP bolt + external ventricular drain in appropriate patients
	Cerebral Neurotrend probe and microdialysis
	Jugular bulb oximetry (retrograde RIJ)
	MCA velocities (transcranial Doppler)
	Pulmonary artery catheter (moderate/severe lung injury, cardiac contusion or cardiac disease)
	EEG recording

Despite it not being clear in the literature what the precise threshold for red blood cell transfusion in traumatic brain injury should be, a target of 70–90 g/L is reasonable, as any lower haemoglobin concentration is associated with an increased incidence of brain tissue hypoxia and increased mortality.[28,29]

Anticonvulsants are indicated in patients at risk of seizures. According to the most recent TBI guidelines[18] general prophylactic use of phenytoin or valproate is not recommended, but phenytoin is recommended to decrease the incidence of early post-traumatic seizures (within 7 days of injury). At present, there is insufficient evidence to recommend levetiracetam over phenytoin with regard to the efficacy in preventing early post-traumatic seizures and toxicity. However, it is not inferior in its efficacy and has a more favourable side effect profile.

The use of steroids is not recommended for improving outcome or reducing ICP. Moreover, in patients with severe TBI, high-dose methylprednisolone is associated with increased mortality and is contraindicated.[18] Finally, tight blood sugar control is recommended and a tight control of temperature is required to avoid hyperpyrexia.

Brain Chemistry

Brain chemistry monitoring through brain tissue PO_2 (PbO_2) and microdialysis probes can be used as subsidiary targets. PbO2 is the partial pressure of oxygen in the extracellular fluid of the brain and reflects the availability of oxygen for oxidative energy production. It represents the balance between oxygen delivery and consumption, and is influenced by changes in cerebral perfusion. Cerebral microdialysis provides localised analysis of brain tissue biochemistry in neurointensive care. The microdialysis catheter has a tip with a semi-permeable dialysis membrane which is placed into brain tissue and perfused via an inlet tube with fluid isotonic to the tissue interstitium. Diffusion drives the passage of molecules across the membrane along their concentration gradients.[30] The most common assays for bedside use are those for glucose, lactate, pyruvate, glycerol and glutamate, which reflect the metabolic state of the brain. Both tools are becoming an established part of multi-modality monitoring during the management of acute brain injury in some research centres. Targets may vary depending on whether the probe is in normal or perilesional tissue.[30]

The aim is to keep $PbO_2 > 15$ mmHg, and lactate/pyruvate ratio (LPR) < 25. If these limits are exceeded, in the first instance, it is important to ensure that CPP targets are met; if brain chemistry remains unsatisfactory, it would be usual to increase F_IO_2 augmenting oxygen delivery. Conversely, if PbO_2 suggests a good oxidative energy production state such as $PbO_2 \gg 35$ mmHg and LPR is $\ll 25$, this would be corroborative evidence that CPP levels that may be considered otherwise marginal (~60 mmHg) are probably adequate, and would support a decision not to escalate CPP augmentation therapy. However, it is less clear whether these thresholds provide any confidence when deciding whether to treat moderate elevations in ICP (~ 25 mmHg) or not when the CPP is in the target range.

Intracranial Hypertension and Staircase Approach

The level of therapy in patients with raised intracranial pressure is usually increased in a stepwise manner, with use of progressively aggressive interventions (Table 13.2). The sequence of interventions may vary amongst different institutions and the escalation of treatment can potentially be associated with adverse effects (Figure 13.1). However in general, ICP lowering strategies include appropriate sedation, analgesia and paralysis, osmotic therapy, mechanical ventilation and $PaCO_2$ manipulation, and in more severe cases, the use of temperature control, barbiturate coma and surgical decompression.[31]

Sedation, Analgesia and Muscle Relaxants

Adequate sedation and analgesia are cornerstones of post-traumatic ICP control. Inadequate sedation and analgesia are associated with waves of elevated ICP, partly related to an increased cerebral metabolic rate for oxygen ($CMRO_2$). Furthermore, many sedative drugs have additional benefits in terms of seizure reduction/control. Muscle relaxants are important to optimise ventilation in patients with severe TBI as well as to minimise ventilator asynchrony, which may be associated with increased ICP. The ideal sedative agent has a rapid onset and recovery, allowing assessment of neurological status; is easily titrated to achieve the desirable level of sedation; reduces ICP, cerebral blood flow (CBF) and $CMRO_2$ whilst maintaining flow-metabolism coupling; and enables cerebral

Table 13.2 Initial management goals and settings

Early evacuation of intracranial space occupying lesions
Cerebral spinal fluid drainage to manage intracranial hypertension wherever possible
Sedation, analgesia, paralysis; head elevation to 30°

    Ventilation: PEEP 5–10 cm H_2O, $FIO_2 \leq 0.5$
    Target $PaO_2 = \geq 82$ mmHg (11 kPa) (or $SpO_2 \geq 95\%$)
    Target $PaCO_2 = 33.7$–37.5 mmHg (4.5–5.0 kPa) (avoid $PaCO_2 < 30$ mmHg (4.0 kPa))
    Aim for normocapnoea ($PaCO_2$ 37.5–40 mmHg; /5–5.3 kPa if no ICP elevation)

$ICP \leq 20$ mmHg
$CPP \geq 70$ mmHg (at least $CPP \geq 60$ mm Hg)

    Core temperature 36°–37°C
    Optimal haemodynamic and volume status
    Tight control of seizures. Consider anticonvulsant if significant head injury on CT, patient
       sedated and/or paralysed, EEG unavailable, and ICP rises suggest fits
    Early enteral feeding (within 24 hours)
    Tight blood sugar control (at least daily blood sugars: 4–10 mmol/L, avoiding hypoglycaemia at
       all costs)
    Maintain SjO2 $\gg$ 55% by increasing PaCO2 and elevating CPP
    Use brain chemistry monitoring as subsidiary targets. Aim to keep brain tissue pO_2 (PbO_2) > 15
       mmHg (2 kPa), and lactate/pyruvate ratio (LPR) <25

autoregulation and normal cerebral vascular reactivity to $PaCO_2$. Moreover, it should have minimal cardiovascular effects and predictable clearance, independent of end organ function.[32] No single available agent has all the desirable characteristics needed for sedation and analgesia in patients with severe TBI.

Propofol is the most common induction and maintenance agent for the haemodynamically stable neurosurgical patients for the reduction of intracranial pressure. It is commonly used along with opioids for a general anaesthesia and it has a fast onset of action and plasma clearance, which allows rapid assessment of neurological status. Propofol exhibits potential neuroprotective effects by reducing ICP and cerebral metabolic requirements, with dose dependent reductions in $CMRO_2$ and CBF, whilst flow metabolism coupling, cerebrovascular CO_2 reactivity and autoregulation remain intact.[33] Propofol can also produce EEG and metabolic suppression. However, from cardiopulmonary bypass data, burst suppression with propofol does not seem to decrease the number of 'jugular desaturation episodes' ($SjVO_2$) during cardiopulmonary bypass nor the ischaemic burden in brain-injured patients with a normal ICP.[34]

Propofol is administered by continuous infusion (2–4 mg/kg/h), and the duration of action is dependent on the redistribution of propofol into the peripheral compartments.

A number of problems have been associated with propofol, including precipitous cardiovascular collapse and propofol infusion syndrome.[35] Therefore, it is recommended not to exceed a dose of 4 mg/kg/h for more than a few hours and also to avoid its use in patients with profound hypothermia and at risk of hyperlipidaemia.

Propofol can be replaced by midazolam (0.1–0.2 mg/kg/hr) for long-term sedation. Benzodiazepines exhibit sedative, hypnotic, anxiolytic, anticonvulsant and amnestic effects.

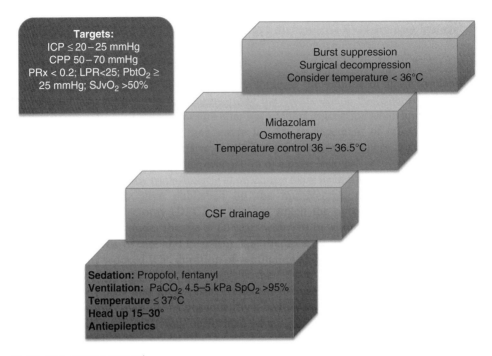

Figure 13.1 Staircase approach.

In particular, the relatively short context sensitive half-time (CS $t_{1/2}$) of midazolam makes it the benzodiazepine of choice used alongside other drugs for sedation of brain-injured patients. It reduces cerebral metabolic rate, cerebral blood flow and ICP without impairing autoregulation.[36] In the absence of any randomised trials and due to uncertainties over its effect on cerebral blood flow and haemodynamic side effects, dexmedetomidine is not currently recommended for use in TBI.

Adequate analgesia is generally provided with an infusion of opioids. Opioids have a key role in neurocritically ill patients with the added benefit of minimal effects on cerebrovascular haemodynamics. However, at higher doses, they can induce hypotension resulting in cerebral hypoperfusion and increased ICP.[37] The context-sensitive half-time (CS $t_{1/2}$) of opioid infusions would determine the time to offset. Fentanyl has a long CS $t_{1/2}$ and hence prolonged infusions could potentially delay waking, but remains a popular choice for sedation. Remifentanil has unique pharmacodynamic properties exhibiting reliable quick offset, as it is rapidly hydrolysed by tissue and plasma esterases prevent accumulation.[32] Therefore, it is useful for rapid and reliable reversal of sedation with preservation of good airway reflexes and patient alertness. Morphine is not the drug of choice due to its prolonged duration of action and its proconvulsant metabolite normeperidine.

The use of ketamine in patients with intracranial hypertension has been traditionally discouraged;[38] however, recent clinical trials have confirmed that ketamine[39,40] could have neuroprotective and anticonvulsant properties, with minimal effects on ICP. Therefore it is considered to be the induction agent of choice for the brain-injured patient at risk of haemodynamic compromise.

Assessment of the depth of sedation can be problematic in patients with severe TBI. Patients who have appropriate sedation and analgesia should not elicit responses of raised ICP waveforms on ICP monitoring, in response to stimulation such as endotracheal suctioning. The use of bi-spectral index monitoring (BIS) or processed EEG may be a useful adjunct for monitoring the depth of sedation in such patients. The use of a 'sedation hold' to assess levels of sedation in patients in whom ICP control is critical is contraindicated.

Ventilation

Mechanical ventilation is often necessary in the brain-injured patient, and respiratory failure could result from multiple aetiologies (aspiration pneumonia, pulmonary contusion related to chest trauma, neurogenic pulmonary oedema, etc.). The main goals of mechanical ventilation in TBI are to avoid hypoxaemia and to maintain tight control of $PaCO_2$, avoiding hypoxaemia- and hypercapnoea-related exacerbations of intracranial hypertension. Therefore, mechanical ventilation should be instituted early in the management of TBI. Normal values of arterial oxygen and carbon dioxide partial pressure tensions (PaO_2 >80 mmHg/10 kPa $PaCO_2$ = 35–40 mmHg/5–5.3 kPa) should be aggressively maintained.

Current evidence[41] suggests that lung protective ventilation is useful in certain subgroups of patients.[42] However, low tidal volume and permissive hypercapnoea are associated with cerebral vasodilation and increased cerebral blood volume with consequent increase in intracranial pressure.

Striking a balance between ensuring adequate brain protection with hyperventilation driven control of ICP against prevention of ventilator induced lung injury remains difficult. In neurocritical care patients these strategies remain somewhat controversial and on occasion contraindicated; the resultant rise in ICP from permissive hypercapnoea and/or use of high airway pressures during lung recruitment manoeuvers may be very hazardous.[43]

Carbon dioxide is a potent arterial vasodilator with hypocapnoea leading to cerebral vasoconstriction and subsequent reduction of cerebral blood volume.[44] Cerebral blood flow decreases in a linear relationship to $PaCO_2$ tension with the range from 75 to 20 mmHg (2.5–10 kPa). The reduction in CBF and the concomitant reduction in cerebral blood volume is the most likely explanation for the potent reduction in ICP seen with hyperventilation, and the original basis for its use as an integral part of TBI management.

Cerebral blood volume is linearly related to $PaCO_2$[45] and therefore in patients with TBI, strict attention must be paid to $PaCO_2$ control. Overzealous hyperventilation with lower tensions of $PaCO_2$ (<30 mmHg) is potentially dangerous, with severe hypocapnoea inducing consequent cerebral vasoconstriction leading to inadvertent worsening of cerebral ischemia.[44]

As per the most recent BTF guidelines,[18] prolonged prophylactic hyperventilation with $PaCO_2$ of 25 mm Hg is not recommended. Hyperventilation is recommended as a temporising measure for the reduction of elevated ICP, but it should be avoided during the first 24 hours after injury when CBF is often critically reduced. If hyperventilation is used early, $SjVO_2$ or PbO_2 monitoring is recommended to monitor cerebral oxygen delivery. In the absence of intracranial hypertension, the initial $PaCO_2$ target should be ~37.5 mmHg (5 kPa)

Positive end expiratory pressure (PEEP) and recruitment manoeuvers (RM) are both useful strategies to improve oxygenation and alveolar recruitment and optimise ventilation –

perfusion matching. However, high PEEP (>10 cm H_2O) and RM could potentially have dangerous effects on ICP and their use is therefore controversial. They potentially lead to an increase in intrathoracic pressure and impaired cerebral venous return to the right atrium, particularly in an underfilled patient. The resulting elevation of ICP in patients with critical cerebral tissue perfusion could be deleterious.[46] Some literature argues that if PEEP is less than ICP, then the associated augmentation of intrathoracic pressure and pulmonary dynamics does not result in an increase in ICP. Numerous studies show that in patients with acute stroke and subarachnoid haemorrhage, high PEEP leads to a reduced CPP and consequently an indirect decrease in CBF, rather than from a direct effect from increased intrathoracic pressure.[43,47] Some authors debate that whilst PEEP and RM have a significant effect on ICP and intracranial haemodynamics, ensuring optimal oxygen carriage is important and hence PEEP and/or RM may be used cautiously in some selected patients. The absolute effects of PEEP and RM on cerebrovascular haemodynamics continue to be debated.

Ventilation in a prone position in patients with ARDS has been demonstrated to be an effective method to improve oxygenation (better PaO_2:FiO_2 ratios)[50] and to reduce mortality. It should be used cautiously in TBI patients as it raises ICP in patients with reduced intracranial compliance.[48,49] Prone position ventilation can impair jugular venous return and hence raise ICP. Significant intracranial hypertension (>25 mmHg) may preclude full prone ventilation in most instances. The effect of prone position on ICP should be monitored continuously in real time, with additional treatment interventions for any increased ICP or de-escalation to a different ventilatory strategy if the increase in ICP becomes refractory to intervention. We would not recommend turning patients prone where the increased local pressure or gravitational position related to being prone may compromise the perfusion in the perilesional areas such as in frontal contusions.

Osmotic Therapy

Osmotic agents have long been used to manage acute rises in ICP. Brain volume is extremely responsive to changes in parenchymal water content. When plasma osmolality is rapidly increased by solutes that do not easily diffuse across the blood-brain barrier, the brain-plasma osmotic gradient results in net water diffusion from the brain parenchyma into the circulation volume. However, when plasma osmolality decreases, free water diffuses across the blood-brain barrier from the circulation volume into the brain parenchyma, precipitating brain oedema.[51] Solutes able to generate clinically relevant osmotic gradients across the blood-brain barrier include mannitol and hypertonic saline.

Mannitol is a sugar alcohol with osmotic diuretic properties, that does not cross the intact blood-brain barrier or cellular membranes. Controversy still exists over the exact mechanism of action of mannitol in reducing ICP. Its immediate effect is likely to arise from improved blood rheology due to a reduction in viscosity, and a plasma–expanding effect which increases cerebral blood flow and oxygen delivery.[52] Mannitol dehydrates erythrocytes, reducing blood viscosity, improving cerebral perfusion and oxygenation irrespective of its effects on ICP. Mannitol also creates an osmotic gradient across the intact blood-brain barrier, reducing cerebral oedema by drawing water into the vascular compartment.[52] An effect of mannitol on ICP is usually seen within 10–20 minutes of a bolus administration and lasts variably from 90 min up to 6 hours. The effectiveness of repeated administration of mannitol is not established. The diuretic properties of mannitol cause systemic dehydration and a sustained increase in plasma osmolality. It is contraindicated in patients whose serum osmolality is > 320 mOsm/L due to its association with an increased incidence of neurological and renal side effects.[53]

Other side effects of mannitol include systemic hypotension, intravascular volume depletion, profound diuresis, hyperkalaemia and rebound increase in ICP.[54]

Mannitol is most frequently prescribed as a single bolus dose of 0.25–1.0 g/Kg body weight, administered often as a 20% w/v solution, and is supported by the most recent TBI guidelines.[18] This is effective in reducing ICP, provided that arterial hypotension (systolic blood pressure <90 mm Hg) is avoided. The use of mannitol *prior* to ICP monitoring should be restricted to patients with signs of transtentorial herniation or progressive neurological deterioration not attributable to extracranial causes.

The effect of hypertonic saline on ICP depends on a direct increase in plasma osmolality, resulting in a net flow of water from the brain parenchyma into the circulation volume. Similar to mannitol, an added effect is from the rheological effect from dehydration of erythrocytes with subsequent reduction in blood viscosity, improved cerebral blood flow and a reduction in cerebral blood volume. Hypertonic saline has an osmotic effect with water extracted down an osmotic gradient from the brain parenchyma to the intravascular space, so reducing tissue turgor pressure and cell size, and hence brain volume.

Hypertonic saline causes intravascular volume expansion (whereas mannitol causes an osmotic diuresis). Mobilisation of fluid into the vascular compartment helps maintain blood pressure and CPP. Effects on the vascular endothelium and erythrocytes are also of relevance. Vasodilatation and reduction of endothelial oedema may improve cerebral perfusion and reduce leukocyte adherence.[55]

Hypertonic saline is available as a 3%, 5%, 7.5% and 23.4% w/v solutions. It has a rapid onset of action and numerous regimes have been described, making it difficult to draw conclusions about optimal doses, concentrations or treatment. Sodium and chloride levels can be routinely measured at the bedside as part of serial blood gas sampling, facilitating titration of treatment. When serum sodium concentration exceeds 160 mmol/L, it is unlikely that additional doses of hypertonic saline will have further beneficial effects on ICP.[56]

Compared to mannitol, hypertonic saline can achieve similar or better reductions in ICP following TBI, and it has proven to be effective in the management of intracranial hypertension refractory to mannitol.[57] Moreover unlike mannitol, rebound intracranial hypertension is not a problem observed with repeated administration.[58]

In response to brain dehydration, astrocytes and neurons produce polyols, amino acids and other osmotically active molecules. This contributes to a gradual re-equilibration of the osmotic gradient between extracellular space and brain parenchyma. When a state of serum hyperosmolality has been maintained over a number of days, care should be taken to prevent a rapid reversal of brain-plasma water gradient, in order to prevent subsequent rebound brain oedema.

Treatment with hypertonic saline is generally well tolerated. In contrast to mannitol, it is effective as a volume expander without the risks of inducing hyperkalaemia or acute kidney injury. The main risk associated with hypertonic saline administration is in precipitating or aggravating pulmonary oedema in patients with underlying cardiac or pulmonary dysfunction.[59]

Hypothermia

Homeostasis normally maintains the human body at a core temperature of 36.5°–37.5°C. Therapeutic hypothermia is defined as an intentional reduction of core temperature.

A number of experimental and clinical studies describe the effects of mild (34°–36°C) moderate (32°–34°C) and deep hypothermia (30°–32°C), and it has long been hypothesised that cooling patients may have a neuroprotective effect.

The neuroprotective properties of therapeutic hypothermia include the inhibition of excitotoxicity and neuronal apoptosis,[60] the suppression of the inflammatory cascade, with reduction of blood-brain barrier disruption, preserved cell membrane integrity and reduced cytotoxic oedema.[61]

Mild to moderate hypothermia (32°–36°C) is effective in decreasing intracranial pressure and control of fever for prevention and treatment of neurological injuries. But the effects of hypothermia are complex and several adverse effects can occur in patients with traumatic brain injury who receive cooling to control refractory intracranial hypertension.

Several single centre trials investigated the neuroprotective effect of hypothermia after severe head injury. These mostly demonstrated a benefit in those patients who were cooled, especially in patients who had Glasgow Coma Scale (GCS) of 4–7 on admission.[62,63] Results from a large multi-centre randomised controlled trial in 2001 demonstrated a reduction in ICP for those patients who were 'prophylactically' cooled but with no benefit in terms of neurological outcome or survival,[64] along with an increase in 'days with complications' in this group. Proponents of induced hypothermia have criticised this study because some of the units involved had little prior experience in the use of therapeutic hypothermia, the speed at which hypothermia was induced was slow and there were significant differences in results between individual centres. It is hence possible that benefits of hypothermia are only seen when it is performed by experienced units with expertise in the management of the hypothermic period.

A more recent randomised control trial demonstrated that early hypothermia (32°–35°C) as a therapeutic intervention in response to raised ICP does not improve outcome following TBI,[65] suggesting no evidence to support the use of hypothermia as a primary neuroprotective strategy following severe TBI. Recruitment to the trial was stopped when there were signs of harm in the hypothermia group. The current BTF guidelines[18] state that early (within 2.5 h), prophylactic hypothermia maintained short term (less than 48 hrs) is not recommended, as it does not improve outcomes in patients with diffuse injury.

However, there are some centres that continue to use staged hypothermia therapy in patients with otherwise refractory intracranial hypertension.

The induction of hypothermia is not without complications,[66] although these become more pronounced as core temperature decreases below 29°C. Shivering may be seen with temperature as high as 35°C. This causes an increase in oxygen consumption, CO_2 production and cardiac output and potentially arterial oxygen desaturation and haemodynamic instability.[67,68] The use of muscle relaxants limits these effects in cooled patients. Blood pressure and cardiac output drop at temperatures below 32°C. This is partly a function of the reduced metabolic rate and oxygen consumption, but it is also due to a direct effect on the myocardium and is the basis of 31°–32°C being the lower limit for therapeutic hypothermia. The reduction of cardiac output also leads to a reduction in renal perfusion and glomerular filtration rate. Tubular reabsorption of water also declines, as a combined effect of reduced cellular activity and probable resistance to antidiuretic hormone. In mild to moderate hypothermia tubular dysfunction tends to predominate and large volumes of hypo-osmolar urine is produced (so-called cold-diuresis), which may render the patient both hypovolaemic and hypokalaemic. The former particularly becomes evident on rewarming to normothermia. Prolonged bleeding times and platelet dysfunction tend only to be seen in patients who are profoundly hypothermic. Moderate hypothermia is also not devoid of adverse effects, including time and temperature dependent coagulopathy, immunological suppression, electrolyte and volume disturbances. The adverse effects associated with moderate hypothermia tend to develop over periods of hours and days, and are usually treatable and rarely considered to be life threatening.[69]

There are several devices available to facilitate cooling. These include external/surface cooling devices (ice packs, sponge water baths, air cooled circulating blankets, ice water circulating blankets) and endovascular/body cavity cooling devices (infusion of cooled fluids, peritoneal lavage, extracorporeal circuits and intravascular catheter-based heat exchange systems). Endovascular cooling devices have the advantages of having a shorter time to target temperature and the ability to maintain a relatively more stable temperature. However, they are associated with potentially severe complications, such as deep venous thrombosis and catheter-related infections.[70] Surface cooling techniques seem to offer a superior safety profile when hypothermia needs to be maintained for a more protracted period such as for greater than 24 hours.

Barbiturate Coma

Barbiturates include a broad family of central nervous system depressants. Their neuro-protective properties include profound cerebral metabolic suppression and reduction of ICP. Many laboratory and clinical studies demonstrate a beneficial effect of barbiturates in lowering ICP in severe TBI. Despite this, the use of barbiturates in TBI remains controversial because of a high incidence of serious side effects.[71] High-dose barbiturates such as thiopentone can be administered as bolus doses of 250 mg up to 3–5 g until burst suppression is achieved on EEG monitoring, followed by an infusion of 3–8 mg/kg to maintain burst suppression. Barbiturates have a long half-life due to their slow hepatic metabolism combined with high lipid solubility. Therefore, a prolonged residual sedative effect is often seen after the cessation of barbiturate infusions and is particularly disadvantageous following TBI, since clinical assessment becomes difficult.[72]

Barbiturates lower ICP by a number of mechanisms, including reduced cerebral metabolism, altered cerebral vascular haemodynamics, reduced intracellular acidosis, inhibition of excitoxicity and inhibition of free radical-mediated lipid peroxidation.[73] However, their use is associated with a number of complications with potentially significant consequences. Hypotension is due to a combination of impaired venous return, inhibition of baroreflexes and direct myocardial depression. A pronounced fall in serum potassium is common during barbiturate infusions, but significantly, this is not associated with increased urinary losses, and it is likely to represent increased intracellular uptake of potassium. Sudden cardiovascular collapse and severe hyperkalaemia have been reported following cessation of barbiturate infusions. Other complications of barbiturates include immunosuppression and hepatic dysfunction. Renal dysfunction has been described, but it is difficult to explain and may be a function of other concomitant elements of critical illness.

The use of barbiturates either prophylactically, or as first line sedative agents, is not recommended.[74,75] The most recent BTF guidelines suggest that administration of barbiturates to routinely induce burst suppression measured by EEG as prophylaxis against the development of intracranial hypertension is not recommended. However, high-dose barbiturate administration is recommended to control elevated ICP refractory to maximum standard medical and surgical treatment and hence its use should be confined to the management of refractory intracranial hypertension, unresponsive to other therapies. Haemodynamic stability is essential before, during and upon cessation of barbiturate therapy.[18]

ICP and Surgical Management

The surgical management of intracranial hypertension includes the evacuation of space-occupying masses, drainage of cerebrospinal fluid, and decompressive craniectomy and are described in detail in other chapters of this book.

Intracranial lesions including epidural and acute subdural haematomas should be rapidly detected and evacuated in a timely manner. This is especially important when there is clinical or radiological evidence of mass effect.[76,77] The surgical management of intraparenchymal haemorrhage and contusions is more controversial; in such cases, the surgical indication depends on the size, location and the presence of any intraventricular extension of blood.[78]

Recently, the STICH 1 and 2 trials suggested that early surgical evacuation of spontaneous intraparenchymal masses has no benefit when compared with medical management.[79,80]

CSF drainage is a simple and effective strategy to reduce intracranial pressure, and insertion of an external ventricular drain (EVD) can be also considered as second-tier therapy for the treatment of intracranial hypertension. Also, an EVD can enable continuous or intermittent monitoring of ICP.

Decompressive craniectomy (DC) can rapidly control ICP in patients with intracranial hypertension refractory to maximal medical treatment. Several different techniques for decompressive craniectomy have been described depending on location and technique; bifrontal decompression is utilised in patients with diffuse cerebral oedema, whereas unilateral decompression is usually performed in patients with unilateral lesions and midline shift.

There is little doubt regarding the effectiveness of a large decompression for the control of intracranial hypertension, but the major concern is that although this may improve survival, it would be at the cost of surviving with severe residual long-term disability. The DECRA trial[81] demonstrated that early decompressive craniectomy has no benefit upon mortality. However, patients undergoing decompressive craniectomy had a significantly higher proportion of unfavourable neurologic outcomes. The Randomized Evaluation of Surgery with Craniectomy for Uncontrollable Elevation of Intracranial Pressure (RESCUE-ICP)[82] study compared medical therapy with decompressive craniectomy in patients with intracranial hypertension not responding to medical treatment. The results demonstrated that decompressive craniectomy in traumatic brain injury reduces the mortality in patients with refractory intracranial hypertension, but with higher rates of neurological disability.

The recent TBI guidelines[18] suggest that bifrontal decompressive craniectomy is not recommended in severe TBI patients with diffuse injury (without mass lesions), and for those with ICP values of ≥ 20 mmHg for more than 15 min within a given 1 hour period, that remain refractory to first-tier therapies. However, this procedure has been demonstrated to reduce ICP and to minimise ICU length of stay. Overall decompressive craniectomy should be considered only after a considered multidisciplinary discussion and an appropriately nuanced discussion with the patients next of kin.

Finally, BTF guidelines favour a larger decompressive craniectomy over a limited one. A frontotemporoparietal decompression (not less than 12 cm diameter) is preferred over a small frontotemporoparietal decompressive craniectomy to help reduce mortality and improve neurological outcomes in patients with severe TBI.

References

1. Elf K, Nilsson P, Enblad P. Outcome after traumatic brain injury improved by an organized secondary insult program and standardized neurointensive care. *Crit Care Med* 2002;30(9):2129–34.

2. Patel HC, Menon DK, Tebbs S, Hawker R, Hutchinson PJ, Kirkpatrick PJ. Specialist neurocritical care and outcome from head injury. *Intensive Care Med* 2002;28 (5):547–53.

3. Clayton TJ, Nelson RJ, Manara AR. Reduction in mortality from severe head injury following introduction of a protocol for intensive care management. *Br J Anaesth* 2004;93(6):761–7.

4. Patel HC, Bouamra O, Woodford M, King AT, Yates DW, Lecky FE. Trends in head injury outcome from 1989 to 2003 and the effect of neurosurgical care: an observational study. *Lancet* 2005;366 (9496):1538–44. Erratum in Lancet 2006;367(9513):816.

5. Rosner MJ, Rosner SD, Johnson AH. Cerebral perfusion pressure: management protocol and clinical results. *J Neurosurg* 1995;83(6):949–62.

6. Eker C, Asgeirsson B, Grände PO, Schalén W, Nordström CH. Improved outcome after severe head injury with a new therapy based on principles for brain volume regulation and preserved microcirculation. *Intensive Care Med* 2006;32(10):1475–84.

7. Grände PO. The 'Lund Concept' for the treatment of patients with severe traumatic brain injury. *J Neurosurg Anesthesiol* 2011;23(4):358–62.

8. Asgeirsson B, Grände PO, Nordström CH. A new therapy of post-trauma brain oedema based on haemodynamic principles for brain volume regulation. *Intensive Care Med* 1994;20 (4):260–7.

9. Grände PO, Asgeirsson B, Nordström CH. Volume-targeted therapy of increased intracranial pressure: the Lund concept unifies surgical and non-surgical treatments. *Acta Anaesthesiol Scand* 2002;46(8):929–41.

10. Grande PO, Möller AD, Nordström CH, Ungerstedt U. Low-dose prostacyclin in treatment of severe brain trauma evaluated with microdialysis and jugular bulb oxygen measurements. *Acta Anaesthesiol Scand* 2000;44(7):886–94.

11. Eker C, Asgeirsson B, Grände PO, Schalén W, Nordström CH. Improved outcome after severe head injury with a new therapy based on principles for brain volume regulation and preserved microcirculation. *Intensive Care Med* 2006;32(10):1475–84.

12. Naredi S, Olivecrona M, Lindgren C, Ostlund AL, Grände PO, Koskinen LO. An outcome study of severe traumatic head injury using the 'Lund therapy' with low-dose prostacyclin. *Acta Anaesthesiol Scand* 2001;45(4):402–6.

13. Elf K, Nilsson P, Ronne-Engström E, Howells T, Enblad P. Cerebral perfusion pressure between 50 and 60 mm Hg may be beneficial in head-injured patients: a computerized secondary insult monitoring study. *Neurosurgery* 2005;56 (5):962–71.

14. Chesnut RM, Marshall LF, Klauber MR, Blunt BA, Baldwin N, Eisenberg HM, et al. The role of secondary brain injury in determining outcome from severe head injury. *J Trauma* 1993;34(2):216–22.

15. Chesnut RM, Marshall SB, Piek J, Blunt BA, Klauber MR, Marshall LF. Early and late systemic hypotension as a frequent and fundamental source of cerebral ischemia following severe brain injury in the Traumatic Coma Data Bank. *Acta Neurochir Suppl* 1993;59:121–5.

16. Clifton GL, Miller ER, Choi SC, Levin HS. Fluid thresholds and outcome from severe brain injury. *Crit Care Med* 2002;30 (4):739–45.

17. Aries MJ, Czosnyka M, Budohoski KP, Steiner LA, Lavinio A, Kolias AG, et al. Continuous determination of optimal cerebral perfusion pressure in traumatic brain injury. *Crit Care Med* 2012;40 (8):2456–63.

18. Carney N, Totten AM, O'Reilly C, Ullman JS, Hawryluk GW, Bell MJ, et al. Guidelines for the management of severe traumatic brain injury, fourth edition. *Neurosurgery* 2017 Jan 1;80(1):6-15.

19. Gupta AK, Hutchinson PJ, Al-Rawi P, Gupta S, Swart M, Kirkpatrick PJ, Menon DK, Datta AK. Measuring brain tissue oxygenation compared with jugular venous oxygen saturation for monitoring cerebral oxygenation after traumatic brain injury. *Anesth Analg* 1999;88(3):549–53.

20. Coles JP, Fryer TD, Smielewski P, Chatfield DA, Steiner LA, Johnston AJ, et al. Incidence and mechanisms of cerebral ischemia in early clinical head injury. *J Cereb Blood Flow Metab* 2004;24 (2):202–11.

21. Coles JP, Fryer TD, Smielewski P, Rice K, Clark JC, Pickard JD, Menon DK. Defining ischemic burden after traumatic brain injury using 15O PET imaging of cerebral physiology. *J Cereb Blood Flow Metab* 2004;24(2):191–201.

22. Czosnyka M, Smielewski P, Kirkpatrick P, Menon DK, Pickard JD. Monitoring of cerebral autoregulation in head-injured patients. *Stroke* 1996;27(10):1829–34.

23. Howells T, Elf K, Jones PA, Ronne-Engström E, Piper I, Nilsson P, Andrews P, Enblad P. Pressure reactivity as a guide in the treatment of cerebral perfusion pressure in patients with brain trauma. *J Neurosurg* 2005;102(2):311–17.

24. Bratton SL, Chestnut RM, Ghajar J, McConnell Hammond FF, Harris OA, Hartl R, et al. Guidelines for the management of severe traumatic brain injury. XIV. Hyperventilation. *J Neurotrauma* 2007;24(Suppl 1):S87–90.

25. Muizelaar JP, Marmarou A, Ward JD, Kontos HA, Choi SC, Becker DP, Gruemer H, Young HF. Adverse effects of prolonged hyperventilation in patients with severe head injury: a randomized clinical trial. *J Neurosurg* 1991;75(5):731–9.

26. Moppett IK, Sherman RW, Wild MJ, Latter JA, Mahajan RP. Effects of norepinephrine and glyceryl trinitrate on cerebral haemodynamics: transcranial Doppler study in healthy volunteers. *Br J Anaesth* 2008;100(2):240–4.

27. Talmor D, Shapira Y, Artru AA, Gurevich B, Merkind V, Katchko L, Reichenthal E. 0.45% saline and 5% dextrose in water, but not 0.9% saline or 5% dextrose in 0.9% saline, worsen brain edema two hours after closed head trauma in rats. *Anesth Analg* 1998;86 (6):1225–9.

28. Oddo M, Milby A, Chen I, Frangos S, MacMurtrie E, Maloney-Wilensky E, et al. Hemoglobin concentration and cerebral metabolism in patients with aneurysmal subarachnoid hemorrhage. *Stroke* 2009;40 (4):1275–81.

29. Sekhon MS, McLean N, Henderson WR, Chittock DR, Griesdale DE. Association of hemoglobin concentration and mortality in critically ill patients with severe traumatic brain injury. *Crit Care* 2012;16 (4):R128.

30. Helmy A, Carpenter KL, Hutchinson PJ. Microdialysis in the human brain and its potential role in the development and clinical assessment of drugs. *Curr Med Chem* 2007;14(14):1525–37.

31. Stocchetti N, Maas AI. Traumatic intracranial hypertension. *N Engl J Med* 2014;371(10):972.

32. Citerio G, Cormio M. Sedation in neurointensive care: advances in understanding and practice. *Curr Opin Crit Care* 2003;9(2):120–6.

33. Johnston AJ, Steiner LA, Chatfield DA, Coleman MR, Coles JP, Al-Rawi PG, Menon DK, Gupta AK. Effects of propofol on cerebral oxygenation and metabolism after head injury. *Br J Anaesth* 2003;91 (6):781–6.

34. Karabinis A, Mandragos K, Stergiopoulos S, Komnos A, Soukup J, Speelberg B, Kirkham AJ. Safety and efficacy of analgesia-based sedation with remifentanil versus standard hypnotic-based regimens in intensive care unit patients with brain injuries: a randomised, controlled trial. *Crit Care* 2004;8(4):R268–80.

35. Krajčová A, Waldauf P, Anděl M, Duška F. Propofol infusion syndrome: a structured review of experimental studies and 153 published case reports. *Crit Care* 2015;19: 398.

36. Fleischer JE, Milde JH, Moyer TP, Michenfelder JD. Cerebral effects of high-dose midazolam and subsequent reversal with Ro 15–1788 in dogs. *Anesthesiology* 1988;68(2):234–42.

37. Hocker SE, Fogelson J, Rabistein AA. Refractory intracranial hypertension due to fentanyl administration following closed head injury. *Front Neurol* 2013; 4:3.

38. Sheth RD, Gidal BE. Refractory status epilepticus: response to ketamine. *Neurology* 1998;51(6):1765–6.

39. Kolenda H, Gremmelt A, Rading S, Braun U, Markakis E. Ketamine for analgosedative therapy in intensive care treatment of head-injured patients. *Acta Neurochir (Wien)* 1996;138(10):1193–9. Erratum in: Acta Neurochir (Wien) 1997;139(12):1193.

40. Filanovsky Y, Miller P, Kao J. Myth: ketamine should not be used as an induction agent for intubation in patients with head injury. *CJEM* 2010;12(2):154–7.

41. Slutsky AS, Ranieri VM. Mechanical ventilation: lessons from the ARDSNet trial. *Respir Res* 2000;1(2):73–7.

42. Neto AS, Simonis FD, Barbas CS, Biehl M, Determann RM, Elmer J, et al. Lung-protective ventilation with low tidal volumes and the occurrence of pulmonary complications in patients without acute respiratory distress syndrome: a systematic review and individual patient data analysis. *Crit Care Med* 2015;43(10):2155–63.

43. Borsellino B, Schultz MJ, Gama de Abreu M, Robba C, Bilotta F. Mechanical ventilation in neurocritical care patients: a systematic literature review. *Expert Rev Respir Med* 2016;10 (10):1123–32.

44. Coles JP, Fryer TD, Coleman MR, Smielewski P, Gupta AK, Minhas PS, et al. Hyperventilation following head injury: effect on ischemic burden and cerebral oxidative metabolism. *Crit Care Med* 2007;35(2):568–78.

45. Grubb RL Jr, Raichle ME, Eichling JO, et al. The effects of changes in PaCO2 on cerebral blood volume, blood flow, and vascular mean transit time. *Stroke* 1974;5:630–9.

46. Serpa Neto A, Filho RR, Cherpanath T, Determann R, Dongelmans DA, Paulus F, et al. Associations between positive end-expiratory pressure and outcome of patients without ARDS at onset of ventilation: a systematic review and meta-analysis of randomized controlled trials. *Ann Intensive Care* 2016;6(1):109.

47. Lovas A, Szakmány T. Haemodynamic effects of lung recruitment manoeuvres. *Biomed Res Int* 2015;2015:478970.

48. Robba C, Bragazzi NL, Bertuccio A, Cardim D, Donnelly J, Sekhon M, et al. Effects of prone position and positive end-expiratory pressure on noninvasive estimators of ICP: a pilot study. *J Neurosurg Anesthesiol* 2016;29.

49. Thelandersson A, Cider A, Nellgård B. Prone position in mechanically ventilated patients with reduced intracranial compliance. *Acta Anaesthesiol Scand* 2006;50(8):937–41.

50. Guérin C, Reignier J, Richard JC, Beuret P, Gacouin A, Boulain T, et al. Prone positioning in severe acute respiratory distress syndrome. *N Engl J Med* 2013;368 (23):2159–68.

51. Ropper AH. Hyperosmolar therapy for raised intracranial pressure. *N Eng J Med* 2012;367(8):746–52.

52. Nath F, Galbraith S. The effect of mannitol on cerebral white matter water content. *J Neurosurg* 1986;65(1):41–3.

53. Bullock R. Mannitol and other diuretics in severe neurotrauma. *New Horiz* 1995;3 (3):448–52.

54. Manninen PH, Lam AM, Gelb AW, Brown SC. The effect of high-dose mannitol on serum and urine electrolytes and osmolality in neurosurgical patients. *Can J Anaesth* 1987;34(5):442–6.

55. Rallis D, Poulos P, Kazantzi M, Chalkias A, Kalampalikis P. Effectiveness of 7.5% hypertonic saline in children with severe traumatic brain injury. *J Crit Care* 2016;38:52–6.

56. Burgess S, Abu-Laban RB, Slavik RS, Vu EN, Zed PJ. A systematic review of randomized controlled trials comparing hypertonic sodium solutions and mannitol for traumatic brain injury: implications for emergency department management. *Ann Pharmacother* 2016;50(4):291–300.

57. Vialet R, Albanèse J, Thomachot L, Antonini F, Bourgouin A, Alliez B, Martin C. Isovolume hypertonic solutes (sodium chloride or mannitol) in the treatment of refractory posttraumatic intracranial hypertension: 2 mL/kg 7.5% saline is more effective than 2 mL/kg 20% mannitol. *Crit Care Med* 2003;31(6):1683–7.

58. Horn P, Münch E, Vajkoczy P, Herrmann P, Quintel M, Schilling L, Schmiedek P, Schürer L. Hypertonic saline solution for control of elevated intracranial pressure in patients with exhausted response to mannitol and barbiturates. *Neurol Res* 1999;21(8):758–64.

59. Qureshi AI, Suarez JI. Use of hypertonic saline solutions in treatment of cerebral edema and intracranial hypertension. *Crit Care Med* 2000;28(9):3301–13.

60. Suehiro E, Fujisawa H, Ito H, Ishikawa T, Maekawa T. Brain temperature modifies glutamate neurotoxicity in vivo. *J Neurotrauma* 1999;16(4):285–97.

61. Kimura A, Sakurada S, Ohkuni H, Todome Y, Kurata K. Moderate hypothermia delays proinflammatory cytokine production of human peripheral blood mononuclear cells. *Crit Care Med* 2002;30(7):1499–502.

62. Clifton GL, Allen S, Barrodale P, Plenger P, Berry J, Koch S, Fletcher J, Hayes RL, Choi SC. A phase II study of moderate hypothermia in severe brain injury. *J Neurotrauma* 1993;10 (3):263–71.

63. Marion DW, Penrod LE, Kelsey SF, Obrist WD, Kochanek PM, Palmer AM, Wisniewski SR, DeKosky ST. Treatment of traumatic brain injury with moderate hypothermia. *N Eng J Med* 1997;336 (8):540–6.

64. Clifton GL, Miller ER, Choi SC, Levin HS, McCauley S, Smith KR Jr, et al. Lack of effect of induction of hypothermia after acute brain injury. *N Engl J Med* 2001;344 (8):556–63.

65. Andrews PJD, Sinclair L, Rodriguez A, Harris BA, Battison CG, Rhodes JKJ, Murray GD. Hypothermia of intracranial hypertension after traumatic brain injury. *N Engl J Med* 2015;373:2403–12.

66. Polderman KH, Ely EW, Badr AE, Girbes AR. Induced hypothermia in traumatic brain injury: considering the conflicting results of meta-analyses and moving forward. *Intensive Care Med* 2004;30(10):1860–4.

67. Polderman KH. Application of therapeutic hypothermia in the ICU: opportunities and pitfalls of a promising treatment modality. Part 1: Indications and evidence. *Intensive Care Med* 2004;30(4):556–75.

68. Cook CJ. Induced hypothermia in neurocritical care: a review. *J Neurosci Nurs* 2017;49(1):5–11.

69. Polderman KH. Mechanisms of action, physiological effects, and complications of hypothermia. *Crit Care Med* 2009;37(7 Suppl):S186–202.

70. Polderman KH, Herold I. Therapeutic hypothermia and controlled normothermia in the intensive care unit: practical considerations, side effects, and

cooling methods. *Crit Care Med* 2009;37 (3):1101–20.

71. Helmy A, Vizcaychipi M, Gupta AK. Traumatic brain injury: intensive care management. *Br J Anaesth* 2007;99 (1):32–42.

72. Shein SL, Ferguson NM, Kochanek PM, Bayir H, Clark RS, Fink EL, et al. Effectiveness of pharmacological therapies for intracranial hypertension in children with severe traumatic brain injury – results from an automated data collection system time-synched to drug administration. *Pediatr Crit Care Med* 2016;17(3):236–45.

73. Goodman JC, Valadka AB, Gopinath SP, Cormio M, Robertson CS. Lactate and excitatory amino acids measured by microdialysis are decreased by pentobarbital coma in head-injured patients. *J Neurotrauma* 1996;13 (10):549–56.

74. Schwartz ML, Tator CH, Rowed DW, Reid SR, Meguro K, Andrews DF. The University of Toronto head injury treatment study: a prospective, randomized comparison of pentobarbital and mannitol. *Can J Neurol Sci* 1984;11 (4):434–40.

75. Roberts I, Sydenham E. Barbiturates for acute traumatic brain injury. *Cochrane Database Syst Rev* 2012;12:CD000033.

76. Bullock MR, Chesnut R, Ghajar J, Gordon D, Hartl R, Newell DW, Servadei F, Walters BC, Wilberger JE. Surgical management of acute subdural hematomas. *Neurosurgery* 2006;58(3 Suppl):S16–24.

77. Bullock MR, Chesnut R, Ghajar J, Gordon D, Hartl R, Newell DW, Servadei F, Walters BC, Wilberger JE. Surgical management of acute epidural hematomas. *Neurosurgery* 2006;58(3 Suppl): S7–15.

78. Bullock MR, Chesnut R, Ghajar J, Gordon D, Hartl R, Newell DW, Servadei F, Walters BC, Wilberger J. Surgical management of traumatic parenchymal lesions.*Neurosurgery* 2006;58 (3 Suppl):S25–46.

79. Mendelow AD, Gregson BA, Rowan EN, Murray GD, Gholkar A, Mitchell PM, STICH II Investigators. Early surgery versus initial conservative treatment in patients with spontaneous supratentorial lobar intracerebral haematomas (STICH II): a randomised trial. *Lancet* 2013;382 (9890):397–408.

80. Gregson BA, Rowan EN, Mitchell PM, Unterberg A, McColl EM, Chambers IR, McNamee P, Mendelow AD. Surgical trial in traumatic intracerebral hemorrhage (STITCH(Trauma)): study protocol for a randomized controlled trial. *Trials* 2012;13:193.

81. Cooper DJ, Rosenfeld JV, Murray L, Arabi YM, Davies AR, D'Urso P, et al. Decompressive craniectomy in diffuse traumatic brain injury. *N Engl J Med* 2011;364(16):1493–502.

82. Hutchinson PJ, Kolias AG, Timofeev IS, Corteen EA, Czosnyka M, Timothy J, et al. Trial of decompressive craniectomy for traumatic intracranial hypertension. *N Engl J Med* 2016;375(12):1119–30.

Therapeutic Options in Neurocritical Care
Beyond the Brain

Aggie Skorko, Matthew J. C. Thomas, Elfyn Thomas and Richard Protheroe

Cardiorespiratory Issues in Patients with a Head Injury

Systemic Complications of Head Injury

It has long been recognised that a neurological injury can elicit profound systemic complications, from Harvey Cushing who in 1903 described strategies to limit fatal haemodynamic dysfunction during surgical CNS surgery to reports of pulmonary oedema post-seizures in 1908.[1]

Studies of patients admitted to intensive care with traumatic brain injury (TBI) showed that up to 89% developed non-neurological organ dysfunction, worsening their outcome.[2,3] Most commonly patients develop sepsis, respiratory or cardiovascular complications with rates of 75%, 41% and 44% respectively in one cohort.[3] Renal and hepatic system involvement is much less common.[4] The presence of hypotension, severe respiratory failure or sepsis has been shown to be independent predictors of death and mortality rates rise from 31%–40% for single organ failure to 47%–91% with two organ system failures and up to 100% in cases with three or more organ system failures.[2,3,5]

The reasons for increased incidence of complications after TBI may be due to systemic effects of the brain injury itself, the presence of other associated injuries or as a complication of treatment. The implications of systemic complications following head injury are increasingly being recognised.

Cardiovascular Complications

Cardiac dysfunction is well documented following subarachnoid haemorrhage and can result in subendocardial changes, regional wall abnormalities and global dysfunction.[1] The mechanism behind this is presumed to be as a result of an acute catecholamine surge related to the primary insult. Conduction abnormalities are near ubiquitous following SAH.[6] Most commonly QRS, ST segment or T-wave abnormalities are demonstrated, but life-threatening arrhythmias such as asystole and ventricular fibrillation also occur in 5% of patients.[4,7,8] ECG abnormalities correlate poorly with presence of cardiac dysfunction, with only 14% of those with myocardial dysfunction exhibited ECG abnormalities in one cohort.[9] Regional wall motion abnormalities post-SAH occur in 8%–28% of patients and are often atypical for coronary artery disease and instead more closely followed the pattern of sympathetic innervation to the myocardium.[1,8] Myocyte damage is likely to be as a result of coronary vasoconstriction in the face of increased sympathetic stimulation and so oxygen demand, leading to subendocardial ischaemia, and if severe enough may lead to pulmonary oedema.[4] Post-mortem studies show a characteristic pattern of myocardial damage with contraction band necrosis and myocytolysis, a pattern that is distinct from that seen in myocardial ischaemia.[4] Pathological findings at autopsy however correlate poorly to echocardiographic findings.[9]

Studies of echocardiograms following TBI show that 22.3%–28% of patients had evidence of myocardial dysfunction.[10,11] The acute echocardiograph and echocardiogram changes are often reversible but may persist for several weeks.[4,7] The phenomenon of neurogenic stunned myocardium has been advocated by some authors, being a triad of transient left ventricular dysfunction, electrocardiogram changes and elevation in cardiac enzymes, to distinguish the catecholamine-driven changes in cardiac function from other causes of acute coronary syndrome.[12] Indirect ventricular dysfunction has also been postulated to occur as catecholamine-driven systemic and pulmonary vasoconstriction occurs such that the ventricles are no longer able to pump effectively against the high vascular resistances.[1] This is proposed as the neuro-haemodynamic mechanism for the development of neurogenic pulmonary oedema.

Neurogenic pulmonary oedema (NPO) has long been recognised as a complication of many neurological insults in 2%–40% of cases but most commonly following SAH where it is recognised in 25%–50% of cases.[1,7,13] It is characterised by dyspnoea, tachypnoea and pink frothy sputum and is associated with generalised sympathetic hyperactivity which includes fever, tachycardia, and hypertension with bilateral infiltrates on imaging.[13] NPO may be self-limiting and resolve within 24 hours but in profound brain injury may be far more persistent. Age, disease severity and time to surgery increase the risk of NPO, and its presence worsens survival.[1] NPO has a bimodal distribution, occurring either immediately or 12–24 hours post-insult.

Several theories as to the development of NPO have been postulated: neuro-cardiac, neuro-haemodynamic, 'blast theory' and pulmonary venule adrenergic hypersensitivity.[1] The neuro-haemodynamic theory has been described above as a possible mechanism of causing pulmonary oedema. The neuro-cardiac hypothesis describes pulmonary oedema developing as a result of neurogenic stunned myocardium.[1] The 'blast theory' postulates that sudden catecholamine-driven systemic and pulmonary hypertension induce direct endothelial damage and the associated permeability defect causes the development of transudative pulmonary oedema.[13] This also explains why the oedema persists after restoration of normal pressures. Finally, it has been suggested that direct injury to the pulmonary vascular bed is caused by profound activation of adrenergic receptors ubiquitous to lung tissue. Animal studies have demonstrated that blockade of the adrenoreceptors may mitigate against the development of pulmonary oedema via this mechanism.[1] Treatment of NPO is mainly supportive using oxygen and mechanical ventilation with positive end expiratory pressure (PEEP), as clinical condition allows. It differs from the treatment of cariogenic pulmonary oedema in that although dobutamine may be beneficial in improving ventricular function, blanket use of diuretics or nitrates may lead to a reduction in blood pressure and potentially in cerebral perfusion.

Neurogenic hypotension as a result of disruption to brain stem pathways complicates 13% of head injury cases, often in those with diffuse axonal injury.[4] This relatively rare diagnosis should be one of exclusion, made after causes such as haemorrhage have been investigated. More commonly a period of hypotension follows the initial hyperdynamic phase following brain injury. This usually responds to fluid resuscitation but may require vasoactive infusions to maintain MAP in refractory cases.[4]

Vasoactive Drugs Following TBI

Vasoactive drugs are frequently used in head-injured patients, most commonly to increase MAP and cerebral perfusion pressure (CPP), but occasionally they are required in patients who develop neurogenic pulmonary oedema, myocardial dysfunction or multiple organ failure where they seem effective at normalising ventricular work and oxygenation.[7] It may seem counter-intuitive to treat the cardiac and respiratory complications of an endogenous catecholamine surge with exogenous sympathomimetics, but it is postulated that the massive levels of endogenous catecholamines decline rapidly and subsequent depletion necessitates exogenous supplementation.[7]

No vasoactive drug can be given without risk of side effects, and all drug that increase blood pressure by vasoconstriction will increase CPP but at the possible expense of cerebral blood flow. Before using vasoactive drugs to augment MAP and CPP in head-injured patients, it is important to ensure that hypovolaemia is excluded, and adequate circulating volume is achieved. The 2016 guidelines from the Brain Trauma Foundation (BTF) recommend a target SBP at ≥100 mm Hg for 50 to 69 years old patients, with a higher goal of ≥110 mm Hg for younger and older patients as potentially leading to better outcomes, with the caveat that aiming for a CPP above 70 mmHg may be harmful. Excess fluid and vasoactive drugs required to achieve a high CPP may themselves increase the incidence of acute respiratory distress syndrome (ARDS).[14]

The commonly used drug infusions in neurosurgical intensive care practice are norepinephrine, epinephrine and dobutamine. All are sympathomimetic agents acting by stimulating naturally occurring adrenoreceptors to exert an effect. Newer therapeutic options are increasingly being introduced.

Epinephrine

Epinephrine is a naturally occurring hormone that acts on α1, β1 and β2 adrenergic receptors. It increases the heart rate and force of cardiac contraction by its β1 effect and increases peripheral vasoconstriction by its α1 effect. The result is an increase in cardiac output (CO), systemic vascular resistance (SVR) and MAP. However, its use is associated with ventricular arrhythmias and the development of lactic acidosis. For this reason, although it reliably increases MAP, it is not usually the first-line drug in intensive care. The use of epinephrine for CPP control has been shown to be an independent risk factor for developing ARDS, although the authors make the point that raising blood pressure by any means increases the risk of ARDS.[15]

Norepinephrine

Norepinephrine is primarily an α1 adrenergic agonist, increasing SVR and MAP with little effect on cardiac contractility. Indeed, by increasing SVR, norepinephrine can worsen cardiac failure. Whilst norepinephrine is the most reliable vasoactive drug for increasing CPP, and is used most commonly in TBI, some authors suggest that it may play a part in worsening multi-organ failure, possibly due to its adverse effects on thrombocytes and leukocytes.[16,17]

Occasionally other α1 agonists are used, particularly the synthetic drug metaraminol since it can be administered peripherally in the short term and has similar effects to norepinephrine. All adrenergic agents show tachyphylaxis requiring increasing doses to achieve the same effect.

Dobutamine

Dobutamine is a synthetic catecholamine that exerts its effect primarily β1 adrenergic receptors, increasing cardiac contractility and heart rate. Peripheral β2 stimulation can also cause vasodilatation with the resulting effect that, whilst dobutamine improves blood flow, it may cause hypotension and tachycardia. Dobutamine is a useful drug in the management of cardiac failure, sepsis and NPO, where it improves myocardial function, but it is less reliable than other drugs at increasing CPP in head-injured patients and therefore is used less frequently for this purpose.[18]

Other Vasoactive Agents

Dopamine, a naturally occurring substance that exerts its effects via α1, β1 and β2 adrenergic receptors as well as specific dopaminergic receptors. It has a similar effect to epinephrine in increasing both CO and SVR with a resultant rise in CPP. However since the SOAP study demonstrated an increase in mortality in patients with sepsis receiving dopamine and evidence of norepinephrine's superiority at delivering more predictable blood pressure control, dopamine's use has waned in European ICUs.[17,19]

Vasopressin, also known as antidiuretic hormone (ADH) or arginine vasopressin (AVP) has a twofold action; increasing free water reabsorption into the circulation from renal tubules and of arterial vasoconstriction. Both of these mechanisms lead to a rise in MAP. The addition of vasopressin to norepinephrine is a technique advocated by some authors, particularly in the setting of sepsis-related hypotension but large-scale studies have failed to demonstrate a definitive benefit from this strategy.[20] Concerns regarding the potential of vasopressin to induce unwanted cerebral ischaemia and cerebral oedema limits its use in brain-injured patients.[4]

Newer drugs to improve cardiac output are of increasing interest.[8] The phosphodiesterase-3 inhibitor Milrinone and myocardial calcium-sensitising Levosimendan are both indodilators that improve contractility, increase heart rate and cause peripheral vasodilatation without increasing myocardial oxygen consumption. So far their use in brain-injured patients has been limited to animal studies and case reports but they may have a role to play in selected individuals with underlying cardiac dysfunction or those developing florid cardiac dysfunction as a complication of their head injury.[21] Their indodilating properties may also have additional neuroprotective benefits on cerebral vasospasm.[22,23]

Given that the common thread underlying the systemic effects in brain-injured patients is the catecholamine surge, interest in the prophylactic inhibition of the autonomic nervous system with α and β antagonists has been proposed as a therapeutic strategy, in patients whose blood pressure will tolerate this.[7] Small-scale studies have examined the effects of exposure to α- and/or β-blocker such as clonidine and propranolol respectively. Such pharmacological targets may reduce the damaging effects of excessive catecholamine and potentially improve survival.[4,7,24] However, at present, robust evidence of such promising effects is lacking.

Respiratory Complications

It is well recognised that pulmonary and particularly infective complications due to altered conscious state, invasive ventilation and reduced airway protective mechanism following brain injury are the most common non-neurological complications in brain-injured patients.[2–4]

Pneumonia

Early onset pneumonia (within 5 days) is the commonest non-neurological complication of brain injury, occurring in 41%–60% of head trauma and is associated with poorer neurological outcomes.[4,25] Typical organisms often implicated are *Staphylococcus aureus*, *Haemophilus influenzae* and *Streptococcus pneumoniae* so empirical treatment whilst awaiting culture and sensitivities should cover against local strains of these pathogens.[4,25] All patients who are comatose following TBI are likely to aspirate substantial quantities of oropharyngeal secretions and these may contain potentially pathogenic commensal organisms. Aspiration pre-intubation, older age, nasal carriage of *S. aureus* and barbiturate use worsen the neurological prognosis.[4,25] Prophylactic antibiotic use was protective against early onset pneumonia.[25] It is interesting to note that interventions commonly used in TBI as part of CPP management increase the risk of pneumonia. Sedative infusions and barbiturates are immunosuppressive and have been shown to increase the incidence of pneumonia, as has the use of induced hypothermia.[25,26]

Since most aspiration occurs before the airway is protected with a cuffed endotracheal tube it can be difficult to prevent early onset pneumonia in head-injured patients. Manoeuvres to reduce further aspiration in patients being mechanically ventilated, including semi-recumbent positioning, selective digestive decontamination, early feeding, subglottic suctioning and the use of low-volume, low-pressure tracheal tube cuffs that stop microaspiration around the cuff but do not cause tracheal necrosis, have all been recommended in this patient population.[4,25,26]

The use of antibiotic prophylaxis to prevent early onset pneumonia remains controversial. Patients who receive antibiotics for other reasons such as open fractures develop less pneumonia.[4,25,26] Despite this, prophylactic antibiotics are not routinely used after head injury as they have not been shown to reduce mortality and they increase the risk of subsequent colonisation with resistant organisms.[4] The updated 2016 BTF guidelines have removed the previous level 2 recommendation for prophylactic antibiotics, due to lack of mortality benefit and instead advocate the adherence to established pneumonia-reducing protocols.[14] The use of selective decontamination of the digestive tract has been reviewed in multiple trials but its implementation remains low due to fear of multi-resistant organisms.[27] Oral decontamination with antibiotics and antiseptics without parenteral drugs has been shown to reduce the risk of pneumonia but failed to demonstrate a mortality benefit.[28]

Acute Respiratory Distress Syndrome (ARDS)

The 2012 Berlin definition of Acute Respiratory Distress Syndrome (ARDS) describes a clinical syndrome of acute onset bilateral opacities on chest imaging, not fully explained by cardiac failure or fluid overload with hypoxia despite the application of positive end expired pressure (PEEP). ARDS is further stratified into three categories depending on the degree of hypoxia: mild (PaO_2/FiO_2 ratio of 300–200 mmHg), moderate (PaO_2/FiO_2 ratio of 200–100 mmHg) and severe (PaO_2/FiO_2 ratio less than 100 mmHg).[29] This definition has replaced the 1994 American European Consensus Conference definition of acute lung injury (ALI) and ARDS.

Rates of ARDS post-TBI are estimated to be 20%–30% and confer a mortality of up to 40%.[2,13] ARDS may develop as a result of the initial insult with 48 hours of admission or in the weeks following as a result of nosocomial insults such as pneumonia, vasoactive drug infusion or as part of a systemic inflammatory response picture.[4] Multivariate analyses have identified severity of injury and administration of dopamine and norepinephrine as risk factors for developing ARDS post-TBI and suggest that aggressive CPP-targeted therapy, rather than ICP-targeted, is associated with higher rates of ARDS.[4,15]

The outcomes of patients with ARDS is improved if a lung protective ventilation strategy is used.[13] This includes the use of low tidal volumes and low inspiratory pressures combined with the use of high levels of PEEP to maintain oxygenation, and permissive hypercarbia. The latter and other aspects of current ARDS management such as fluid restriction are at odds with CPP/ICP management goals in head-injured patients where normocarbia and adequate volume status are of vital importance.[4] Techniques to improve oxygenation such as PEEP up to 12 cmH$_2$0 do not affect ICP and in fact decrease it by improving cerebral oxygenation provided an adequate fluid status is maintained.[4] The use of prone position ventilation is controversial, with conflicting reports as to whether the beneficial impact of improvement in PaO$_2$/FiO$_2$ ratio overcomes the deleterious increase in IC.[3,30] Evidence is emerging that aggressive ventilation with the use of high driving pressures may be a risk factor for the development of ARDS in TBI patients, in a 'double hit phenomenon' where lungs damaged by the catecholamine surge are further injured by high-pressure ventilation.[31] Given the conflicting evidence as to the optimal ventilatory strategy for brain-injured patients, close physiological monitoring of ventilated patients is warranted.[3]

Ventilatory strategies aiming to provide low pressure whilst allowing effective oxygenation and carbon dioxide removal include the use of high-frequency oscillatory ventilation (HFOV), extra-corporeal carbon dioxide removal and extra-corporeal membrane oxygenation (ECMO). Since the publication of the OSCAR trial which failed to demonstrate a survival benefit from the use of HFOV this mode of ventilation has largely fallen out of favour, and no evidence exists of its benefit in TBI patients.[32] Extra-corporeal carbon dioxide removal has the advantage over ECMO in that it does not require the same degree of systemic anticoagulation, a major drawback to its use in the vast majority of brain-injured patients. The use of non-anticoagulated ECMO circuits in high-risk patients has been published and this technique may continue to develop.[33] Better evidence is emerging as to the safety and efficacy of extra-corporeal carbon dioxide removal and this may prove to be a useful adjunct to the management of brain-injured patients.[13,34] However, at present the impact on survival of extra-corporeal techniques cannot be appraised.

The conflicting therapeutic requirements of maintaining CPP and lowering ICP versus those required to manage concomitant systemic organ dysfunction remain the most challenging aspect of the intensive care management of patients with TBI and must be weighed on an individual patient basis.

Venous Thromboembolism

Thromboprophylaxis is effective and has been repeatedly shown to reduce the risk of deep vein thrombosis (DVT), pulmonary embolism (PE) and fatal PE which is the most common cause of preventable hospital death. There is grade 1 evidence that DVT prophylaxis with low molecular weight heparin improves outcome in the general intensive care population. In cases of TBI up to 54% of patients may develop DVT if not treated with thromboprophylaxis, and in 25% of those treated only with sequential compression devices.[14] Predictors for DVT include age, subarachnoid haemorrhage, injury severity score of >15 and increasing severity of injury.[14]

It is important to acknowledge that the recommendations for treatment for patients following trauma and head injury are different to those undergoing elective neurosurgery.

The latter should be managed using intermittent pneumatic compression (grade 1A recommendation) with additional pharmacological prophylaxis in those at particularly high risk (grade 2A).[35] The increased risk of thrombosis post-trauma has historically led to a recommendations of LMWH when it is safe to do so.[35] However a Cochrane review in 2013 found a paucity of literature to enable a subgroup analysis of brain-injured trauma patients, but concluded that in the overall trauma population the use of LMWH reduced rates of DVT with no reduction in PE rates or mortality benefit.[36] Subsequently, the 2016 BTF guidelines have downgraded the use of pharmacological prophylaxis in combination with mechanical prophylaxis to grade 3 evidence, accepting that there is an increase in the risk of intracranial haemorrhage and so a risk/benefit balance must be struck.[14] The use of compression stockings is supported by this guideline being as they are considered a general standard of care in hospitalised non-mobile individuals and despite there being no body of evidence specific to brain injury in this regard.

Tracheostomy in Head Injury

Tracheostomy is a procedure undertaken commonly in the ICU, with up to a third of patients requiring long-term mechanical ventilation having a tracheostomy worldwide.[37] This is not surprising considering many intensivists believe that tracheostomy facilitates nursing care, improves comfort and mobility, allows speech and oral nutrition and speeds weaning from mechanical ventilation.[37] Many patients with a head injury will undergo tracheostomy, occasionally because they require prolonged mechanical ventilation, but more commonly as a means of securing the airway, allowing pulmonary toilet and preventing aspiration in patients who breathe spontaneously and adequately but who continue to have a reduced level of consciousness, poor bulbar function or associated facial trauma.

Percutaneous dilatation technique (PDT) has become the technique of choice in the UK, with two thirds of tracheostomies performed in this manner.[38] The procedure can be performed rapidly on the ICU, as safely as open surgical tracheostomy, without the need for surgical staff or a transfer to an operating theatre. Various meta-analysis show that although PDT may be associated with more early complications it does however lead to reduced rates of stoma site infections and scarring when compared to open surgical techniques.[39,40] It should be remembered that PDT is a semi-elective procedure and not an emergency one and should only be undertaken when the patient is stable. Although relatively safe, PDT is not a risk-free procedure, causing periods of hypoventilation, hypercarbia and occasionally hypoxaemia potentially leading to a rise in ICP and fall in CPP.[41] However surgical tracheostomy may also lead to periods of depressed cerebral perfusion.[41] When PDT is undertaken with bronchoscopic guidance, the hypercarbia may be more pronounced and the potential for cerebral ischaemia potentially more significant. Bronchoscopy should therefore be used for as short a time as possible to confirm correct position of the needle, guidewire and tube, and meticulous care should be taken to maintain MAP and CPP during the procedure.[42] On current evidence there is little to suggest that one technique of PDT is superior to another in terms of early complications, but the guide wire dilator technique may be associated with a higher risk of bleeding.[43]

Concern has been raised about the incidence of long-term complications such as tracheal stenosis following PDT and that stenosis may occur at a higher level and be more difficult to treat.[44] Most follow-up studies so far have shown rates of asymptomatic stenosis in the order of 10% and authors feel that long-term follow-up is unwarranted.[45,46] Patients with brain injuries who have undergone tracheostomy because of prolonged coma are considered by some to have a worse prognosis, but an observational study of 277 brain-injured patients showed that whilst prolonged coma was associated with poor outcome, tracheostomy *per se* was not.[47] Furthermore, less than 10% of patients continue to require tracheostomy after 3 months and 66% of patients who have undergone tracheostomy were discharged from hospital and able to return to their previous vocation.[47]

Early tracheostomy had been proposed as a strategy to decrease the incidence of pneumonia, shorten the duration of mechanical ventilation and reduce the length of ICU stay but this has not been definitively borne out in the published literature.[14,37,48] The TracMan study, a large multi-centre UK trial that recruited 909 mechanically ventilated patients, hoped to answer whether early tracheostomy is of benefit but failed to demonstrate that a tracheostomy at day 4 was associated with a survival benefit.[37] A subsequent meta-analysis focusing on tracheostomy timing in brain-injured patients demonstrated a reduction in mechanical ventilation by 2.7 days and length of ICU stay by 2.5 days in those who received a tracheostomy within 10 days of admission, but again did not demonstrate a clear impact on mortality.[49]

The latest BTF guidelines make a level 2A recommendation that early tracheostomy be undertaken when the benefits outweigh the risk of the procedure itself, with the aim of reducing the duration of mechanical ventilation.[14] The guideline authors acknowledge that early tracheostomy has no impact on mortality or rates of nosocomial pneumonia. Many aspects of tracheostomy management remain unresolved in intensive care practice and decisions regarding the indications and timing will continue to be made on an individual patient basis.

Nutrition in Brain Injury

Patients with severe brain injury have altered metabolic homeostasis, resulting in increased energy expenditure and increased protein catabolism. In the early 1980s, several studies were conducted to assess the metabolic effect of severe head injury compared to patients without TBI.[50–52] Hypermetabolism and nitrogen wasting were well documented, and early feeding was found to reduce the mortality rate. The observed depletion of muscle mass and depressed immuno-function was reported to increase complication rates and worsen long-term outcome. One suggested preventive approach is to provide nutrition in accordance with the accelerated metabolism, but evidence-based guidelines in this respect are lacking.[53–56]

A systematic Cochrane review in 2008 based on 11 RCTs concluded that early feeding may be associated with a trend towards better outcomes in terms of survival and disability.[57] A further review in 2013 found early feeding was associated with better neurological outcomes.[58] The 2016 fourth edition BTF guidelines conducted its own literature analysis and based on the current evidence make a level II A recommendation that TBI patients should feed to attain basal caloric replacement at least by the fifth day and at most by the seventh day post-injury to decrease mortality.[54]

Tight glycaemic control has not been shown to significantly improve outcome in TBI and appears to be associated with an increased incidence of hypoglycaemic episodes. The fourth BTF guidelines concluded there was insufficient evidence to make any recommendations with regard to tight glycaemic control.[54]

Nitrogen balance is usually defined as the difference between nitrogen intake and nitrogen excretion. For each gram of nitrogen measured in urine, 6.25 g of protein is catabolised. Optimal protein use has been found to be heavily dependent on the adequacy of caloric intake. After severe brain injury, energy requirements rise and nitrogen excretion increases. In severely brain-injured patients, nitrogen catabolism is 14–25 g N/d and the average nitrogen loss of a fasting head-injured patient is double or triple that of a normal patient. This loss will produce a 10% decrease in lean mass in 7 d, and underfeeding for 2–3 weeks could result in a 30% weight loss, which is potentially deleterious.[59,60]

Data suggest that, at a high range of nitrogen intake (>17 g/d), less than 50% of administered nitrogen is retained after head injury. Therefore, the level of nitrogen intake that generally results in less than 10 g of nitrogen loss per day is 15 to 17 g N/d, or 0.3 to 0.5 g N/kg/d. This value is about 20% of the caloric composition of a 50 kcal/kg/d feeding protocol (2 g protein/kg/d). Twenty per cent is the maximal protein content and amino-acid content of most enteral and parenteral formulations, respectively, in a hypermetabolic patient. Nitrogen equilibrium is seldom achieved; however, increasing the nitrogen content of feeding from 14% to 20% does result in improved nitrogen retention. Thus, the survival rate is better when an increased protein diet is begun within 1–10 days of injury versus the same diet administered more gradually or after a longer period.[60–62]

There is inconclusive data on the benefits of immune enhancing diets or vitamins and supplements to make any recommendations.[54]

Enteral feeding via the nasogastric route (after exclusion of base of skull fracture) is preferred in intensive care settings. The advantages of enteral nutrition are less risk of hyperglycaemia, lower risk of infection and reduced cost. Increased intracranial pressure and the severity of the brain injury may affect the ability to begin enteral feeding. This delay in feeding has been attributed to increased gastric residuals, delay in gastric emptying, prolonged paralytic ileus, abdominal distention, aspiration pneumonitis and diarrhoea.[63–65] Upper gastrointestinal dysfunction is common after severe TBI with a reported frequency ranging from 44% to 100%. The initiation and absorption of enteral feeds in the clinical setting are determined by measurements of gastric residual volume along with other clinical signs of impairment. The reported criteria of gastrointestinal intolerance used in the nutritional protocols varied between studies, most studies recommending a residual volume below 200 ml and checking every 2–8 hours or a total amount residual volumes per day of 500–700 ml. In such circumstances, supplementary partial or total parenteral nutrition may be required.[66,67] Some investigators believe that early parenteral-nutritional support improves the outcome after head injury. Other studies have shown that the mode of administration has no effect on neurologic outcome and either parenteral or enteral support is equally effective when prescribed according to individually measured energy expenditure and nitrogen excretion. The BTF make a level IIB recommendation to use transgastric jejunal feeding (to reduce the incidence of ventilator associated pneumonia).[54]

There are several options available to administer longer term enteral support beyond the nasogastric/jejunal route. Percutaneous endoscopic gastrotomy or jejunostomy tube is the usual; however, percutaneous gastrojejunostomy tubes are gaining favour.[65,68–69]

Nutrition – Conclusion

Current recommendations for nutritional support in severe head injury include a high-protein diet (2 g/kg/d, or about 15% of the total calorie value), which helps with nitrogen retention. Enteral feeding is the preferred mode of nutritional support, but data suggest that both parenteral and enteral modes are equally effective. Initiation of early feeding within the first 24 hours of head injury and attainment of 'full feed' no later than day 7 seems to reduce the relative risk of morbidity and mortality.

Fluid Balance in TBI

Fluid, electrolyte and metabolic consequences of severe head injury are profound. The goal of fluid management is homeostasis, that is to provide appropriate parenteral and/or enteral fluid to maintain intravascular volume, left ventricular filling pressure, cardiac output, blood pressure and ultimately oxygen delivery (DO_2) to tissues, when normal physiological functions are often altered by surgical and traumatic stress and by anaesthetic agents. A specific aim is to prevent secondary neuronal damage due to inadequate oxygen delivery to the brain; this requires adequate ventilation and oxygenation as well as cardiac output.

Effects of Intravenous Fluids on the Brain

Historically, fluid restriction has been the buzzword of head injury management due to inherent fears about the possibilities of development of cerebral oedema due to damage of the blood-brain barrier and alteration of cerebral auto-regulation. The reduction of oedema formation has been the mainstay of the 'Lund protocol' of head injury management with its emphasis on reduction of capillary hydrostatic pressure by reducing MAP, cerebral blood volumes and negative fluid balance by use of diuretics.[70,71] Clifton's work looked at critical factors associated with poor outcomes as a post-hoc analysis of the NABISH study. It found that fluid balance less than −594 ml in a 24 hour period exerted significant poorer outcome.[72] Step-wise logistic regression showed effects of negative fluid balance were similar to GCS at admission when looking at outcome measures. There are few data apart from the Lund protocol to support dehydration in brain injuries. Maintenance of euvolaemia may avoid predisposition to problems with elevated ICPs, but there is no good evidence supporting fluid restriction as a means of limiting cerebral oedema after brain injury. Dehydration increases sympathetic stimulation, metabolism and O_2 demand.

Extremes of hydration may be necessary to maintain plasma volume in conditions where capillaries are leaky such as the systemic inflammatory response (SIRS) but this strategy is not without pitfalls. The administration of large volumes of fluid may be associated with other medical complications, that is pulmonary oedema, and the therapeutic aim recommended by the BTF is to maintain euvolaemia and normal physiological indices.[54]

Hypernatraemia in TBI

Abnormal homeostasis with impairment of sodium regulation is one of the most common and significant abnormalities following TBI. Hypernatraemia is defined as plasma sodium greater than 145 mmol/L. It is always associated with hyperosmolality and may be caused by water depletion, excessive administration of sodium salts or both. Hypernatraemia has been shown to be an independent predictor of early mortality in all classes of TBI.[73]

Thirst mechanisms are absent in (unintubated) brain-injured patients leading to water-depleted states (renal, enteral and insensible). Excessive administration of sodium salts may cause hypernatraemia through therapeutic misadventure or over-zealous administration of sodium in isotonic or hypertonic intravenous fluids.[74–77] Head-injured patients may have diabetes insipidus because of pituitary or hypothalamic dysfunction causing hypernatraemia. Increased insensible loss from central fever is also a contributing factor. In patients with raised intracranial pressure, hypernatraemia frequently results from the therapeutic use of osmotic diuretics (mannitol or hypertonic saline) and is an independent predictor of mortality when the peak serum sodium exceeded 160 mmol/L. Other causes of polyuria include use of iodinated contrast-medium, severe hyperglycaemia and fluid overload.

Central diabetes insipidus (DI) due to brain injury leads to complete or partial failure of anti diuetetic hormone (ADH) secretion. A very early onset is characteristic of major hypothalamic damage and is associated with a high mortality. Head-injured patients with fractures involving the base of the skull and sella turcica appear to be at increased risk of DI. The time of onset is variable, but it usually appears after 5–10 days.[78–79] In most cases, onset is characterised by polyuria, hypernatraemia and plasma hyperosmolality, sometimes as early as 12–24 hours after injury. If the damage is limited to the pituitary or lower pituitary stalk, the DI may only be transient, and this is usually the case. High stalk lesions or injury to the hypothalamus usually cause permanent DI. Pituitary dysfunction has been reported to occur in up to 37.5%, 57.1% and 59.3% in the patients with mild, moderate and severe TBI, respectively.[80]

Diagnosis of hypernatraemia is made by measuring paired serum and urinary osmolalities. Normal concentration of urine (urine osmolality > 700 mosmol/L) suggests insufficient water intake, with or without excessive extra-renal water loss. Urine osmolality between 700 mosmol/L and plasma osmolality suggests partial central DI, osmotic diuresis, diuretic therapy, nephrogenic DI or renal failure. A urine osmolality below that of plasma suggests either complete central DI or nephrogenic DI. In milder cases urine osmolality may not be below that of plasma, and may be 300–600 mosmol/L. Patients with central DI remain sensitive to exogenous ADH. Patients with partial DI have urinary volumes much less than those with complete DI. In contrast to DI, a solute diuresis is usually accompanied by a higher urinary osmolality (between 250 and 320 mosmol/L).[81]

Treatment of Hypernatraemia

A correction rate of hypernatraemia of about 10–12 mmol/L/d is recommended to avoid rebound cerebral oedema. Hypernatraemia leads to increased plasma osmolarity that leads to shrinkage of brain cells due to loss of water. With prolonged high plasma osmolarity, brain cells accumulate organic osmolytes such as polyols (e.g. sorbitol and myo-inositol), amino acids (e.g. alanine, glutamine, glutamate, taurine) and methylamines (e.g. glyceryl-phosphorylcholine and betaine). Rapid correction of chronic hypernatraemia can lead to shift of water into the hyperosmolar brain cells and thus exacerbate cerebral oedema.

Pure water depletion is treated by water administration (NG route or intravenous fluids 5% dextrose). The rate of increase in osmolality should be no greater than 2 mosmol/kg/h. Hypernatraemia due to excess sodium, is treated by water/dextrose and diuretic administration.[82,83]

1 Replace free water deficit:

Free H_2O deficit (litres) $= 0.6 * $ (body weight [kg]) $ * $ ([Na+/140] $- 1$)

2 Parenteral replacement of half of deficit immediately; rest over 24–36 hours. Use 5% dextrose, *not* saline solutions

3 Calculate maintenance fluid requirements and hourly urine output and replace with 5% dextrose

4   Aqueous vasopressin (AVP): if urine output remains excessive (>200–250 ml/h) in the absence of diuretics, or if maintenance of fluid balance is difficult or hyperosmolality is present, give 5–10 U s.c. or i.m.

5   Desmopressin (DDAVP) synthetic analogue of AVP with longer half-life and fewer vasoconstrictive effects: 1–2 μg s.c. or i.v. every 12–24 hours or by nasal insufflation of 5–20 μg every 12 hours

Hyponatraemia in TBI

Hyponatraemia (plasma Na+ < 135 mmol/L) is seen in 5%–12% of patients with severe head injury. Significant hyponatraemia (<120 meq) can cause significant and permanent neurologic injury and death. Hyponatraemia may be isotonic, hypertonic or hypotonic, based on the measured plasma osmolality. The risk of hyponatraemia seems greater in those with severe head injuries, chronic subdural haematoma and basal skull fracture. Deterioration in levels of consciousness, new focal deficits, myoclonus, seizures or increasing ICP could indicate possibility of hyponatraemia in the patient with a severe brain injury.[84,85]

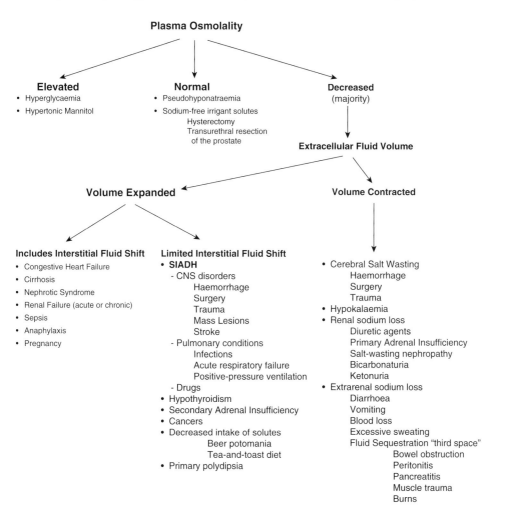

Hypertonic Hyponatraemia

Hyperglycaemia is common after brain injuries and mannitol use is frequently used to treat increased intracranial pressure. In patients with an increased amount of an impermeant solute, such as glucose or mannitol, osmotic equilibration occurs by water shifting from the ICF to the ECF, thus diluting the ECF sodium. In such circumstances, hyponatraemia is often associated with an elevated measured osmolality.[86]

The corrected sodium value is derived from the formula

Corrected Na value = measured plasma Na+ 0.288 * (plasma glucose value in mmol/ L – 5.6)

Hypotonic Hyponatraemia

Hyponatraemia may be due to excessive infusion of hypotonic intravenous fluids such as 5% dextrose, 0.45% saline, particularly when administered rapidly or in the presence of high circulating ADH levels. Less water is needed to produce hyponatraemia in brain injuries where there is an increase in stimulation of ADH by hypovolaemia, hypotension, pain, nausea or postoperative stress. Low plasma osmolality causes osmotic pressure gradient across the brain cell membranes resulting in water entering the brain leading to cellular swelling which may lead to contusional expansion, diffuse axonal injury and herniation due to limited space. Hyponatraemic encephalopathy and cerebral oedema may eventually occur; many changes in brain architecture are irreversible and therefore prevention is the key. See Figure 14.1.

Normally the brain partially adapts to the hypo-osmolality within 24 hours, reducing the cerebral water excess by losing or inactivating intracellular osmotically active solutes. However in brain-injured patients this re-adaption may take more time (5–7 days).[87]

Syndrome of Inappropriate Antidiuresis (SIADH)

This syndrome is defined as hypotonic hyponatraemia due to an elevated level of ADH non-commensurate with the prevailing osmotic or volume stimuli. ADH secretion from the neurohypophysis is no longer under normal regulatory influences. SIADH is a form of dilutional hyponatraemia; ECF volume is usually increased by 3–4 litres, but interstitial shifts do not occur and peripheral oedema is not seen due to unknown reasons. Because of the expanded ECF volume, it is hypothesised that glomerular filtration rate is increased and the renin–angiotensin–aldosterone mechanism is suppressed, resulting in a decrease in the renal reabsorption of sodium.[84]

Cerebral Salt Wasting Syndrome (CSW)

The term cerebral salt wasting was introduced in 1950,[88] although many subsequent authors have considered the existence of a condition of CSW to be dubious.[84,89] It is described in medical literature in the form of case series and anecdotal reports. CSW may be caused by a defect in direct neural regulation of renal tubular activity in the presence of intact hypothalamic-pituitary-adrenal axis. Patients were also noted to be hypovolaemic as compared to euvolaemic or hypervolaemic. Cerebral infarction may occur in patients who are fluid restricted due to hyponatraemia. The mechanism by which intracranial disease leads to

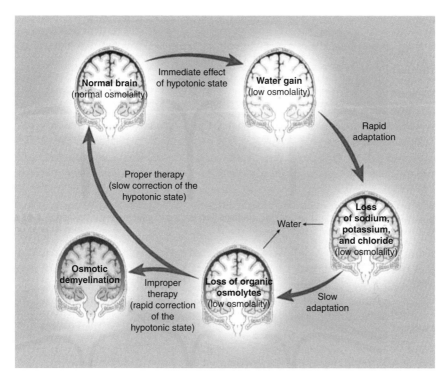

Figure 14.1 Effects of hyponatraemia on the brain. Minutes after the development of hyponatraemia, the decreased osmolality causes swelling of the brain. Rapid adaption occurs within hours as a result of the cellular loss of electrolytes. Slow adaption occurs over several days through the loss of organic osmolytes from brain cells to normalise brain volume. Aggressive correction of hyponatraemia may lead to irreversible brain damage (osmotic demyelination); however, proper correction of hyponatraemia re-establishes normal osmolality without the risk of brain damage. From Adrogue HJ, Madias NE: Hyponatraemia. *N Engl J Med* 2000;342:1581–9; reprinted with permission.

CSW is not well understood. Many physicians have postulated that the most probable process involves the disruption of neural input into the kidney and/or the central elaboration of a circulating natriuretic factor.[90,91] Decreased sympathetic input to the kidney directly and indirectly alters salt and water management and may explain the natriuresis and diuresis seen within CSW. A decrease in sympathetic tone leads to a decreased glomerular filtration rate, a decreased renin release and a decreased renal tubular sodium resorption. In addition to a decreased neural input to the kidney, an ouabain-like compound in the brain may play a role in renal salt wasting though studies have shown that they may not be the sole intermediary of CSW. Circulating ANP and BNP could contribute to the picture and other mediators producing natriuresis are being investigated for their role in CSW.

Diagnosis of Hyponatraemia

The evaluation of hyponatraemia with hypo-osmolality requires clinical assessment of volume status and measurement of urinary indices. However, volume status can be difficult to assess clinically in a critically ill patient. Fall in body weight, large negative fluid balance, decrease in skin turgor and increase of urea/creatinine ratio > 20:1 may reflect fluid depletion. However, ECF volume may be affected by blood loss, the amount and type of fluid administered and the use of diuretics. Urinary Na+ measurements are affected by the use of osmotic and non-osmotic diuretics. When making the diagnosis of SIADH, it is essential to exclude other causes of hyponatraemia that commonly occur in neurological diseases such as oedematous states, recent diuretic therapy, and hypovolaemic states. Moreover, the diagnosis of SIADH cannot be made in the presence of severe pain, nausea, stress or hypotension, because these conditions can stimulate ADH secretion even in the presence of serum hypotonicity. All the changes in electrolyte imbalances observed in SIADH have also been described in CSW; however, the presence of signs of volume depletion (e.g. decreased skin turgor, or low central venous pressure) with salt wasting distinguishes CSW from SIADH. In essence, the primary distinction between SIADH and CSW lies in the clinical assessment of the ECV. SIADH is an expanded state of ECV due to an ADH-mediated renal water retention, whereas CSW is characterised by a contracted state of ECV due to renal salt wasting. Additional laboratory evidence that relates to the ECV may also help distinguish SIADH from CSW. These include haemoconcentration, albumin concentration, blood urea nitrogen/creatinine ratio, potassium concentration, plasma renin, aldosterone levels, atrial natriuretic factor, plasma urea concentration and central venous pressure.[92–94]

Criteria for Diagnosing the Syndrome of Inappropriate Secretion of Antidiuretic Hormone (SIADH)

- Hypotonic hyponatraemia
- Urine osmolality greater than plasma osmolality
- Urine sodium excretion greater than 20 mmol/l
- Normal renal, hepatic, cardiac, pituitary, adrenal and thyroid function
- Absence of hypotension, hypovolaemia, oedema and drugs that can stimulate

ADH release

- Correction by water restriction

Management of SIADH

Management of hyponatraemia is dependent on documentation of its presence and assessment of severity of symptoms (acute, chronic) and determination of most appropriate treatment strategy based on volume status:

- Fluid restrict to 500 ml/d or less if possible
- Hypertonic saline 1.8%–3% (50–70 mmol/h)
- Diuresis of 160 ml/h or greater
- Rate of correction: no greater than 8–12 mmol/L/d
- Seizures: 100–250 mmol hypertonic saline over 10 min

The rate of correction of acute hyponatraemia should be no greater than 1–2 mmol/L/hr of sodium until the plasma level has increased to 120 mmol/L or by a maximum of 8–12 mmol/L during the first 24 hours. This is achieved initially by intravenous administration of hypertonic saline given at 50–70 ml/h. It is important to note that the purpose of using hypertonic saline is not to correct a saline deficit, since there is no deficiency, but rather the hypertonic saline draws water into the intravascular compartment and reduces brain oedema. A spontaneous or frusemide-induced diuresis (e.g. by 20–40 mg intravenously) is then required to excrete the water excess.

If the hyponatraemia presents with convulsions, then urgent correction of the cerebral oedema using 250 mmol of hypertonic sodium chloride over 10 minutes (equivalent to 500 ml of 20% mannitol) has been used. This will immediately elevate the plasma sodium in adults by about 7 mmol.

If fluid deprivation is difficult to sustain in patients with SIADH, then patients with hyponatraemia and chronic CCF may benefit from an ACE inhibitor added to furosemide. This will inhibit the stimulation of thirst and ADH release by angiotensin II. However, in these patients a direct ADH inhibitor such as phenytoin may be of greater value. Pharmacologic treatment has been tried with demeclocycline which inhibits ADH action on renal tubules and increases excretion of solute-free urine but is slow and associated with nephrotoxicity. Lithium has been considered but is associated with numerous side effects.

Tolvaptan a V2 receptor antagonist acts by stimulating free water excretion and has been shown to improve plasma sodium concentration. The SALT-1 and SALT-2 trails excluded TBI patients from the studies. Its role in the management of TBI associated hyponatraemia is yet to be defined; however, there are case reports describing its safe use in brain-injured patients.[95–97]

Management of CSW

The objectives of treatment of CSW are volume replacement and maintenance of positive salt balance. Intravenous hydration with normal saline hypertonic saline or oral salt may be used alone or in combination. A cautious approach is to raise it by 0.5–1 mmol/L/hr for a maximum total daily change not exceeding 12 mmol/L. Management aims primarily at repletion of plasma volume. It should be kept in mind that signs of volume depletion may be masked by the high catecholamine state of the patient. Volume restriction (as for SIADH) is definitely contraindicated. The hypotonic state should be treated with additional sodium, often requiring the administration of hypertonic saline. The concomitant administration of furosemide and saline is rarely adequate.[84,85,87,90]

Increasing salt intake during CSW enhances salt excretion as well and therefore, use of fludrocortisone to enhance renal tubular sodium reabsorption would be beneficial. However, fludrocortisone is strongly associated with pulmonary oedema, hypokalaemia and hypertension.

Complications of Treatment of Hyponatraemia

The complications reported with the use of hypertonic saline include congestive cardiac failure and cerebral haemorrhage – intracerebral and subdural, presumed due to tearing of bridging veins. Rapid correction of hyponatraemia may lead to central pontine and extrapontine myelinolysis. The lesions of central pontine myelinolysis (CPM) are caused by the destruction of myelin sheaths in the centre of the basilar portion of the pons and may extend from the midbrain to the lower pons. The clinical features range from coma, flaccid quadriplegia, facial weakness and pseudobulbar palsy to minor behavioural changes without focal findings. The onset may be from one to several days after the hyponatraemia has been corrected and may require MRI to confirm the diagnosis.[97]

References

1.   Davison DL, Terek M, Chawla LS. Neurogenic pulmonary edema. *Crit Care* 2012;16(2):212.

2.   Zygun D. Non-neurological organ dysfunction in neurocritical care: impact on outcome and etiological considerations. *Curr Opin Crit Care* 2005;11(2):139–43.

3.   Corral L, Javierre CF, Ventura JL, Marcos P, Herrero JI, Mañez R. Impact of non-neurological complications in severe traumatic brain injury outcome. *Crit Care* 2012;16(2):R44.

4.   Lim HB, Smith M. Systemic complications after head injury: a clinical review. *Anaesthesia* 2007;62(5):474–82.

5.   Zygun DA, Kortbeek JB, Fick GH, Laupland KB, Doig CJ. Non-neurologic organ dysfunction in severe traumatic brain injury. *Crit Care Med* 2005;33(3):654–60.

6.   Brouwers PJ, Wijdicks EF, Hasan D, Vermeulen M, Wever EF, Frericks H, et al. Serial electrocardiographic recording in aneurysmal subarachnoid hemorrhage. *Stroke* 1989;20(9):1162–7.

7.   Macmillan C, Grant I, Andrews P. Pulmonary and cardiac sequelae of subarachnoid haemorrhage: time for active management? *Intens Care Med* 2002;28(8):1012–23.

8.   Bruder N, Rabinstein A. Cardiovascular and pulmonary complications of aneurysmal subarachnoid hemorrhage. *Neurocrit Care* 2011;15(2):257.

9.   Dujardin KS, McCully RB, Wijdicks EFM, Tazelaar HD, Seward JB, McGregor CGA, et al. Myocardial dysfunction associated with brain death: clinical, echocardiographic, and pathologic features. *J Heart Lung Transpl* 2001;20(3):350–7.

10. Prathep S, Sharma D, Hallman M, Joffe A, Krishnamoorthy V, Mackensen GB, et al. Preliminary report on cardiac dysfunction after isolated traumatic brain injury. *Crit Care Med* 2014;42(1):10.1097/CCM.0b013e318298a890.

11. Hasanin A, Kamal A, Amin S, Zakaria D, El Sayed R, Mahmoud K, et al. Incidence and outcome of cardiac injury in patients with severe head trauma. *Scand J Trauma Resuscitation Emerg Med* 2016;24:58.

12. Biso S, Wongrakpanich S, Agrawal A, Yadlapati S, Kishlyansky M, Figueredo V. A review of neurogenic stunned myocardium. *Cardiovasc Psychiatr Neurol* 2017;2017:5842182.

13. Hu PJ, Pittet JF, Kerby JD, Bosarge PL, Wagener BM. Acute brain trauma, lung injury, and pneumonia: more than just altered mental status and decreased airway protection. *Am J Physiol Lung Cell Molecul Physiol* 2017;313(1):L1–l15.

14. Carney N, Totten AM, O'Reilly C, Ullman JS, Hawryluk GW, Bell MJ, et al. Guidelines for the management of severe traumatic brain injury, fourth edition. *Neurosurgery* 2017;80(1):6–15.

15. Contant CF, Valadka AB, Gopinath SP, Hannay HJ, Robertson CS. Adult respiratory distress syndrome: a complication of induced hypertension after severe head injury. *J Neurosurg* 2001;95(4):560–8.

16. Stover JF, Steiger P, Stocker R. Controversial issues concerning norepinephrine and intensive care following severe traumatic brain injury. *Eur J Trauma* 2006;32(1):10–27.

17. Steiner LA, Johnston AJ, Czosnyka M, Chatfield DA, Salvador R, Coles JP, et al.

Direct comparison of cerebrovascular effects of norepinephrine and dopamine in head-injured patients. *Crit Care Med* 2004;32(4):1049–54.

18. Deehan SC, Grant IS. Haemodynamic changes in neurogenic pulmonary oedema: effect of dobutamine. *Intens Care Med* 1996;22(7):672–6.

19. Sakr Y, Reinhart K, Vincent J-L, Sprung CL, Moreno R, Ranieri VM, et al. Does dopamine administration in shock influence outcome? Results of the Sepsis Occurrence in Acutely Ill Patients (SOAP) study. *Crit Care Med* 2006;34(3):589–97.

20. Gordon AC, Mason AJ, Thirunavukkarasu N, et al. Effect of early vasopressin vs norepinephrine on kidney failure in patients with septic shock: the vanish randomized clinical trial. *JAMA* 2016;316(5):509–18.

21. Mrozek S, Srairi M, Marhar F, Delmas C, Gaussiat F, Abaziou T, et al. Successful treatment of inverted Takotsubo cardiomyopathy after severe traumatic brain injury with milrinone after dobutamine failure. *Heart Lung* 2016;45 (5):406–8.

22. Farmakis D, Alvarez J, Gal TB, Brito D, Fedele F, Fonseca C, et al. Levosimendan beyond inotropy and acute heart failure: evidence of pleiotropic effects on the heart and other organs: An expert panel position paper. *Int J Cardiol* 2016;222:303–12.

23. Romero CM, Morales D, Reccius A, Mena F, Prieto J, Bustos P, et al. Milrinone as a rescue therapy for symptomatic refractory cerebral vasospasm in aneurysmal subarachnoid hemorrhage. *Neurocrit Care* 2009;11 (2):165–71.

24. Alali AS, McCredie VA, Golan E, Shah PS, Nathens AB. Beta blockers for acute traumatic brain injury: a systematic review and meta-analysis. *Neurocrit Care* 2014;20 (3):514–23.

25. Esnault P, Nguyen C, Bordes J, D'Aranda E, Montcriol A, Contargyris C, et al. Early-onset ventilator-associated pneumonia in patients with severe traumatic brain injury: incidence, risk factors, and consequences in cerebral oxygenation and outcome. *Neurocrit Care* 2017;27(2):187–98.

26. Bronchard MDR, Albaladejo MDPDP, Brezac MDG, Geffroy MDA, Seince MDP-F, Morris MDW, et al. Early onset pneumoniarisk factors and consequences in head trauma patients. *Anesthesiology* 2004;100(2):234–9.

27. Daneman N, Sarwar S, Fowler RA, Cuthbertson BH. Effect of selective decontamination on antimicrobial resistance in intensive care units: a systematic review and meta-analysis. *Lancet Infectious Dis* 2013;13(4):328–41.

28. Chan EY, Ruest A, Meade MO, Cook DJ. Oral decontamination for prevention of pneumonia in mechanically ventilated adults: systematic review and meta-analysis. *Br Med J* 2007;334 (7599):889.

29. Force ADT. Acute respiratory distress syndrome. *JAMA* 2012;307(23):2526–33.

30. Roth C, Ferbert A, Deinsberger W, Kleffmann J, Kästner S, Godau J, et al. Does prone positioning increase intracranial pressure? A retrospective analysis of patients with acute brain injury and acute respiratory failure. *Neurocrit Care* 2014;21 (2):186–91.

31. Tejerina E, Pelosi P, Muriel A, Peñuelas O, Sutherasan Y, Frutos-Vivar F, et al. Association between ventilatory settings and development of acute respiratory distress syndrome in mechanically ventilated patients due to brain injury. *J Crit Care* 2017;38:341–5.

32. Young NH, Andrews PJD. High-frequency oscillation as a rescue strategy for brain-injured adult patients with acute lung injury and acute respiratory distress syndrome. *Neurocrit Care* 2011;15 (3):623–33.

33. Hssain AA, Raza TM. ECMO in trauma patients: future may not be bleak after all! *Qatar Med J* 2017;2017(1):6.

34. Munoz-Bendix C, Beseoglu K, Kram R. Extracorporeal decarboxylation in patients with severe traumatic brain injury and ARDS enables effective control of

intracranial pressure. *Crit Care* 2015;19
(1):381.

35. Geerts WH, Bergqvist D, Pineo GF,
Heit JA, Samama CM, Lassen MR, et al.
Prevention of venous thromboembolism.
Chest 2008;133(6):381S–453S.

36. Barrera LM, Perel P, Ker K, Cirocchi R,
Farinella E, Morales Uribe CH.
Thromboprophylaxis for trauma patients.
Cochrane Database Syst Rev 2013(3).

37. Prophylaxis of venous thrombosis in
neurocritical care patients: an
evidence-based guidelines: a statement for
healthcare professionals from the
neurocritical care society. P Nyquist et at.
Neurocrit Care 2016;24:47–60.

38. Young D, Harrison DA, Cuthbertson BH,
Rowan K, TracMan Collaborators. Effect of
early vs late tracheostomy placement on
survival in patients receiving mechanical
ventilation: the TracMan randomized trial.
JAMA 2013;309(20):2121–9.

39. Death NCEiPOa. *On the right Trach?
A review of the care of patients who
underwent a tracheostomy.* London; 2014.

40. Oliver ER, Gist A, Gillespie MB.
Percutaneous versus surgical tracheotomy:
an updated meta-analysis. *Laryngoscope*
2007;117(9):1570–5.

41. Brass P, Hellmich M, Ladra A, Ladra J,
Wrzosek A. Percutaneous techniques
versus surgical techniques for
tracheostomy. *Cochrane Database Syst Rev*
2016(7).

42. Stocchetti N, Parma A, Lamperti M,
Songa V, Tognini L. Neurophysiological
consequences of three tracheostomy
techniques: a randomized
study in neurosurgical patients.
J Neurosurg Anesthesiol 2000;12
(4):307–13.

43. Reilly PM, Sing RF, Giberson FA,
Anderson III HL, Rotondo MF,
Tinkoff GH, et al. Hypercarbia during
tracheostomy: a comparison of
percutaneous endoscopic, percutaneous
Doppler, and standard surgical
tracheostomy. *Intens Care Med* 1997;23
(8):859–64.

44. Putensen C, Theuerkauf N, Guenther U,
Vargas M, Pelosi P. Percutaneous and
surgical tracheostomy in critically ill adult
patients: a meta-analysis. *Crit Care* 2014;18
(6):544.

45. Koitschev A, Simon C, Blumenstock G,
Mach H, Graumuller S. Suprastomal
tracheal stenosis after dilational and
surgical tracheostomy in critically ill
patients. *Anaesthesia* 2006;61(9):
832–7.

46. Law RC, Carney AS, Manara AR. Long-
term outcome after percutaneous
dilational tracheostomy. *Anaesthesia*
1997;52(1):51–6.

47. Young E, Pugh R, Hanlon R,
O'Callaghan E, Wright C, Jeanrenaud P,
et al. Tracheal stenosis following
percutaneous dilatational tracheostomy
using the single tapered dilator: an MRI
study. *Anaesth Intens Care* 2014;42
(6):745–51.

48. Keren C, Lazar-Zweker G. Tracheotomy in
severe TBI patients: sequelae and relation
to vocational outcome. *Brain Injury*
2001;15(6):531–6.

49. McCredie VA, Alali AS, Scales DC,
Adhikari NKJ, Rubenfeld GD,
Cuthbertson BH, et al. Effect of early versus
late tracheostomy or prolonged intubation
in critically ill patients with acute brain
injury: a systematic review and
meta-analysis. *Neurocrit Care* 2017;26
(1):14–25.

50. Norton JA, Ott LG, McClain C. The
metabolic response to brain injury. *JPEN*
1987;11:488.

51. Clifton GL, Robertson CS,
Grossman RG. et al. The metabolic
response to severe head injury.
J Neurosurg 1984;60:687.

52. Deutschman CS, Konstantinides FN,
Raup S, Cerra FB. Physiological and
metabolic response to isolated
closed-head injury: part 1: basal metabolic
state: correlation of metabolic and
physiologic parameters with fasting and
stressed controls. *J Neurosurg*
1986;64:89.

53. Twyman D. Nutritional management of the critically ill neurologic patient. *Crit Care Clin* 1997;13:39.

54. https://braintrauma.org/uploads/03/12/Guidelines_for_Management_of_Severe_TBI_4th_Edition.pdf

55. Yanagawa T, Bunn F, Roberts I, Wentz R, Pierro A. Nutritional support for head-injured patients. *Cochrane Database Syst Review* 2003;CD001530.

56. Borzotta AP, Pennings J, Papasadero B, Paxton J, Mardesic S, Borzotta R, Parrott A, Bledsoe F. Enteral versus parenteral nutrition after severe closed head injury. *J Trauma* 1994;37:459–68.

57. Perel P, Yanagawa T, Bunn F, Roberts I, Wentz R, Pierro A. Nutritional support for head-injured patients. *Cochrane Database Syst Rev* 2006;4: CD001530.

58. Wang X, Dong Y, Han X, Qi XQ, Huang CG, Hou LJ. Nutritional support for patients sustaining traumatic brain injury: a systematic review and meta-analysis of prospective studies. *PLoS One* 2013;8(3): e58838.

59. Hadley MN, Grahm TW, Harrington T, et al. Nutritional support and neurotrauma: a critical review of early nutrition in forty-five acute head injury patients. *Neurosurgery* 1986;19: 367.

60. Duke JH Jr, Jorgensen SD, Broell JR. Contribution of protein to caloric expenditure following injury. *Surgery* 1970;68:168.

61. Clifton GL, Robertson CS, Constant DF. Enteral hyperalimentation in head injury. *J Neuro-surg* 1985;62:186.

62. Young B, Ott L, Twyman D, et al. The effect of nutritional support on outcome from severe head injury. *J Neurosurg* 1987;67:668.

63. Glaesener JJ, Fredebohm M. Percutaneous endoscopic gastrostomy in the rehabilitation of neurological disorders. *J Suisse Med* 1992;122:1600.

64. Norton JA, Ott LG, McClain C, et al. Intolerance to enteral feeding in the brain-injured patient. *J Neurosurg* 1998;68:62.

65. Ott L, Young B, Phillips R, et al. Altered gastric emptying in the head injured patients: relationship to feeding intolerance. *J Neurosurg* 1991;74:738.

66. Marino LV, Kiratu EM, French S, Nathoo N. To determine the effect of metoclopramide on gastric emptying in severe head injuries: a prospective, randomized, controlled clinical trial. *Br J Neurosurg* 2003;17:24–8.

67. Kao CH, Changlai SP, Chieng PU, Yen TC. Gastric emptying in head-injured patients. *Am J Gastroenterol* 1998;93:1108–12.

68. Akkersdijk WL, Roukema JA, van der Werken C. Percutaneous endoscopic gastrostomy for patients with several cerebral injury. *Injury* 1998;29:11.

69. Kirby DF, Clifton GL, Turner H, et al. Early enteral nutrition after brain injury by percutaneous endoscopic gastrojejunostomy. *JPEN* 1991; 15:298.

70. Wahlstrom MR, Olivecrona M, Koskinen LO, Rydenhag B, Naredi S. Severe traumatic brain injury in pediatric patients: treatment and outcome using an intracranial pressure targeted therapy - the Lund concept. *Intensive Care Med* 2005;31 (6):832–9.

71. Grande PO. Pathophysiology of brain insult: Therapeutic implications with the Lund Concept. *Schweiz Med Wochenschr* 2000;130(42):1538–43.

72. Clifton GL, Miller ER, Choi SC, Levin HS. Fluid thresholds and outcome from severe brain injury. *Crit Care Med* 2002;30 (4):739–45.

73. Vedantam A, Robertson CS, Gopinath SP. Morbidity and mortality associated with hypernatremia in patients with severe traumatic brain injury. *Neurosurg Focus* 2017;43(5):E2.

74. Adrogue H, Madias N. Hypernatremia. *N Engl J Med* 2000;342: 1493–9.

75. Milionis HJ, Liamis G, Elisaf MS. Hypernatremia in hospitalised patients: a sequel of inadvertent fluid administration. *Arch Intern Med* 2000;160:1541–2.

76. Polderman KH, Schreuder WO, Strack van Schijndel RJ, Thijs LG. Hypernatremia in the intensive care unit: an indicator of quality of care? *Crit Care Med* 1999;27:1105–8.

77. Aiyagari V, Deibert E, Diringer MN. Hypernatremia in the neurologic intensive care unit: how high is too high? *J Crit Care* 2006;21:163–72.

78. Crompton MR. Hypothalamic lesions following closed head injury. *Brain* 1971;94:165–72.

79. Kern K, Meislin H. Diabetes insipidus: occurrence after minor head trauma. *J Trauma* 1984;24:69–72.

80. Bondanelli M, De Marinis L, Ambrosio MR, et al. Occurrence of pituitary dysfunction following traumatic brain injury. *J Neurotrauma* 2004; 21:685-96.

81. Capatina C, Paluzzi A, Mitchell R, Karavitaki N. Diabetes insipidus after traumatic brain injury. *J Clin Med* 2015;4 (7):1448–62.

82. Stern RH. Disorders of plasma sodium. *N Engl J Med* 2015;372:55–65.

83. Maggiore U, Picetti E, Antonucci E, Parenti E, Regolisti G, Mergoni M, Vezzani A, Cabassi A, Fiaccadori E. The relation between the incidence of hypernatremia and mortality in patients with severe traumatic brain injury. *Crit Care* 2009;13:R110.

84. Grant P, Ayuk J, Bouloux P-M, Cohen M, Cranston I, Murray RD, Rees A, Thatcher N, Grossman G. The diagnosis and management of inpatient hyponatraemia and SIADH. *Eur J Clin Invest* 2015;45(8):888–94.

85. Rajagopal R, Swaminathan G, Nair S, Joseph M. Hyponatremia in traumatic brain injury: a practical management protocol. *World Neurosurg* 2017;108:529–33.

86. Katz MA. Hyperglycemia-induced hyponatraemia – calculation of expected serum sodium depression. *N Engl J Med* 1973;289:843–4.

87. Adrogue HJ, Madias NE. Hyponatremia. *N Engl J Med* 2000; 342: 1581–1589.

88. Peters JP, Welt LG, Sims EA, Orloff J, Needham J. A salt-wasting syndrome associated with cerebral disease. *Trans Assoc Am Physicians* 1950;63:57–64.

89. Oh MS, Carroll HJ. Disorders of sodium metabolism: hypernatraemia and hyponatraemia. *Crit Care Med* 1992; 20:94–103.

90. Palmer BF. Hyponatremia in patients with central nervous system disease: SIADH versus CSW. *Trends Endocrinol Metab* 2003;14(4):182.

91. Harrigan MR. Cerebral salt wasting syndrome. *Crit Care Clin* 2001;17:125–38.

92. Hannon MJ, Thompson CJ. Neurosurgical hyponatremia. *J Clin Med* 2014;3 (4):1084–104.

93. Cole CD, Gottfried ON, Liu JK, Couldwell WT. Hyponatremia in the neurosurgical patient: diagnosis and management. *Neurosurg Focus* 2004;16 (4):E9.

94. Schrier RW, Gross P, Gheorghiade M, Berl T, Verbalis JG, Czerwiec FS, Orlandi C. Tolvaptan, a selective oral vasopressin v2-receptor antagonist, for hyponatremia. *N Engl J Med* 2006;355:2099–112.

95. Human T, Onuoha A, Diringer M, Dhar R. Response to a bolus of conivaptan in patients with acute hyponatremia after brain injury. *J Crit Care* 2012:27(6):745.

96. Jeon S-B, Choi HA, Lesch C, Kim MC, Badjatia N, Claassen J, Mayer SA, Lee K. Use of oral vasopressin V_2 receptor antagonist for hyponatremia in

acute brain injury. *Eur Neurol* 2013;70:142–8.

97. Brunner JE, Redmond JM, Haggar AM, Kruger DF, Elias SB. Central pontine myelinolysis and pontine lesions after rapid correction of hyponatraemia: a prospective magnetic resonance imaging study. *Ann Neurol* 1990;27:61–6.

Brain Stem Death and Organ Donation

Mark Sair and Martin B. Walker

Introduction

Death is the end point of a process of irreversible and progressive loss of vital organ function leading to certain and irreversible cessation of the characteristics that define life. Perhaps surprisingly, there is no globally accepted definition of what constitutes death, and in the UK, there is no statutory definition. However, successive working parties of the medical Royal Colleges have produced guidance for the diagnosis and confirmation of neurological death and these have been revised more recently to include death after cardiorespiratory arrest.[1] The irreversible loss of consciousness with the irreversible loss of the capacity to breathe produced by brain stem death (BSD) is accepted in the UK as the death of the individual and can be diagnosed using clinical tests of brain stem function. Diagnosis of BSD allows the discontinuation of treatment, which is no longer in the patient's best interest and thereby reduces distress to relatives, carers and positively impacts on the costs of health care. Diagnosing BSD on these ethical, humanitarian and utilitarian grounds also facilitates organ donation when patients and families choose to donate.

Brain Stem Death

History

Mollaret and Goulon described brain death in 1959.[2] *Coma dépassé* (beyond coma) was described as irreversible coma with loss of reflexes and electrical brain activity and was differentiated from *coma prolongé* (persistent vegetative state). In 1968, the Harvard Committee defined brain death using the criteria of unreceptivity and unresponsiveness with no movements or respirations and no reflexes during disconnection from the ventilator occurring in the presence of an isoelectric electroencephalogram (EEG).[3] In 1976, the Conference of Medical Royal Colleges stated that permanent functional death of the brain stem constituted brain death. This memorandum provided the foundations for the current UK code of practice for BSD testing, delineating the inclusion and exclusion criteria and describing the clinical tests of BSD function.[4]

Anatomy and Physiology

The brain stem is located between the cerebral hemispheres and the spinal cord; it comprises the mid-brain, pons and medulla. It contains the cranial nerve nuclei and transmits ascending and descending motor and sensory nerve impulses. Pontine reticular nuclei are vital for cortical arousal and conscious awareness. The medulla and pons (under influence of the hypothalamus) control and maintain cardiorespiratory function. Loss of brain stem controls and cranial nerve function form the basis of BSD testing.

Table 15.1 Common causes of brain stem death

Aetiological condition	Features
Traumatic brain injury	Most common cause
Intracranial haemorrhage	e.g. subarachnoid haemorrhage
Tumours	
Infection	
Metabolic encephalopathy	e.g. hepatic
Hypoxaemia	More likely to result in persistent vegetative state
Ischaemia	

Pathophysiology

Brain tissue tolerates hypoxaemia and ischaemia poorly. The overlying brain tissue and skull provide some physical protection to the centrally located brain stem. However, the rigid cranium causes intracranial pressure to rise as brain swelling develops, regardless of the traumatic or non-traumatic aetiology of the primary brain injury. Secondary brain injury readily occurs with a vicious cycle of brain swelling causing tissue hypoxaemia from impaired oxygen delivery leading to worsening intracranial hypertension and ischaemia. Ultimately, this can cause downward pressure on the brain stem resulting in coning through the foramen magnum and BSD. The common causes of BSD are summarised in Table 15.1.

Profound brain stem injury results in unconsciousness, impaired homeostasis and variable cranial nerve lesions. Cushing's reflex (systemic hypertension and bradycardia) is not always observed. Indeed, almost any combination of cardiac rhythm and systemic pressure abnormality may occur. After BSD, systemic hypotension and tachycardia usually ensue with loss of all cranial nerve function. Loss of thermostatic homeostasis results in hypothermia. Cranial diabetes insipidus is common and results in profound polyuria, hypovolaemia and hypernatraemia unless treated vigorously.

Devastating Brain Injury

Devastating brain injury (DBI) can be defined as 'any neurological condition at the time of hospital admission that is an immediate threat to life or incompatible with good functional recovery and where early limitation or withdrawal of therapy is being actively considered'. It is often the result of intracranial haemorrhage or infarction and is usually associated with profound loss of consciousness (Glasgow Coma Score <4) with loss of one or more cranial reflexes. Historically patients with DBI were often intubated for CT imaging of the brain and were palliated in the Emergency Department following consultation with the neurosurgical or neurology team. There are however reports that a small number of these patients when admitted to the intensive care unit and reassessed 24–72 hours later have better than expected neurological outcomes.[5] Prognostication at a very early stage can be unreliable and it may be appropriate to admit these patients to critical care for a period of physiological stabilisation and observation to improve the quality of decision-making.[6] At the end of this period of observation the emphasis of care may subsequently change to more active treatment or more likely to end-of-life care and consideration of end-of-life wishes including consideration of organ donation. Inevitably some of these patients will progress to BSD and will require formal BSD testing to confirm death. In the UK a joint working party of the Intensive Care Society and Faculty of Intensive Care Medicine with members from a range of stake-holder professional organisations has recently produced a consensus statement and a number of pragmatic recommendations concerning optimal care and prognostication in DBI.[7]

Brain Stem Death Testing

The UK Code of Practice for BSD Testing

The 2008 code of practice for the diagnosis of death encompasses the diagnosis and confirmation of brain stem death in severely brain-injured ventilated patients using neurological criteria.[1] Regardless of the cause of brain stem death, the irreversible cessation of brain stem function results in irreversible cessation of the integrative functions of the brain with absent cranial nerve reflexes, coma and apnoea. Prior to BSD testing, mandatory inclusions and exclusions have to be considered (Table 15.2). Other reversible causes including electrolyte and metabolic disturbances must also be corrected.

It is necessary to maintain relatively normal cardiovascular and respiratory physiological parameters in the preceding hours prior to testing. The timing of BSD testing is not mandated and, whilst it may be appropriate to test a few hours after an intracranial catastrophe (e.g. traumatic brain injury or spontaneous intracranial haemorrhage), it is preferable to wait for more than 24 hours when the period of insult is more uncertain (e.g. cardiac arrest, circulatory insufficiency, hypoxaemia or air and fat embolism). The tests are performed by two medical practitioners who have been registered with the General Medical

Table 15.2 Mandatory inclusions and exclusions to be considered prior to BSD testing

Prerequisite inclusions

1 Patient is deeply unconscious (Glasgow Coma Score of 3)

2 Presence of severe irremediable brain damage of certain aetiology

3 Patient is on a ventilator – spontaneous respiratory efforts are absent

Mandatory exclusions

1 Presence of sedative agents that might result in the comatose state of the patient
Therapeutic or recreational drug effects can persist in critically ill patients

2 Primary hypothermia causing unconsciousness. It is recommended that there is a 24 hour observation period post-warming to normothermia.
Core temperature >35°C

3 Reversible circulatory, metabolic and endocrine abnormalities causing unconsciousness
It is recognised that changes may occur as a result of BSD, but these effects rather than causes of the condition do not prevent BSD testing

4 Muscle relaxants or other drugs causing profound muscular weakness
Determined by using a nerve stimulator or eliciting deep tendon reflexes

Table 15.3 BSD tests and the cranial nerves they examine

BSD test	Cranial nerves
Pupils are fixed and unresponsive to light (direct and consensual)	II and III
Pupils may be unequal or not fully dilated	
Absence of corneal reflex	V and VII
Avoiding corneal injury	
Absence of vestibulo-ocular reflexes	III, VI and VIII
Absent eye movements on instillation of >50 ml ice-cold water over 1 min in to each external auditory meatus in turn.	
Head flexed to 30° plus access to tympanic membrane is confirmed with an otoscope (removing wax or debris first if needed)	
Local injury or disease may prevent this test being performed on one or other side, but this does not prevent or invalidate the diagnosis of BSD	
Absent motor response in the cranial nerve or somatic distribution with supra-orbital pressure	V and VII
Absence of gag reflex	IX, X
Using orange stick or flat spatula to stimulate soft palate and oropharynx	
Absence of cough or reflex response to tracheal stimulation with suction catheter	IX, X
Absence of spontaneous respiratory effort on disconnection from the ventilator	IX, X
Preoxygenation, allow $PaCO_2$ to rise to 6.0 kPa before test	
Use CPCP circuit or disconnect from the ventilator and administer oxygen via a catheter at a rate > 6 L/min	
Observe 5 min for respiratory effort, PCO_2 must rise by at least 0.5 kPa	

Council for over 5 years, are competent in the practice of the tests and are not members of the transplant team. At least one practitioner should be a consultant. Two sets of tests are performed. These may be carried out by the two practitioners separately or together. Repetition of the tests avoids observer error. The time interval between tests is discretionary, dependent on the patient's pathology and clinical course. Although death is not pronounced until the second set of tests has been completed, the legal time of death is when the first set of tests was performed. The clinical BSD tests comprise a detailed assessment of cranial nerve function and a test of respiratory drive (Table 15.3).

The Diagnosis of BSD in Special Situations

Paediatric Considerations

In children aged over 2 months the criteria for BSD are similar to adults.[1] Between a gestational age of 37 weeks and 2 months, the diagnosis of BSD can be difficult to make and below 37 weeks BSD criteria cannot be applied. For anencephalic infants, organ donation can proceed if two clinicians (not in the transplant team) agree that spontaneous respirations have ceased.

Chronic Lung Disease

Patients with significant pre-existing chronic lung disease may need greater levels of hypercarbia to produce maximal stimulation of the respiratory centre. These special cases should be discussed with a specialist in respiratory disease.

High Spinal Cord Injury

The presence of high spinal cord injury prevents full BSD testing being performed.

Presence of Long-Acting Sedative Agents

Diagnosing BSD is problematical following sedation. When small doses of short-acting agents are used during resuscitation and evaluation of the patient, clinical judgement alone can be used to time the performance of BSD tests. Due to the unpredictable pharmacokinetics and pharmacodynamics of sedative agents in the critically ill, more prolonged use causes uncertainty. Indeed, considerable variation exists in UK clinical practice for the delay following cessation of sedation of all types and in the use of antagonists (naloxone and flumazenil).[8,9] Measurement of drug levels can be time consuming, is not invariably available and causes further uncertainty in interpretation. This has led to proposals that confirmatory tests should gain clinical and legal acceptance.

Confirmatory Tests

The code of practice states that the safety of BSD testing has been confirmed and that confirmatory tests (neurophysiological or radiological) are not justified. Uncertainty in diagnosing BSD may arise in the special situations described previously or when local facial, pharyngeal and aural trauma prevents full BSD testing. Using confirmatory tests remains an attractive prospect in uncertain cases and when residual sedation, hypothermia or metabolic disturbances prevent routine BSD diagnosis. It speeds up BSD diagnosis and reduces the duration of futile treatment and the deterioration of multi-organ function that occurs over time following BSD.[10] There is inadequate evidence to recommend one specific confirmatory test over another and more studies are needed to evaluate their precise role. Techniques demonstrating cerebral circulation or brain tissue perfusion offer most promise and the total absence of cerebral circulation may become acceptable for diagnosing BSD. Cerebral arterial blood flow can persist after clinical BSD and repeated tests of the circulation may be needed for individual patients. [11]

Features of various confirmatory tests are detailed in Table 15.4.[12–14]

Currently, if confounding factors prevent clinical BSD testing, the sole use of confirmatory tests in the UK is not sanctioned in law or by any national guidelines. However, on a case-by-case basis close involvement of the relatives, early referral to HM Coroner, use of second opinions from neurologists or neurosurgeons and legal opinions from hospital legal departments and medical defence organisations may facilitate BSD diagnosis using such tests without ethical or legal risk.

International Variation in Diagnosing Brain Death

Significant international variation exists in BSD testing. A survey has demonstrated differences between guidelines of 80 countries.[15] Marked variation occurs in such

Table 15.4 Features of confirmatory tests for BSD testing

Confirmatory test	Potential for BSD testing	Availability	Bedside use?	Safety and level of invasiveness
Four-vessel angiography	Good	Limited	No	Risks to patient and donor organs
Transcranial Doppler ultrasonography	Poor access to posterior circulation	Variable	Yes	Non-invasive
Magnetic resonance imaging and angiography	Good	Variable	No	Low risk
Radioisotope scintigraphy	Good	Poor	Yes	Low risk
Xenon-enhanced computerised tomography (CT)	Good	Poor	No	Low risk
CT angiography	Good	Good	Yes	Low risk
Positron emission tomography	Good	Very poor	No	Low risk
EEG	Not useful for BSD	Variable	Yes	Non-invasive
Multimodality evoked potentials	Good	Variable	Yes	Non-invasive

fundamental areas as apnoea testing (targeting $PaCO_2$, using ventilator disconnection alone or not even examining for apnoea), the number of physicians mandated (varying from one to three), using confirmatory tests (mandatory, optional or not permissible) and the time between tests (0–24 hours). There appear to be no cultural or religious attitudes that influence the variations. In the USA brain death is defined using the concept of whole brain death. Brain death testing in the USA includes use of a negative atropine test (1–2 mg intravenous atropine resulting in a heart rate rise of less than 5 bpm). Confirmatory testing is also permissible in conditions that might confound brain death testing (such as brain stem encephalitis or persistence of sedative agents). There is variation between individual states, but most mandate separation of the sets of tests by 12–24 hours.

Organ and Tissue Donation within Critical Care

The National Institute for Clinical Excellence[16] and the UK General Medical Council[17] state that organ donation should be considered as a usual part of 'end of life' care. Potential donors are identified by being on the Organ Donor Register (ODR) or by family or friends knowing their wishes. There is no strict framework over the timing and manner of requesting assent for donation. Most practitioners wait until BSD is confirmed (i.e. after the second set of tests) unless the relatives raise the issue earlier. Very few contraindications to organ donation are absolute and so all potential donors should be referred for consideration.

Despite this the demand for organ transplantation outstrips the supply of donor organs, whether from living donor or cadaveric donation programmes. Cadaveric organ donation can be from brain stem dead (donation following brain death or DBD) or less commonly from asystolic (non-heart beating or DCD) donors. Currently, most of the UK employs an opt-in system for cadaveric organ and tissue donation, but since 2015 Wales has successfully operated a deemed consent or 'opt-out' system and in 2020 this will be introduced in England.

In 2008 the Organ Donation Taskforce published a report making a number of recommendations in key areas such as donor identification and referral, donor co-ordination and organ retrieval. This aimed to increase the number of deceased organ donors by 50% over a 5 year period.[18] Despite achieving this target these initiatives have yet to meet the current need and more than 7000 individuals remain on the transplant waiting list. The latest strategy aimed at increasing assent rates to over 80% by 2020 (26 deceased donors per million population) would result in the UK comparing favourably with the top performing countries in the world.[19]

Ethical and Legal Considerations Relating to BSD and Organ Donation

It has been argued that BSD testing is flawed by the lack of controlled studies assessing the true prognosis of the clinical signs of BSD. However, series comprising more than 1000 BSD patients receiving organ support have been published. Asystole (usually occurring within a few days) was the invariable outcome after BSD. Although the concept of BSD evolved before organ transplantation could occur from cadaveric donors (limited by surgical techniques and immunosuppression), concerns persist about an apparent linkage of BSD to organ donation. Difficulties arise because the withdrawal of futile multiorgan support does not require formal declaration of BSD. It is argued that the only reason to perform the tests is to facilitate organ donation. However, it remains usual practice in the UK not to withdraw ventilatory support of an apnoeic patient without BSD testing.

Cases proceeding to donation that would normally be referred to the coroner should still be referred so that coronial permission can be granted for donation. The coroner may refuse permission for donation of an organ if that organ may have caused death, if the coroner's enquiries might be obstructed by the organ's removal or if the organ may have evidential value. Therefore, close co-operation between clinicians, the specialist nurse for Organ Donation (SNOD), the coroner, the police and the pathologist is required for some coroner's cases.

The UK Human Tissue Act 2004 (HTA) regulates storage and use of organs and tissues from living and deceased patients. Consent underpins the Act, which defines a hierarchy of consent with the patient (or a person with parental responsibility for a child) being at the top, above a new status of a nominated representative and lastly a further hierarchy of qualifying relatives. The HTA states that the known wishes of the deceased take precedence (over relatives' objections) for donation, but falls short of making donation obligatory in this situation and retains a case-by-case basis for decision-making, involving consultation with the relatives. The HTA states the ODR should always be checked so that registered patients' wishes can be followed.

Management of the Potential DBD Donor

Active management of the patient should continue to facilitate BSD testing. If BSD is confirmed the emphasis changes to optimising organ function in those patients who are to become organ donors or cessation of ventilatory support and other therapies in those who are not. The pathophysiological changes occurring with BSD can present significant challenges from cardiorespiratory instability and hypothalamic failure. The actual DBD donor donates 3.9 organs with number or organs falling sharply over the age of 50. There is evidence that standardised donor management protocols increase the number of retrieved organs and particularly thoracic organs. The basic principles of donor management are summarised in Table 15.5. Consensus

Table 15.5 Optimal donor management

Management goal	Clinical intervention	Comments
Organ perfusion	Optimise preload	Correct hypovolaemia
	Use advanced cardiac monitoring in labile patients	Evidence for choice of monitor remains unclear
	Minimise pressor support	Use vasopressin, avoiding noradrenaline when possible
	Inotropes if indicated	Dopamine <10 mcg/kg/min
	Treat diabetes insipidus	Bolus and/or infusion of intravenous 1-desamino-D-arginine vasopressin
	Administer methylprednisolone	
Lung function	Maintain normal ABGs	
	Minimise PEEP	Target 5 cm H_2O
	Ensure lung protective strategy	Target tidal volume 4–7 ml/kg
	Frequent pulmonary physiotherapy and endotracheal suction	Recruitment manoeuvres
Biochemistry	Maintain strict normoglycaemia	Target 4.0–10.0 mmol/L
	Maintain potassium levels	Target 4.0–5.0 mmol/L
	Maintain sodium levels	Target 130–150 mmol/L
Haematology	Treat coagulopathy	
	Maintain haemoglobin concentration	>7.0 g/dl in stable patients and 9.0–10.0 g/dl in unstable patients
Temperature	Maintain normothermia	
Other priorities	Treat infection with appropriate antimicrobials	Keep SNOD informed
	Continue enteral feeding	
	Continue thromboprophylaxis	

guidelines on optimal donor management have been published alone[20,21] or as an extended care bundle.[22] Collaboration between the critical care team at the local hospital and the cardiothoracic centre may also improve donor rates. A pilot scheme deploying cardiothoracic 'scouts' to attend local hospitals and aid with delivery of extended care bundles may also be of benefit.

Relatives of the Potential Donor

The family should be supported and kept fully informed throughout their relative's critical illness. As BSD supervenes, this need becomes greater rather than reduces. A senior clinician should inform the relatives of the grave clinical outlook and the clinical reasons for conducting brain stem death tests. Early and prompt referral to the Specialist Nurse Organ Donation (SNOD) should facilitate a collaborative approach in counselling relatives and seeking consent for organ donation. Audit data from NHS Blood and Transplant (NHSBT) has shown collaborative approaches improve assent rates. Family refusals are minimised when requests are made by staff experienced in requesting. The SNOD obtains fully informed assent from the family explaining the details of the process and collecting information necessary for retrieval to proceed.

Organ Donation after BSD

Organ donation following BSD should proceed without delay to prevent deteriorating organ function. Optimal donor management continues from the critical care unit throughout the operative procedure. The clinical team's aspiration should be to achieve multiorgan donation; however, this is usually limited by organ and recipient suitability. Anaesthetic drugs such as muscle relaxants and volatile anaesthetic agents may be administered during organ retrieval to prevent spinal reflexes and autonomic surges. It is important that all members of staff involved in the procedure are aware of the rationale. The anaesthetist will be required until the aorta is cross-clamped, extra-corporeal organ perfusion is commenced and ventilation is stopped.

Donation Following Cardiac Death (DCD)

DCD previously referred to as non-heart beating donation is the donation of organs from asystolic patients. In 1994 a workshop in Maastricht categorised the situations when this may occur (Table 15.6).[23] In the UK this is usually in the setting where asystole follows planned withdrawal of multiorgan support on the grounds of futility It requires rapid pronouncement of death (5 min after asystole) and immediate transfer of the patient to the operating theatre where a rapid laparotomy is performed and organ retrieval is performed after cold perfusion

Table 15.6 Categories of non-heart-beating organ donation

Category	Description of process	Status of potential donor	Location
1	Uncontrolled	Dead on arrival	Emergency department
2	Uncontrolled	Unsuccessful resuscitation	Emergency department
3	Controlled	Planned withdrawal of futile treatment	Intensive care unit
4	Controlled	Cardiac arrest after BSD	Intensive care unit

of the organs. Best results are obtained when both cold and warm ischaemic times are minimised. The results of kidney transplantation from DCD are excellent[24] and progress has been made with new methods such as normothermic regional perfusion and ex vivo lung perfusion enabling improved liver, lung and even heart retrieval.[25-27]

Tissue Donation

Patients in intensive care units can be tissue and organ donors or be solely tissue donors. The most commonly retrieved tissues are heart valves and corneas. Depending on local transplant programmes, other tissues such as skin, bone, tendons, cartilage and pericardium may also be retrievable. Local SNODs are able to provide any necessary advice.

Conclusion

Patients admitted to critical care with devastating brain injury have a poor prognosis, but inaccuracies in prognostication can lead to premature withdrawal of treatment. Many of these patients however do progress to become BSD. Clinical testing to diagnose BSD remains a valid and legally acceptable method to determine death of an individual. It facilitates both a dignified death and organ donation in appropriate patients. Future developments in this challenging field may see a considered increase in the use of confirmatory tests, which will speed up the process and potentially improve donor organ function.

References

1. Academy of Royal Medical Colleges. A code of practice for the diagnosis and confirmation of death; 2008.

2. Mollaret P, Goulon M. Le coma dépassé. *Rev Neurol* 1959;101:3–15.

3. Anon. A definition of irreversible coma. Report of the ad hoc Committee of the Harvard Medical School to examine the definition of brain death. *J Am Med Assoc* 1968;205:337–40.

4. Conference of Medical Royal Colleges and their Faculties (UK). Diagnosis of brain death. *Br Med J* 1976;2:1187–8.

5. Manara AR, Thomas I, Harding R. A case for stopping the early withdrawal of life sustaining therapies in patients with devastating brain injuries. *J Intensive Care Soc* 2016;17(4):295–301.

6. Souter MJ, Blissitt PA, Blosser S, et al. Recommendations for the critical care management of devastating brain injury: prognostication, psychosocial, and ethical management: a position statement for healthcare professionals from the Neurocritical Care Society. *Neurocrit Care* 2015;23 (1):4–13.

7. Harvey D, Butler J, Groves J, et al. Management of perceived devastating brain injury after hospital admission: a consensus statement from stakeholder professional organizations. *Br J Anaes* 2018;120(1):138–45.

8. Pratt OW, Bowles B, Protheroe RT. Brain stem death testing after thiopental use: a survey of UK neuro critical care practice. *Anaesthesia* 2006;61:1075–8.

9. Lopez-Navidad A, Caballero F, Domingo P, et al. Early diagnosis of brain death in patients treated with central nervous system depressant drugs. *Transplantation* 2000;70:131–5.

10. Young GB, Shemie SD, Doig CJ. Brief review: the role of ancillary tests in the neurological determination of death. *Can J Anesth* 2006;53:620–7.

11. Flowers WM Jr, Patel BR. Persistence of cerebral blood flow after brain death. *South Med J* 2000;93:364–70.

12. Monteiro LM, Bollen CW, van Huffelen AC, et al. Transcranial Doppler ultrasonography to confirm brain death: a meta-analysis. *Intens Care Med* 2006;32:1937–44.

13. Yatim A, Mercatello A, Coronel B, et al. 99 mTc-HMPAO cerebral scintigraphy in the diagnosis of brain death. *Transpl Proc* 1991;23:2491.

14. de Tourtchaninoff M, Hantson P, Mahieu P, et al. Brain death diagnosis in misleading conditions. *Q J Med* 1999;92:407–14.

15. Wijdicks EFM. Brain death worldwide: accepted fact but no global consensus in diagnostic criteria. *Neurology* 2002;58:20–5.

16. NICE. Organ donation for transplantation CG135; 2011.

17. GMC. Treatment and care towards end of life: good practice in decision making; 2010.

18. Department of Health (UK) Report of the Organ Donation Taskforce. Organs for transplants; 2008.

19. NHSBT. Taking organ transplantation to 2020: a detailed strategy; 2014.

20. Intensive Care Society. *Guidelines for adult organ and tissue donation*. London: Intensive Care Society; 2004.

21. Shemie SD, Ross H, Pagliarello J, et al. Organ donor management in Canada: recommendations of the forum on medical management to optimise donor organ potential. *Can Med Associ J* 2006;174: S13–30.

22. NHSBT. Donation after brainstem death (DBD) donor optimisation extended care bundle; 2014.

23. Koostra G, Daemen JHC, Oomen APA. Categories of non-heart beating donors. *Transpl Proc* 1995;27:2893–4.

24. Summers DM, Watson CJ, Pettigrew GJ, et al. Kidney donation after circulatory death (DCD): state of the art. *Kidney Int.* 2015 Aug;88(2):241–9.

25. Reeb J, Cybel M. Ex vivo lung perfusion. *Clin Transplant.* 2016;30 (3):183–94.

26. Morrissey PE, Monaco AP. Donation after circulatory death: current practices, ongoing challenges, and potential improvements *Transplantation* 2014;97 (3):258–64.

27. Macdonald PS, Chew HC, Connellan M, Dhital K. Extracorporeal heart perfusion before heart transplantation: the heart in a box. *Curr Opin Organ Transplant.* 2016; 21 (3):336–42

Chapter 16

Anaesthesia for Emergency Neurosurgery

Nicola Pilkington and W. Hiu Lam

Introduction

An estimated 1.4 million people per year attend Emergency Departments in the UK following head trauma.[1] Approximately 10% of these patients have a moderate or severe Traumatic Brain Injury (TBI) with a Glasgow Coma Score (GCS) <12 or <9 respectively. TBI results in more than 3600 Intensive Care admissions per year[2] and remains the leading cause of mortality in patients aged under 25 with 6–10 brain injury deaths per 100 000 of population per annum.[1]

The focus of this discussion is primarily based on adult intracranial neurosurgical pathology and its implications for anaesthesia.

Emergency anaesthesia for neurosurgery follows an algorithm of rapid initial assessment, resuscitation, stabilisation for transfer, investigation of relevant pathology and timely surgical evacuation of compressive lesions. In order to appreciate the rationale and principle of clinical anaesthetic management in these patients, the following areas must be considered.

- The importance of preservation of global neurological status, as assessed by GCS.[3]
- An insight of the pathophysiology of brain injury.
- Awareness of the effects of attenuation of cerebral autoregulation caused by the intracranial pathology.[4]
- The need for target directed management strategies for the prevention of secondary brain injury (SBI) in patients undergoing anaesthesia.[5]

The existence of comorbidities, particularly cervical spine injury (up to 10.3% of moderate to severe TBI[6]) as well as other systems involvement in the context of polytrauma, must be remembered when assessing these patients. Multidisciplinary teamwork is pivotal in optimising outcomes.

There is recent evidence indicating that older patients present with a higher GCS compared to younger patients given the same anatomical severity of TBI,[7] the decision threshold of surgical intervention needs to be considered in this context in this patient group.

Pathophysiology

Neurological deficit caused by primary brain injury (PBI) is dependent on the severity of the initial impact; whereas brain ischaemia (Cerebral Blood Flow (CBF) uncoupled from cerebral metabolic demand) occurs as a result of SBI. Ischaemia is the single most important factor affecting outcome after brain injury and, to a certain extent, is preventable.

Table 16.1 Indications for surgical intervention in TBI

Indications	Notes
Depressed skull fracture	To reduce risk of infection and damage to underlying structures
Acute extradural haematoma	Due to middle meningeal artery (with skull fracture)
Acute subdural haematoma	Cortical venous injury and underlying brain contusion
Intracranial haematoma/contusion	Especially urgent in temporal lobe and/or posterior fossa
Intracranial hypertension	External ventricular drainage or decompressive craniectomy
Hydrocephalus	External ventricular drainage or shunt

Approximately 90% of fatal TBI cases have evidence of cerebral ischaemia at post-mortem examinations.[8] The aims of anaesthetic management are to maintain adequate brain perfusion and to avoid, anticipate and aggressively treat intracranial hypertension (IcHTN).

Cerebral ischaemia is caused by a reduction of arterial blood flow and cerebral perfusion pressure triggered either by direct focal compression and/or IcHTN secondary to expanding lesions. This pressure-volume relationship is the Monro Kelly Doctrine.[9] The common surgical indications for patients with TBI are illustrated in Table 16.1.

The extracranial causes of SBI are predominantly non-surgical. These factors include disturbances in haemodynamics, respiratory insufficiency, seizures and metabolic imbalance.

Cerebral autoregulation, measured by continuous transcranial Doppler velocity, is impaired in 28% of moderate brain injury and 67% of severe brain injury patients.[10] Certain anaesthetic agents also affect cerebral autoregulation, which is essential in maintaining an adequate coupling of CBF and cerebral oxygen metabolism (CMRO2).[11] It is essential to control the fluctuations in systemic arterial blood pressure during anaesthesia in order to ensure adequate cerebral perfusion. Uncoupling of CBF and CMRO2 leads to brain ischaemia.[12] Advances in functional imaging techniques such as Oxygen-15 positron emission tomography allows more accurate regional delineation of CBF, cerebral blood volume (CBV), $CMRO_2$ and oxygen extraction ratio; hence a more precise functional definition of cerebral ischaemia.[13]

At a cellular level, large quantities of the excitatory amino acid neurotransmitters such as glutamate are released. This initiates an excitotoxic cascade via over-activation of the inotropic (N-methyl D-aspartate (NMDA) receptors) and metabotropic (G-protein linked) glutamate receptors.[14]

The result is an intracellular influx of calcium, sodium and potassium, leading to a cascade of catabolic processes which end with neuronal damage and death.[15] A compensatory increase in the Na^+/K^+-ATPase pump activity to restore the cell back to its resting ionic state increases the metabolic demand of the cell, leading to flow-metabolism uncoupling.[4]

Target-Directed Strategy

Haemodynamics

Hypertension, hypotension and hypoxia have all been shown independently to significantly increase morbidity and mortality in both adults[5,16] and children.[17] A single episode of systolic hypotension (<90 mmHg) increases morbidity and doubles mortality rates in adults.[18]

Cerebral Perfusion Pressure (CPP)

CPP is the difference of mean arterial pressure (MAP) and intracranial pressure (ICP). Traditionally a target CPP of 70 mmHg has been used for brain-injured patients,[19] partially based on Rosner's study which demonstrated a low mortality rate of 29% and a good 6 month post-injury recovery rate of 59%.[20] The Lund hypothesis, however, advocating a reduction in microvascular pressure to minimise oedema, reported an impressive 8% mortality rate and 80% recovery rate in their studies.[21,22] Furthermore, a 50% reduction in secondary brain ischaemia was demonstrated by Robertson's study where the CPP threshold was increased from 40 mmHg to 60 mmHg, but this was accompanied by a fivefold increase of adult respiratory distress syndrome.[23,24]

The Brain Trauma Foundation recommends a target CPP between 60 and 70 mmHg in order to optimise survival and favourable outcomes whilst avoiding complications such as adult respiratory distress syndrome, pulmonary and cerebral oedema related to hypervolaemia and hypertension.[25]

Individualising the CPP target for a patient may be estimated using surrogate measures of autoregulation, for example the pressure reactivity index. More detail on this is discussed in Chapters 11 and 13.

Intracranial Pressure (ICP)

It is generally accepted that the treatment threshold for IcHTN should be set at an ICP of 22 mmHg.[25] If an intracranial monitoring device is in situ prior to induction of anaesthesia, it is imperative to treat IcHTN above the set threshold and maintain an adequate MAP to generate the appropriate CPP until the dura is surgically incised when the brain is exposed to atmospheric pressure where the CPP required equals MAP (provided central venous pressure is insignificant).

Perioperative Anaesthetic Management

Preoperative Assessment and Optimisation

In patients with significant TBI requiring urgent surgery, history taking often involves assimilating information from witnesses and emergency services personnel. Further past medical, drug and allergy history can be obtained from relatives and the patient's GP records. The clinical examination must be comprehensive and co-existing injuries and co-morbidities sought.

Anaesthetic assessment must include a global neurological state of the patient. The reduction in GCS from the scene of injury onwards may indicate a progressive deterioration. An accurate documentation of the pupil size and reactivity is essential. Any preoperative motor, sensory and speech deficit should be recorded as a baseline, enabling comparison in the postoperative period. Bulbar function needs to be specifically elicited. An impaired bulbar function may have led to aspiration of gastric contents preoperatively. In addition, the patient may not have sufficient airway protection postoperatively. If lung aspiration is suspected, urgent tracheo-bronchial toileting must be considered prior to surgery. Aspiration pneumonia increases intrathoracic pressure on intermittent positive pressure ventilation, which impedes venous return and can worsen existing IcHTN. The increase in venous pressure may also render surgical haemostasis more arduous. The resulting ventilation-perfusion mismatch could promote hypercapnoea and hypoxaemia, both of which worsen IcHTN.

A spectrum of neurogenic cardiovascular complications following TBI exists. ECG changes, arrhythmias as well as regional wall motion abnormalities resulting in ventricular dysfunction are commonly observed and a thorough preoperative cardiovascular risk assessment is mandatory.[26]

The preoperative arterial blood pressure and heart rate should be noted as they become the target parameters once the patient is under anaesthesia especially when ICP measurement is not available. Fluid balance record, serum and urine electrolytes and osmolality must be examined as complications from TBI such as diabetes insipidus, syndrome of inappropriate antidiuretic hormone secretion and cerebral salt wasting syndrome can cause significant morbidity and mortality.[27] Serum haemoglobin, platelet count, electrolytes, clotting studies and electrocardiograph (ECG) are mandatory investigations. Cross-matched red cells should be readily available. Sedative premedication is rarely indicated and appropriate monitoring and supplementary oxygen therapy must accompany transfer to the operating theatre; such inter- and intra-hospital transfers must be undertaken by trained clinician in accordance to local and national guidelines.

Timing of Anaesthesia

Traditionally, it is recommended that Acute Subdural Haematomas (ASDH) are surgically decompressed within 4 hours.[28] However, Fountain reported that the time interval from injury to surgery for ASDH was not an independent prognostic factor of improved survival when analysing more than 20 years of data from the Trauma Audit and Research Network (TARN).[29] Furthermore, Tien demonstrated a trend towards lower mortality with increased time interval to surgery even when taking into consideration that those with more severe brain injury are frequently operated on more rapidly.[30] This research suggests that age, clot size, post-operative ICP control and the primary underlying TBI are more important than the time-to-theatre interval.[29,30]

Induction of Anaesthesia

The objective is to achieve smooth 'tramline' anaesthesia from induction through to emergence from anaesthesia. Pre-induction monitoring of the patient as per the Association of Anaesthetists standards is manatory.[31] Establishment of pre-induction invasive arterial blood pressure measurement is appropriate in enabling close CPP monitoring at the time of potential haemodynamic instability. Central venous and urinary catheters and a pharyngeal temperature probe may be introduced post-induction if appropriate.[32] Vasopressors such as metaraminol and ephedrine and anticholinergic agents must be readily available to anticipate and prevent hypotension and bradycardia.

No consensus exists as to which induction agent is superior, however Propofol is most frequently used in the UK, possibly due to familiarity.[33] Obtunded patients often require less than the traditional induction dose of 2–3 mg/kg and care must be taken to preserve adequate CPP in view of systemic vasodilatory effects of propofol.

Thiopental (5–7 mg/kg), a barbiturate, is another well-tolerated induction agent with a reliable end point and remains very much in use worldwide. For many years Ketamine has been considered 'contra-indicated' in TBI due to concerns regarding increased CBF and ICP. However, a 2012 review of the use of ketamine in neurosurgical patients suggests that is offers a cardiovascular stable induction without adverse cerebral haemodynamic effects when used in conjunction with controlled ventilation. Doses of 1–2 mg/kg of ketamine are commonly used.[34]

Opioids have a major role in neuroanaesthesia. Remifentanil (1–5 µg/kg/min), an ultra short-acting esterase metabolised mu receptor agonist, has gained wide acceptance as the opioid of choice for intracranial surgery. Similar to other opioids, it has no direct effect on cerebrovasculature and produces rapid intense analgesia with stable, easily adjustable haemodynamics as well as enabling rapid postoperative recovery for neuro-logical assessment.[35] Fentanyl (7–10 µg/kg) can also be used for analgesia and obtund-ing the pressor response of laryngoscopy and is particularly useful for anaesthesia out of the theatre environment as it can be administered as a bolus as well as continuous infusion.

In patients with TBI, co-existing cervical spine injury must be considered. The anterior portion of rigid neck collars should be removed prior to intubation and Manual In-Line Spinal Immobilisation (MILSI) applied.[36,37] Although MILSI minimises cervical movement, it does not completely eliminate it and MILSI itself reduces Cormack-Lehance laryngoscopy grade by >1 in 35% of patients.[36] Video-laryngoscopy reduces cervical spine movement further and is becoming increasingly popular.[36] Rapid sequence induction with an adequate depth of anaesthesia and optimal muscle relaxation is required to facilitate tracheal intuba-tion and avoid bucking on laryngoscopy (which increases ICP) and regurgitation of gastric contents. Prevention of hypoxia and hypercapnoea during intubation are key.

Muscle relaxants such as suxamethonium (1.5 mg/kg), atracurium (0.5 mg/kg), vecur-onium (0.15 mg/kg) and rocuronium (0.6 mg/kg) have all been used satisfactorily. Vocal cord topicalisation with 4% lignocaine may reduce the risk of coughing with the endotra-cheal tube (ETT) in situ. The trachea is intubated with an armoured ETT to ensure its patency throughout the duration of surgery. Particular attention is also needed to ensure the correct length of the ETT placement to avoid accidental bronchial intubation.

Monitoring

In addition to haemodynamic monitoring, arterial CO_2 tension should be maintained between 4.5 and 5 KPa as elective prophylactic hyperventilation has been associated with adverse outcome in TBI.[38]

A single episode of hyperglycaemia (≥11.1 mmol/L) is associated with a 3.6-fold mor-tality increase in severe brain injury[39]; therefore, perioperative blood glucose levels should be monitored to avoid both hypo- and hyperglycaemia (particularly if dexamethasone is used peri-operatively).

Pyrexia is associated with long-term poor outcomes and must be treated aggressively to maintain normothermia.[40] Neuromuscular junction monitoring should be instituted.

Position

The patient should usually be in reverse Trendelenburg position to encourage adequate venous drainage. The head is either on a horseshoe or secured in pins. The haemodynamic and stress response of the pin fixation may be attenuated by scalp blocks[41] which also significantly improve post-operative pain scores following craniotomy.[42]

The arterial and central venous pressure transducers should be level with the tragus and the right atrium to reflect the respective CPP and atrial filling pressure. Eye protection, ETT position/connections, monitoring equipment attachments and accessibility of vascular access devices must be scrutinised again at this point prior to the application of surgical drape. All pressure points must be meticulously padded to avoid skin damage. Due to the high-risk nature of emergency neurosurgical patients, mechanical thromboprophylaxis (graduated compression stockings or intermittent pneumatic devices) should be considered for all cases.[43]

Maintenance

Anaesthesia can be maintained by total intravenous anaesthesia (TIVA) using propofol (and/or remifentanil) or by volatile inhalational anaesthesia. Although propofol usage has theoretical advantages (reducing CBF, ICP and $CMRO_2$ whilst preserving autoregulation and vascular reactivity), anaesthetic agents are not an independent risk factor for intraoperative brain swelling.[44]

Propofol TIVA is often administered using a Target Controlled Infusion model (often a Marsh or Schnider model) whereby an infusion pump with a built-in algorithm infuses propofol at an automated rate to achieve the user defined target site or compartment concentration. Alternatively, propofol TIVA can be delivered using a manual regimen, which is particularly useful when transferring a patient between clinical areas or when programmable infusion pumps are not available.

The Bristol regimen is described in Table 16.2.[45]

All volatile agents cause a dose-related decrease in $CMRO_2$ but an increase in CBF due to vasodilation. At <1 MAC (Minimal Alveolar Concentration) the reduction in $CMRO_2$ balances the vasodilation and CBF remains relatively constant with intact autoregulation.[46]

Maintaining MAC between 0.8 and 1 minimises these effects whilst reducing the risk of awareness.

Sodium chloride 0.9% remains the maintenance fluid of choice (osmolality = 308 mosmol/kg). Hypo-osmolar solutions should be avoided as they increase cerebral oedema formation.[47]

Intra-operative Management

It is important, even for emergency surgery, to ensure patient safety through appropriate team briefing and completion of the World Health Organization checklist. This enables

Table 16.2 The Bristol regimen for administration of propofol total intravenous anaesthesia.

Regimen of propofol	Time (min)
Commence with 1 mg/kg followed by	bolus
10 mg/kg/hour followed by	10
8 mg/kg/hour followed by	10
6 mg/kg/hour	thereafter

multidisciplinary team discussion on patient management such as administration of medications including anticonvulsants, antibiotics, hyperosmolar therapies and steroids, as well as patient positioning.

Anti-seizure prophylaxis should be considered as post-traumatic seizures (PTS) occur clinically in 12% of patients with severe brain injury and subclinically in up to 25%. Phenytoin has traditionally been used as the anticonvulsant of choice to reduce the incidence of PTS. There is insufficient evidence to recommend the use of levetiracetam over phenytoin, but there is an increasing trend towards its use as a first-line anticonvulsant due to its more favourable side effect profile.[25] Antibiotic prophylaxis is recommended according to local antimicrobial guidelines.

Hyperosmolar therapy, mannitol (0.25–1 g/kg) and hypertonic saline (3 ml/kg of 3% NaCl), are both used to reduce ICP, in part, by reducing blood viscosity and improving microcirculatory flow.[25] Evidence is emerging to suggest hypertonic saline may be more effective than manniotol,[48] though clinical uncertainty remains regarding their role in brain injury.[25]

Dexamethasone reduces tumour-associated cerebral oedema and vascular permeability as well as acting as an effective anti-emetic.[49] Concerns regarding increased post-operative infection rates have been refuted following a post-hoc analysis of the ENIGMA-II trial.[50] Of note, steroids have not been recommended for use in brain injury since a systematic review in 2005 demonstrated an increased mortality and morbidity risk.[51]

Extubation and Postoperative Care

Smooth extubation of trachea (in a reverse Trendelenburg position) must only take place if adequate respiration and stable haemodynamics are combined with a GCS comparable with pre-induction level. Pain relief can be adequately provided by paracetamol and judicious administration of intravenous opiates. Non-steroidal anti-inflammatory drugs must only be administered after careful consideration of risk benefit assessment and are avoided in the acute phase.

Postoperative vomiting following intracranial surgery can cause increase in ICP. Ondansetron 4 mg given at dural closure has been shown to reduce incidence of vomiting by 60%.[52] Supplementary oxygen therapy must be continued into the postoperative period. Euvolaemic status is the aim throughout the postoperative period as guided by clinical markers, including hourly urine output and the trend of central venous pressure. After discharge from the post-anaesthesia care unit, the patient must be transferred to a unit with appropriately trained nurses and equipment for close observation and invasive monitoring, such as a level 2 area.

In summary, anaesthesia for emergency neurosurgical patients relies on multidisciplinary teamwork, attention to detail in all aspects of perioperative anaesthetic care and a good knowledge of pathophysiology and management strategy for these patients.

References

1. National Institute for Health and Care Excellence. Head injury: assessment and early management. NICE guideline (CG176). 2014. www.nice.org.uk/guidance/cg176

2. Harrison DA, Prabhu G, Grieve R, Harvey SE, Sadique MZ, Gomes M, Griggs KA, Walmsley E, Smith M, Yeoman P, Lecky FE. Risk Adjustment In Neurocritical care (RAIN) – prospective validation of risk prediction models for adult patients with acute traumatic brain injury to use to evaluate the optimum location and comparative costs of neurocritical care: a cohort study. *Health Technol. Assessment* 2013;17(23).

3. Teasdale G, Jennett B. Assessment of coma and impaired causes: a practical scale. *The Lancet* 1974;2:81–4.

4. Werner C, Engelhard K. Pathophysiology of traumatic brain injury. *Br J Anaes* 2007;99(1):4–9.

5. Ghajar J. Traumatic brain injury. *The Lancet* 2000;356(9233):923–9.

6. Hasler RM, Exadaktylos AK, Bouamra O, Benneker LM, Clancy M, Sieber R, Zimmermann H, Lecky F. Epidemiology and predictors of cervical spine injury in adult major trauma patients: a multicenter cohort study. *J Trauma Acute Care Surg* 2012;72(4):975–81.

7. Kehoe A, Smith JE, Bouamra O, Edwards A, Yates D, Lecky F. Older patients with traumatic brain injury present with a higher GCS score than younger patients for a given severity of injury. *Emerg Med J* 2016;33(6):381–5.

8. Vespa P, Bergsneider, M, Hattori, N, Wu, H-M, Huang, S-C, Martin, NA, Glenn TC, McArthur DL, Hovda, DA. Metabolic crisis without brain ischemia is common after traumatic brain injury: a combined microdialysis and positron emission tomography study. *J Cerebral Blood Flow Metab* 2005;25 (6):763–74.

9. Prabhu M, Gupta AK. Intracranial pressure. In: Gupta AK, Summors A, eds. *Notes in neuroanaesthesia and critical care.* Greenwich Medical Media; 2001.

10. Junger EC, Newell DW, Grant GA, Avellino AM, Ghatan S, Douville CM, Lam AM, Aaslid R, Winn HR. Cerebral autoregulation following minor head injury. *J Neurosurg* 1997;86:425–32.

11. Prabhu M, Gupta AK. Cerebral blood flow. In: Gupta AK, Summors A, eds. *Notes in neuroanaesthesia and critical care.* Greenwich Medical Media; 2001.

12. Coles JP, Fryer TD, Smielewski P, et al. Incidence and mechanisms of cerebral ischaemia in early head injury. *J Cerebral Blood Flow Metab* 2003;24:202–11.

13. Menon DK. Brain ischaemia after traumatic brain injury: lessons from 1502 positron emission tomography. *Curr Opin Crit Care* 2006;12(2):85–9.

14. Robertson CS, Bell MJ, Kochanek PM, Adelson PD, Ruppel RA, Carcillo JA, Wisniewski SR, Mi Z, Janesko KL, Clark RS, Marion DW, Graham SH, Jackson EK. Increased adenosine in cerebrospinal fluid after severe traumatic brain injury in infants and children: association with severity of injury and excitotoxicity. *Crit Care Med* 2001;29:2287–3393.

15. Weber JT. Altered calcium signaling following traumatic brain injury. *Front Pharmacol* 2012;3(60):1–16.

16. Manley G, Knudson MM, Morabito D, Damron S, Erickson V, Pitts L. Hypotension, hypoxia, and head injury: frequency, duration, and consequences. *Arch Surg* 2001;136(10):1118–23.

17. Lam WH, Mackersie A. Paediatric head injury: incidence, aetiology and management. *Paediatr Anaes* 1999;9:377–85.

18. Chestnut RM, Marshall LF, Klauber MR, et al. The role of secondary brain injury in determining outcome from severe head injury. *J Trauma* 1993;34:216–22.

19. Bullock RM, Chestnut R, Clifton GL, Ghajar J, Marion DW, Narayan RK, Newell DW, Pitts LH, Rosner MJ, Walters BC, Wilberger JE. Management and prognosis of severe traumatic brain injury, part 1: Guidelines for management of severe traumatic brain injury. *J Neurotrauma* 2000;17:451–553.

20. Rosner MJ, Rosner SD, Johnson AH. Cerebral perfusion pressure: management protocol and clinical results. *J Neurosurg* 1995;83:949–62.

21. Eker C, Asgeirsson B, Grande PO, Schalen W, Nordstrom CH. Improved outcome after severe head injury with a new therapy based on principles for brain volume regulation and preserved microcirculation. *Crit Care Med* 1998;26:1881–6.

22. Grande PO, Asgeirsson B, Nordstrom CH. Physiologic principles for volume regulation of a tissue enclosed in a rigid

shell with application to the injured brain. *J Trauma Acute Care Surg* 1997;42:23–31.

23. Robertson CS, Valadka AB, Hannay HJ, Contant CF, Gopinath SP, Cormio M, Uzura M, Grossman RG. Prevention of secondary insults after severe head injury. *Crit Care Med* 1999;27:2086–95.

24. Robertson CS. Management of cerebral perfusion pressure after traumatic brain injury. *Anesthesiology* 2001;95(6):1513–17.

25. Carney NL, Totten AM, O'Reilly C, Ullman JS, Hawryluk GW, Bell MJ, Bratton SL, Chesnut R, Harris OA, Kissoon N, Rubiano AM, Shutter L, Tasker RC, Vavilala MS, Wilberger J, Wright DW, Ghajar J. Guidelines for the management of severe traumatic brain injury, fourth edition. *Neurosurgery* 2017;80(1):6–15.

26. Nguyen H, Zaroff JG. Neurogenic stunned myocardium. *Curr Neurol Neurosci Rep* 2009;9(6):486–91.

27. Arieff AI, Ayus JC, Fraser CL. Hyponatraemia and death or permanent brain damage in healthy children. *Br Med J* 1992;304:1218–22.

28. Royal College of Surgeons of England. *Report of the Working Party on the Management of Patients with Head Injuries.* London: Royal College of Surgeons of England; 1999.

29. Fountain DM, Kolias AG, Lecky FE, Bouamra O, Lawrence T, Adams H, Bond SJ, Hutchinson PJ. Survival trends after surgery for acute subdural hematoma in adults over a 20-year period. *Ann Surg* 2017;265(3):590–6.

30. Tien HC, Jung V, Pinto R, Mainprize T, Scales DC, Rizoli SB. Reducing time-to-treatment decreases mortality of trauma patients with acute subdural hematoma. *Ann Surg* 2011;253(6):1178–83.

31. Association of Anaesthetists of Great Britain and Ireland. *Recommendations for standards of monitoring during anaesthesia and recovery*, 4th edition. London: Association of Anaesthetists of Great Britain and Ireland; 2007.

32. Association of Anaesthetists of Great Britain and Ireland. *Recommendations for the safe transfer of patients with brain injury*. London: Association of Anaesthetists of Great Britain and Ireland; 2006.

33. Fukuda S, Warner DS. Cerebral protection. *Br J Anaes* 2007;99:10–17.

34. Bowles E, Gold M. Rethinking the paradigm: evaluation of ketamine as a neurosurgical anesthetic. *Am Assoc Nurse Anaesth* 2012;80(6):445–52.

35. Fodale V, Schifilliti D, Practico C, Santamaria LB. Remifentanil and the brain. *Acta Anaesth Scand* 2008;52:319–26.

36. Jung J. Airway management of patients with traumatic brain injury/C-spine injury. *Kor J Anesth* 2015;68(3):213–19.

37. National Institute for Health and Care Excellence. Spinal injury: assessment and initial management. NICE Guideline (NG41); 2016. www.nice.org.uk/guidance/ng41

38. Kochanek PM, Carney N, Adelson PD, Ashwal S, Bell MJ, Bratton S, Carson S, et al. Cerebral perfusion pressure thresholds. In: Guidelines for the acute medical management of severe traumatic brain injury in infants, children, and adolescents. 3rd edn. *Pediatric Critical Care Medicine* 2012;Supplement:24–9.

39. Griesdale DE, Tremblay MH, McEwen J, Chittock DR. Glucose control and mortality in patients with severe traumatic brain injury. *Neurocrit Care* 2009;11(3):311.

40. Badjatia N. Hyperthermia and fever control in brain injury. *Crit Care Med* 2009;37(7):250–7.

41. Geze S, Yilmaz A, Tuzuner F. The effect of scalp block and local infiltration on the haemodynamic and stress response to skull-pin placement for craniotomy. *Eur J Anaesth* 2009;26(4):298–303.

42. Guilfoyle MR, Helmy A, Duane D, Hutchinson PJ. Regional scalp block for postcraniotomy analgesia: a systematic review and meta-analysis. *Anesth Analg* 2013;116(5):1093–102.

43. Scales DC, Riva-Cambrin J, Le TL, Pinto R, Cook DJ, Granton JT. Prophylaxis against venous thromboembolism in neurointensive care patients: survey of Canadian practice. *J Crit Care* 2009;24(2): 176–84.

44. Rasmussen M, Bundgaard H, Cold GE. Craniotomy for supratentorial brain tumors: risk factors for brain swelling after opening the dura mater. *J Neurosurg* 2004;101:621–6.

45. Roberts FL, Dixon J, Lewis GTR, Tackley RM, Prys Roberts C. Induction and maintenance of propofol anaesthesia. *Anaesthesia* 1988;43: 14–17.

46. Coles J, Summors A. Inhalational anaesthetic agents. In: Gupta AK, Summors A, eds. *Notes in neuroanaesthesia and critical care.* Greenwich Medical Media; 2001.

47. Van Aken HK, Kampmeier TG, Ertmer C, Westphal M. Fluid resuscitation in patients with traumatic brain injury: what is a SAFE approach? *Curr Opin Anaesth* 2012;25 (5):563–5.

48. Kamel H, Navi BB, Nakagawa K, Hemphill III JC, Ko NU. Hypertonic saline versus mannitol for the treatment of elevated intracranial pressure: a meta-analysis of randomized clinical trials. *Crit Care Med* 2011;39(3):554–9.

49. Hockey B, Leslie K, Williams D. Dexamethasone for intracranial neurosurgery and anaesthesia. *J Clin Neurosci* 2009;16(11): 1389–93.

50. Corcoran T, Kasza J, Short TG, O'loughlin E, Chan MT, Leslie K, Forbes A, Paech M, Myles P. Intraoperative dexamethasone does not increase the risk of postoperative wound infection: a propensity score-matched post hoc analysis of the ENIGMA-II trial (EnDEX). *Br J Anaesth* 2017;118(2): 190–9.

51. Alderson P, Roberts IG. Corticosteroids for acute traumatic brain injury. *Cochrane Database Syst Rev* 2005;Issue 1: CD000196.

52. Kathirvel S, Dash HH, Bhatia A, Subramaniam B, Prakash A, Shenoy S. Effect of prophylactic ondansetron on postoperative nausea and vomiting after elective craniotomy. *J Neurosurg Anesthes* 2001;13:207–12.

Surgical Issues in the Management of Head-Injured Patients

Jane Halliday, Peter C. Whitfield and Puneet Plaha

Introduction

This chapter reviews the indications for surgical intervention and operative nuances that may facilitate neurosurgical procedures. We discuss the surgical management of patients with traumatic intracranial haematomas, depressed skull fractures, the placement of external ventricular drains and the application of decompressive craniectomy.

The overall goal of all surgical treatment is to prevent secondary injury by helping to maintain blood flow and oxygen to the brain and minimise swelling and pressure. Survival from traumatic head injury has improved significantly over the last 20 years, reflecting improved pre-hospital and neuro-intensive care management of head-injured patients, as well as the introduction of the NICE head injury guidelines in 2003, which has led to a greater number of trauma patients undergoing computed tomography (CT) of the head.[1] The initial management of patients with small subdural haematomas and/or small contusions may be conservative (see below). For those patients who require intubation and ventilation in the context of traumatic brain injury, intracranial pressure (ICP) monitoring is typically indicated.[2] The peak ICP is a powerful predictor of outcome, especially for frontal lesions.[3] The association between a sustained ICP >30 mmHg and a poor outcome is well established.[4]

Traumatic Intracranial Haematomas

Acute traumatic intracranial haematomas occur in the extradural space, the subdural space or directly into the parenchyma. They can often occur together. Although haematomas are frequently apparent within the first few hours after trauma, delayed presentation is well recognised and may present with deterioration in level of consciousness or elevation of intracranial pressure. After identifying an intracranial haematoma, a number of common factors are considered. Each of these influences decision-making and the patient's functional outcome as discussed below.

Factors Affecting Outcome

Glasgow Coma Score (GCS) at admission or prior to surgery is the single most important predictor of outcome for patients with traumatic intracranial haematoma.[5-7] Of the three GCS components, the preoperative motor score is the most reliable predictor of functional outcome.

In the absence of ocular trauma and mydriatic eye drops, pupil asymmetry is an indicator of mass effect due to compression of the oculomotor nerve. Ipsilateral mydriasis indicates uncal herniation with direct compression of the third cranial nerve. Contralateral mydriasis indicates pressure on the opposite oculomotor nerve at the medial edge of the tentorium. Such pupillary dysfunction is an indicator of brain stem compression and is associated with high mortality.[8–12] Although bilateral fixed dilated pupils and other brain stem reflexes are associated with a poor outcome,[13] exceptions may occur. Rapid surgery in patients with extradural haematomas was associated with survival in 82%: including some with favourable outcomes. No patients with bilateral fixed and dilated pupils for longer than 6 hours survived.[14] A large case series of EDH patients who underwent craniotomy reported a linear correlation between functional outcome and early surgery following the onset of anisocoria. The combined mortality/severe disability rate in 126 patients who underwent decompressive surgery within 1.5 hours was 7.9% as compared to 53.8% with a latency of 3.5–4.5 hours between the onset of pupillary asymmetry and surgery.[7]

CT findings that correlate with poor outcome are haematoma volume greater than 30 to 150 cm^3, midline shift greater than 10 mm and mixed density haematoma indicative of active bleeding.[7,10] Low attenuation regions within a clot indicate a hyperacute bleed, which may be associated with poor outcome presumably as a consequence of rapid, severe and increasing elevation of intracranial pressure.[10,15] The location of a haematoma appears to be less important at determining outcome than the volume and time delay to theatre.[10] The presence of intracranial lesions such as contusions and subarachnoid haemorrhage are understandably associated with poorer outcomes in patients with traumatic brain injuries and intracerebral haematomas.[7,10,16] CT scan findings that suggest surgical intervention should be undertaken are discussed separately for the different intracranial haematomas.

For patients with extradural haematomas that require surgical management, time to surgery affects outcome. An 8.9% mortality is reported if surgery is performed within 2.4 ± 0.6 hours and 33.3% if surgery was delayed by 9.8 ± 6.1 hours from the time of deterioration.[15] The reported outcomes of the effects of different timings for evacuation of acute SDH are variable in the literature. A large study looking at 2498 patients with acute SDH found that the time interval from injury to craniotomy and direct admission to a neurosurgical unit had no significant effect on prognosis.[1] However, historical studies report an improvement in outcomes with shorter time to surgery (2–4 hours).[17,18] The heterogeneity of the primary neurological injuries, may account for the differences in outcomes in these studies.[19,20]

Raised intracranial pressure (ICP) post-operatively is associated with a poorer outcome from surgically managed extradural haematomas, indicating underlying brain injury.[21]

The probability of a good outcome decreases with increasing patient age[8] with mortality rates increasing exponentially and the chance of survival with good functional outcome low in those over 70.[1,22] Evacuation of acute haematomas in this latter age group is therefore probably not justified except in exceptional circumstances.[23]

Pre-existing medical conditions including cardiovascular and respiratory dysfunction have been shown to be associated with poor outcome presumably due to the interplay amongst cerebral perfusion, microcirculatory function and tissue hypoxia leading to secondary brain injury in addition to increased susceptibility to the complications of prolonged immobilisation.[24,25]

Many patients who present with TBI, surgically or conservatively managed, have clotting abnormalities, often secondary to regular anticoagulant/antiplatelet medications. Close discussion with haematologists is necessary to reverse clotting deficiencies in a rapid, timely manner. Patients treated with warfarin are typically administered with intravenous vitamin K and prothrombin complex concentrate (PCC) if surgery is required.[26] Novel oral anticoagulants include dabigatran, a direct thrombin inhibitor and the Xa inhibitors rivaroxaban and apixiban. They have reversal strategies that vary according to their mechanism of action. Four factor PCC can be used for Xa inhibitor reversal and a reversal agent idarcuzimab has been approved for the emergent reversal of dabigatran.[27]

Extradural Haematomas (EDH)

EDHs have a prevalence of 1%–4% of patients in patients with moderate or severe TBI,[28] peaking in the second decade of life.[29] EDH in patients over 60 years of age is rare, due the adherence of the dura to skull. Associated skull fractures are present in 75%–95% of patients. EDH in adults is most commonly due to middle meningeal artery injury (over 80% of cases).[28] More rarely EDH can occur in the anterior cranial fossa due to rupture of the anterior meningeal artery, and in approximately 15% of cases can be secondary to injury to the dural sinuses.[28] The classical presentation of patients with an EDH comprises a lucid interval followed by a rapid neurological deterioration and occurs in about 50% of cases.[28] On computed tomography (CT) of the head, the most widely used imaging study in trauma due to its speed, ease and widespread availability,[30] extradural haematomas have a lens-shaped pattern because collection of blood is limited by dural attachments at the cranial sutures[28] (Figure 17.1). The haematoma volume can be estimated quickly from the head CT scan by using the formula ABC/2, where A is the greatest haemorrhage diameter on the CT slice with the largest area of haemorrhage, B is the diameter at 90° to A on the same CT slice and C the approximate number of CT slices with haemorrhage multiplied by the slice thickness in centimetres.[31]

Neurologically intact patients with small extradural haematomas can be successfully managed conservatively.[32,33] However, most authors would advocate surgery as the safest option if haematoma volume > 30 cm^3,[8,34] clot thickness >15 mm and midline shift exceeds 4 or 5 mm.[34,35] Close neuro-observations should be performed on conservatively managed patients, with a first follow-up CT scan obtained 6 to 8 hours after head injury.[28]

Urgent surgery is recommended for patients with neurological deterioration, a haematoma >30 cm^3 or midline shift >5 mm.

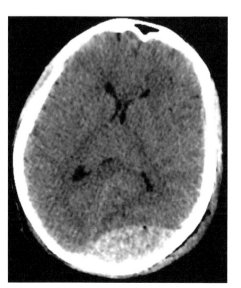

Figure 17.1 CT head scan showing evidence of an occipital extradural haematoma secondary to a head injury from a road traffic accident. The patient required an operation and made a full neurological recovery.

Surgical Technique

Extradural haematomas are most frequently located in the fronto-temporo-parietal and temporal regions and are best accessed via a question mark-shaped scalp flap and craniotomy, whose location and size can be adapted according to the pathology. Reconstruction of any associated vault fractures needs consideration during elevation of the flap. The initial burr hole alone can be used to achieve a rapid initial decompression. Suction and irrigation facilitate removal of an extradural haematoma. Bipolar diathermy controls any continuing middle meningeal bleeding, whilst bleeding at the skull base can be controlled by packing the foramen spinosum region with bone wax and oxidised cellulose followed by placement of dural hitch stitches.

Acute Subdural Haematomas

Acute subdural haematomas (aSDH) form between the dura and the arachnoid membranes, typically caused by tearing of bridging veins from brain surface to dural sinuses (Figure 17.2). Venous bleeding typically stops due to tamponade. Approximately 20% are caused by arterial rupture, typically due to injury of small cortical arteries.[36,37]

aSDH are commonly seen in two settings:

1   High-velocity trauma, associated with severe underlying brain parenchymal injury.
2   Minor trauma in elderly patients on anticoagulants.

Compared to isolated EDH, the degree of underlying brain damage associated with aSDH is typically more severe,[17] in part explaining the poorer outcomes than for EDH.

Conservative Management

Patients with small haematomas of less than 10 mm depth can be managed conservatively, even if they are in a coma, provided that there is no evidence of mass effect or of elevated intracranial pressure (ICP).[38] As there is a high incidence of clot expansion during the first

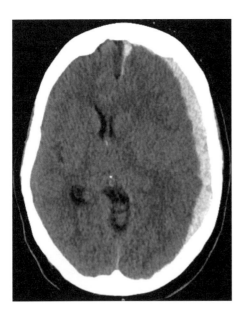

Figure 17.2 A CT head scan revealing evidence of an acute subdural haematoma with midline shift, secondary to a fall down a flight of stairs. The patient required urgent surgical evaluation and decompressive craniectomy due to significant cerebral oedema.

36 hours from injury, it is recommended that a repeat scan be performed after 6–8 hours: in some cases further scans may be required due to clinical concerns.[39,40]

Surgical intervention is recommended for patients with aSDH with clot thickness greater than 10 mm, and/or midline shift greater than 5 mm, regardless of GCS score.[36] Indications for surgery for patients with clot thickness/midline shift less than this include a decline in GCS with no other cause found, ICP greater than 20 mmHg despite medical management and/or asymmetrical or fixed and dilated pupils.[41,42]

Surgical Technique

Surgery for aSDH is typically performed via a large frontotemporoparietal approach, with or without bone flap removal and duraplasty. The technique is similar to that described for the extradural approach, with the exception that the dura must be opened to evacuate the subdural.[41] An intracranial pressure (ICP) monitor should be placed to help guide subsequent neuro-intensive care management. Consideration should be given to decompressive craniectomy if there is significant swelling. The Rescue – aSDH trial aims to evaluate the clinical and cost-effectiveness of decompressive craniectomy versus craniotomy in this group of patients.[43]

Chronic Subdural Haematomas

Five thousand people are diagnosed with chronic subdural haematomas (CSDH) in the UK every year,[44] with a morbidity rate of 10%–14%.[45] Many probably develop from acute subdural haematomas although in some cases such pathology was not evident on an initial scan.[46] As CSDH develop they liquefy and enlarge; the larger the clot the greater the chance of expansion.[47] They are more commonly found in patients with cerebral atrophy who are vulnerable to mild TBI including the elderly and alcoholics.[46] Any lesion causing mass effect (size of 10 mm or more, or greater than 5 mm midline shift) and neurological features warrants surgical treatment in those patients with potential to improve (Figure 17.3). Ideally, for those patients on anti-platelet medications, surgery will be postponed for 5–7 days from stopping the medications to reduce bleeding and recurrence risk. Other anti-coagulants should be reversed prior to operation although for novel anticoagulants this is an incomplete reversal. Conservatively managed patients can be managed with regular review and follow-up scans as necessary. Those on anti-platelet medications are typically advised to stop until resolution of CSDH,[48] but this must be a risk benefit decision. There is a randomised multi-centre trial under way looking at the effects of a 2 week course of dexamethasone for adult patients with a symptomatic (Dex-CSDH trial);[44] some observational studies suggest there may be a benefit.[49]

Surgical Techniques

Two appropriately positioned burr holes placed along the same line as the incision of a trauma flap enable evacuation of most chronic subdural haematomas. Burr-hole evacuation is associated with a low recurrence and complication rate.[50,51] Control of dural bleeding is important. A distinctive grey encapsulating membrane usually requires opening to permit drainage of the liquefied haematoma. This is often under considerable initial pressure. Irrigation of the subdural space, facilitated by the use of a soft Jacques catheter, is effective. Occasionally, conversion to a craniotomy is required if a substantial solid component persists. A craniotomy also permits fluid evacuation and partial removal of the haematoma membrane in patients with recurrent, symptomatic chronic subdural haematomas.[52] A valveless subdural–peritoneal conduit fashioned from a peritoneal catheter with side holes cut for the subdural

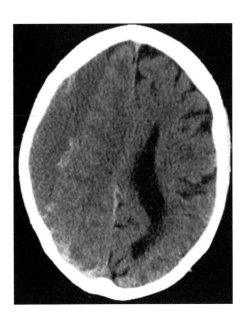

Figure 17.3 CT head demonstrating a large chronic subdural with mass effect and midline shift. The patient underwent burrhole drainage of subdural and made a full neurological recovery.

space and securely anchored to the galea can be useful in the treatment of patients with an atrophic brain where persistence of the subdural collection occurs despite recent drainage.

There is a risk of recurrence of chronic subdurals, reported between 5% and 33% after surgery.[53,54] Consequently there have been many studies looking at factors for recurrence. Older age, thicker haematoma width, bilateral presentation, diabetes mellitus and preoperative seizures have been linked to higher rates of recurrence.[52,55] Evidence supporting the use of intraoperative irrigation to lower the recurrence rate[56] is not universal.[57,58] There is evidence that leaving a postoperative closed subdural drainage system for 24–48 hours is associated with reduced recurrence rates.[54,59] Post-operatively some authors advocate a 30° head up position, others a sitting position and some early mobilisation to minimise the medical complications of bed rest. Overall the balance of evidence seems to support a 30° head up position post-operatively (1–2 days), reducing the complications of flat bed rest while avoiding the increased risks of recurrence with early mobilisation.[60,61] Whether patients can resume antiplatelet and anticoagulant therapy after SDH is a common question. Clinical decision-making relies on analysis of risks and benefits in individual patients, and general recommendations cannot be made.

Intracerebral Haematomas

Intracerebral haematomas (also known as contusions) are common in traumatic brain injury. There is a wide range of severity associated with cerebral contusion from small punctate contusions in mild traumatic brain injuries with no significant clinical effects to large haemorrhagic contusions with significant mass effect which carry high risks of mortality and morbidity (Figure 17.4). Those patients with reduced conscious levels secondary to a contusional brain injury should be monitored with an intracranial pressure (ICP) monitor, as elevated ICP is associated with increased mortality and worsened outcomes.[4] Parenchymal lesions are dynamic. An increase in size of pre-existing lesions or appearance of new non-contiguous lesions commonly occurs especially within the first

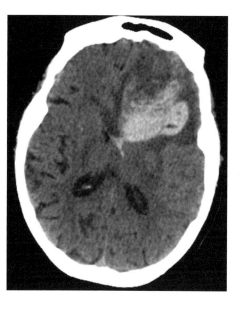

Figure 17.4 CT head demonstrating a large intracerebral haemorrhage secondary to trauma in a patient on anti-platelet medications. The patient was successfully managed with an intracranial pressure monitor and medical management of their intracranial pressure on intensive care.

24–48 hours.[62] In addition, delayed traumatic intracerebral haematoma (DTICH) or space demanding contusions may develop in patients with diffuse injury on the initial scans.[63,64] Clotting abnormalities are associated with this complication.[65] Repeat CT scanning is therefore an important consideration in managing traumatic brain injury patients.[66] If detected early, the high mortality of unrecognised DTICH may be averted.[67]

Given the potential for change, conservative management of traumatic intraparenchymal brain injury requires careful supervision. Given this caveat, a conservative approach is sometimes appropriate:

1. Patients with small parenchymal mass lesions, and no radiological signs of significant mass effect (midline shift <5 mm, no basal cistern effacement) who consistently obey commands and harbour no neurological deficits.
2. ICP monitoring is appropriate for patients who do not obey commands when the initial CT scan shows small parenchymal lesions without significant mass effect.

A mean hourly ICP > 30 mm Hg[68] or a repeat CT scan showing an increase in haematoma/contusion volume with signs of mass effect[3] supports surgical intervention.

Early surgery is recommended for patients with a presenting GCS of > 6 and focal lesion volume > 20 cm^3 and those with temporal contusions with CT scan showing signs of mass effect and GCS >10.[69] It is also indicated for patients with low GCS and with midline shift of at least 5 mm and/or cisternal compression on CT scan[70] and for those intubated patients who fail medical management of their ICP who had significant mass effect from the contusion on their scan. In the posterior fossa surgical evacuation is recommended when there is evidence of significant mass effect; distortion or obliteration of the fourth ventricle or obstructive hydrocephalus.[71]

Surgical Technique

The location and extent of the contusion/haematoma on the CT scan governs the position of the scalp flap. For a supratentorial haemorrhage a large flap provides adequate exposure of contused and haemorrhagic brain and permits an effective decompressive craniectomy, if required. Three-point skull fixation facilitates intra-operative adjustments of head position and provides a more stable platform for undertaking a craniotomy, as well as allowing for use of a fixed retractor system if required. Elevation of the head by 20°–30° helps to control ICP and reduces venous bleeding. Swollen, contused and haemorrhagic brain is removed using gentle suction and bipolar diathermy. For severe polar injury, a temporal or frontal lobectomy (6 cm from the temporal pole and 7 cm from the frontal pole) may enable adequate decompression. Bipolar diathermy coagulates larger bleeding vessels. A monolayer of Surgicel™ coated with cottonoids and packed with saline-soaked cotton balls for 5 min controls small vessel bleeding from exposed dissected brain. The operating microscope facilitates this stage of the procedure. Any uncertainty about haemostasis leads to re-examination of the cavity. Capillary tube drainage of the cavity reliably helps to prevent secondary clots developing in difficult cases. During closure, prophylactic removal of the bone flap to facilitate the management of post-operative brain swelling is considered. In such cases, subgaleal suction drainage may cause brain shift leading to bradycardia and cardiac arrest and should be avoided. A capillary or non-suction drain is preferred in these circumstances. A standard colostomy bag applied over an exiting capillary drain collects drainage products.

Subarachnoid Haemorrhage

Subarachnoid haemorrhage (SAH) is bleeding that occurs between the arachnoid and pia mater, which is normally filled with cerebrospinal fluid (Figure 17.5). Traumatic SAH (tSAH) is typically identified by the clinical setting. Radiologically it often appears as focal bleeding in superficial sulci, is associated with cerebral contusions and external evidence of head injury or the presence of a skull fracture.[72] If there is doubt about the cause of a SAH a CT angiogram may be indicated to rule out an aneurysmal cause. Typically tSAH is managed non-surgically. In the context of mild TBI the recovery is often full. Severe tSAH is a poor prognostic indicator.

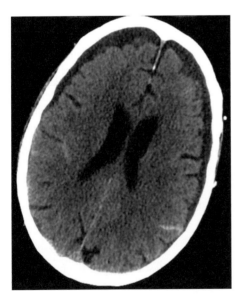

Figure 17.5 CT head in an elderly patient who suffered a minor head injury from a fall, with consequent traumatic subarachnoid blood in a characteristic pattern for traumatic SAH in the superficial sulci. Note the presence of bilateral subdural hygromas.

Intractable Intracranial Hypertension

In adults intracranial pressure is normally ≤15 mmHg, pathologic intracranial hypertension (ICH) is present at pressures ≥20 mmHg. ICP can be elevated even in the setting of a normal initial CT, demonstrating the importance of invasive monitoring in high-risk patients (e.g. those requiring intubation and ventilation for low conscious level following TBI).[73]

Intracranial Pressure Monitor

Intracranial pressure monitors can be intraventricular, intraparenchymal, subarachnoid, and epidural. Intraventricular monitors are regarded as a 'gold standard', but are associated with higher rate of infection, reported at rates of up to 20%.[74] Intraparenchymal devices are most commonly used, consisting of a thin cable with an electronic or fibre-optic transducer at the tip. These monitors can be inserted directly into the brain parenchyma via a small hole drilled in the skull, usually right frontal at Kocher's point. They carry a low risk of infection and haemorrhage (<1%), compared with intraventricular devices[75] and are often placed at the bedside of patients in Intensive Care Units. The ICP normally exhibits a cyclical variation with its waveform a modified arterial pressure trace. When ICP is raised and cerebral compliance reduced its waveform changes, signifying decompensation of autoregulatory mechanisms,[76] and thus the need for intervention.

   The best therapy for intracranial hypertension is resolution of the cause of elevated ICP, as discussed in earlier sections. When there is no such focal target and medical therapy fails, for example in patients with diffuse axonal injury and secondary cerebral oedema, surgical measures include placement of an external ventricular drain to remove cerebrospinal fluid (CSF) or decompressive craniectomy. Both are outlined below. A lumbar drain is generally contraindicated in the setting of high ICP due to the risk of transtentorial herniation.

External Ventricular Drain (EVD)

The reduction of intracranial pressure by placement of a catheter into the frontal horn of the lateral ventricle for cerebrospinal fluid drainage is well established. The technique can be used as an early therapeutic manoeuvre or reserved for patients with refractory intracranial hypertension. In addition, ventricular pressure monitoring is considered the 'gold standard' for ICP measurement. However, the simplicity of intraparenchymal ICP monitoring using robust hardware has superseded ventricular pressure monitoring in many centres.

Surgical Technique

The patient is positioned with 30° head up tilt. Insertion is usually performed on the right side (non-dominant) although, if unilateral hemisphere swelling is evident, ipsilateral placement is advisable to avoid further mid-line shift. A linear incision is performed with a twist drill or burr hole at Kocher's point (1 cm anterior to the coronal suture and in the mid-pupillary line). The catheter, inserted complete with stylet, is directed medially – aiming for the ipsilateral medial canthus – and slightly posteriorly in the sagittal plane – directed at the tragus. A loss of resistance is experienced on entering the ventricle at a depth of 5–6 cm. Withdrawal of the stylet is followed by egress of CSF. If the ventricle is not tapped at a depth of 7 cm, removal and reinsertion in a more medial direction is usually successful. Deeper insertion of the catheter leads to misplacement. Subcutaneous tunnelling for a distance of at least 6 or 7 cm minimises the risk of infection. A '360° loop' of catheter securely anchored to the scalp in two places effectively reduces the risk of inadvertent catheter removal. The distal end is connected to a manometric EVD drainage system.

Decompressive Craniectomy

Decompressive craniectomy is performed to increase the volume of space available for a post-traumatic swollen brain, circumventing the Monro-Kellie doctrine. It may be performed either as a prophylactic measure after haematoma evacuation when brain swelling is anticipated, or as a therapeutic manoeuvre for the management of raised intracranial pressure. Prophylactic decompressive craniectomy is performed where the brain is considered to be at risk of swelling after evacuation of a mass lesion.

There have been many trials looking at outcomes from decompressive craniectomy for TBI. In 2011 results were published on the multicentre, randomised, controlled Decompressive Craniectomy (DECRA) trial, in which the outcomes of decompressive craniectomy in adults under the age of 60 years with TBI in whom ICP was not controlled with first-tier intensive care and neurosurgical therapies. It found that while decompressive craniectomy reduced ICP, duration of ventilation and ICU stay it was associated with a significantly worse outcome at 6 months than those patients medically managed.[77] Concerns were raised that these results reflected the use of decompressive craniectomy as an early-tier intervention.[78] Consequently a further international, multicentre, randomised trial (RESCUE-ICP) was performed, examining outcomes from decompressive craniectomy as a last-tier intervention for severe and refractory intracranial hypertension. It concluded that decompressive craniectomy for severe and refractory intracranial hypertension after TBI, as a last-tier measure, resulted in 22% less mortality at 6 months than with best medical management. Surgically managed patients had higher rates of vegetative state and severe disability than medical management. Rates of moderate disability and good recovery with surgery were similar to those with medical management.[78] Knowledge of the outcome of these trials is important when discussing options with family members.

Surgical Techniques

Therapeutic decompressive craniectomy is most effectively performed as a large bifrontal bone flap, although some recommend a unilateral approach if the CT appearances show swelling of only one hemisphere. A bicoronal skin flap permits exposure of the frontal bone. The craniotomy extends from the supra-orbital ridge to the anterior aspect of the coronal suture. To reduce contamination, entry into the frontal air sinus is avoided by careful study of the pre-operative CT scans. Laterally, the flap extends to the temporal bone. If temporal lobe swelling is evident, the bone flap should extend towards the zygomatic arch. Bleeding from the superior sagittal sinus is not usually problematic and can be controlled with elevation of the head and application of haemostatic sponge. If the dura is opened bilaterally with a medial base on each side, the interhemispheric fissure can be explored to permit division of the falx cerebri and the anterior sagittal sinus. Craniectomy alone has been found to lower ICP by on average 15%, but that additionally opening the dura results in an average decrease in ICP of 70%.[79] A frontal periosteal flap assists closure, although a watertight approximation is not required. A non-suction wound drain can be placed, minimising post-operative subgaleal collections. If a favourable outcome is achieved, a delayed cranioplasty procedure is performed.

Depressed Skull Fractures

Skull fractures are classified by (a) the integrity of the scalp (open or closed), (b) the anatomical location (convexity of skull or basal) and (c) the pattern of fracture (linear, depressed or comminuted). All open fractures require thorough debridement to minimise the risk of infection, and careful patient examination should be performed. In the case of penetrating injury, removal of any accessible debris (e.g. pellets, bullets) minimises the infection risk, as well as closure of the open wound. For patients with bullet wounds aggressive early surgical debridement of entrance and exit wounds, removal of necrotic material and accessible bone and metal fragments is considered mandatory.[80] Cosmesis can be an indication for surgical management. Fractures near the major venous sinuses pose special problems due to the risk of bleeding during disimpaction and the risk of thrombotic sinus occlusion if the depressed fragment remains *in situ*.[81,82] Although the removal of impacted fragments from brain is unlikely to improve any neurological deficit, many consider this a relative indication for surgery. Compound depressed fractures in cosmetically unobtrusive sites may be managed with debridement alone, if there is no clinical or radiological evidence of dural violation (exposed brain/CSF leak or pneumocephalus) and if the degree of depression is less than the depth of the skull.[83] It is now accepted that inaccessible in-driven bone and metallic fragments may be safely left *in situ* to minimise collateral brain damage caused by surgery. Although there are no large randomised trials, antimicrobial prophylaxis is recommended for patients with penetrating craniocerebral trauma. Local microbiology advice should be sought.

Surgical Techniques

Devitalised or contaminated edges of the scalp require excision and thorough debridement. The impacted depressed fragments usually require placement of an adjacent burr hole to permit disimpaction. Fragments are levered upward sufficient to examine the underlying dura. Visualisation of the dura frequently requires removal of the fragments. In the presence of a dural tear the underlying brain requires inspection to permit removal of accessible penetrating bone and fragments of contaminated material. Any cortical bleeding requires attention. A periosteal graft helps repair the dural tear. Bone fragments require thorough irrigation with saline and/or dilute hydrogen peroxide solution. Mini-fixation systems facilitate the re-implantation of large fragments.

References

1. Fountain DM, Kolias AG, Lecky FE, et al. Survival trends after surgery for acute subdural hematoma in adults over a 20-year period. *Ann Surg* 2017;265:590–6. doi:10.1097/SLA.0000000000001682

2. Le Roux P. Intracranial pressure monitoring and management. In: Laskowitz D, Grant G, eds. *Translational research in traumatic brain injury*. Boca Raton, FL: CRC Press/Taylor and Francis Group; 2016. www.ncbi.nlm.nih.gov/books/NBK326713/

3. Bullock R, Golek J, Blake G. Traumatic intracerebral hematoma–which patients should undergo surgical evacuation? CT scan features and ICP monitoring as a basis for decision making. *Surg Neurol* 1989;32:181–7.

4. Badri S, Chen J, Barber J, et al. Mortality and long-term functional outcome associated with intracranial pressure after traumatic brain injury. *Intensive Care Med* 2012;38:1800–9. doi:10.1007/s00134-012-2655-4

5. Uzan M, Yentür E, Hanci M, et al. Is it possible to recover from uncal herniation? Analysis of 71 head injured cases. *J Neurosurg Sci* 1998;42:89–94.

6. Kuday C, Uzan M, Hanci M. Statistical analysis of the factors affecting the outcome

of extradural haematomas: 115 cases. *Acta Neurochir (Wien)* 1994;131:203–6.

7. Lee EJ, Hung YC, Wang LC, et al. Factors influencing the functional outcome of patients with acute epidural hematomas: analysis of 200 patients undergoing surgery. *J Trauma* 1998;45:946–52.

8. van den Brink WA, Zwienenberg M, Zandee SM, et al. The prognostic importance of the volume of traumatic epidural and subdural haematomas revisited. *Acta Neurochir (Wien)* 1999;141:509–14.

9. Bricolo AP, Pasut LM. Extradural hematoma: toward zero mortality: a prospective study. *Neurosurgery* 1984;14:8–12.

10. Rivas JJ, Lobato RD, Sarabia R, et al. Extradural hematoma: analysis of factors influencing the courses of 161 patients. *Neurosurgery* 1988;23:44–51.

11. Cohen JE, Montero A, Israel ZH. Prognosis and clinical relevance of anisocoria-craniotomy latency for epidural hematoma in comatose patients. *J Trauma* 1996;41:120–2.

12. Lobato RD, Cordobes F, Rivas JJ, et al. Outcome from severe head injury related to the type of intracranial lesion. A computerized tomography study. *J Neurosurg* 1983;59:762–74. doi:10.3171/ jns.1983.59.5.0762

13. Caroli M, Locatelli M, Campanella R, et al. Multiple intracranial lesions in head injury: clinical considerations, prognostic factors, management, and results in 95 patients. *Surg Neurol* 2001;56:82–8.

14. Sakas DE, Bullock MR, Teasdale GM. One-year outcome following craniotomy for traumatic hematoma in patients with fixed dilated pupils. *J Neurosurg* 1995;82:961–5. doi:10.3171/jns.1995.82.6.0961

15. Mendelow AD, Karmi MZ, Paul KS, et al. Extradural haematoma: effect of delayed treatment. *Br Med J* 1979;1:1240–2.

16. Haselsberger K, Pucher R, Auer LM. Prognosis after acute subdural or epidural haemorrhage. *Acta Neurochir (Wien)* 1988;90:111–16.

17. Wilberger JE, Harris M, Diamond DL. Acute subdural hematoma: morbidity, mortality, and operative timing. *J Neurosurg* 1991;74:212–18. doi:10.3171/ jns.1991.74.2.0212

18. Seelig JM, Becker DP, Miller JD, et al. Traumatic acute subdural hematoma: major mortality reduction in comatose patients treated within four hours. *N Engl J Med* 1981;304:1511–18. doi:10.1056/NEJM198106183042503

19. Tien HCN, Jung V, Pinto R, et al. Reducing time-to-treatment decreases mortality of trauma patients with acute subdural hematoma. *Ann Surg* 2011;253:1178–83. doi:10.1097/SLA.0b013e318217e339

20. Dent DL, Croce MA, Menke PG, et al. Prognostic factors after acute subdural hematoma. *J Trauma* 1995;39:36–42; discussion 42–3.

21. Heinzelmann M, Platz A, Imhof HG. Outcome after acute extradural haematoma, influence of additional injuries and neurological complications in the ICU. *Injury* 1996;27:345–9.

22. Cagetti B, Cossu M, Pau A, et al. The outcome from acute subdural and epidural intracranial haematomas in very elderly patients. *Br J Neurosurg* 1992;6:227–31.

23. Jamjoom A. Justification for evacuating acute subdural haematomas in patients above the age of 75 years. *Injury* 1992;23:518–20.

24. Choksey M, Crockard HA, Sandilands M. Acute traumatic intracerebral haematomas: determinants of outcome in a retrospective series of 202 cases. *Br J Neurosurg* 1993;7:611–22.

25. Servadei F, Murray GD, Penny K, et al. The value of the 'worst' computed tomographic scan in clinical studies of moderate and severe head injury. European Brain Injury Consortium. *Neurosurgery* 2000;46:70–5; discussion 75–7.

26. Cartmill M, Dolan G, Byrne JL, et al. Prothrombin complex concentrate for oral anticoagulant reversal in neurosurgical

emergencies. *Br J Neurosurg* 2000;14:458–61.

27. Pollack CV, Reilly PA, van Ryn J, et al. Idarucizumab for dabigatran reversal – full cohort analysis. *N Engl J Med* 2017;377:431–41. doi:10.1056/ NEJMoa1707278

28. Bullock MR, Chesnut R, Ghajar J, et al. Surgical management of acute epidural hematomas. *Neurosurgery* 2006;58:S7–15; discussion i–iv.

29. Jones NR, Molloy CJ, Kloeden CN, et al. Extradural haematoma: trends in outcome over 35 years. *Br J Neurosurg* 1993;7:465–71.

30. Grossman RI. Head trauma. In: *Neuroradiology: the requisites.* Philadelphia: Mosby; 2003.

31. Kothari RU, Brott T, Broderick JP, et al. The ABCs of measuring intracerebral hemorrhage volumes. *Stroke* 1996;27:1304–5.

32. Cucciniello B, Martellotta N, Nigro D, et al. Conservative management of extradural haematomas. *Acta Neurochir (Wien)* 1993;120:47–52.

33. Bullock R, Smith RM, van Dellen JR. Nonoperative management of extradural hematoma. *Neurosurgery* 1985;16:602–6.

34. Bejjani GK, Donahue DJ, Rusin J, et al. Radiological and clinical criteria for the management of epidural hematomas in children. *Pediatr Neurosurg* 1996;25:302–8.

35. Servadei F, Faccani G, Roccella P, et al. Asymptomatic extradural haematomas: results of a multicenter study of 158 cases in minor head injury. *Acta Neurochir (Wien)* 1989;96:39–45.

36. Gennarelli TA, Thibault LE. Biomechanics of acute subdural hematoma. *J Trauma* 1982;22:680–6.

37. Maxeiner H, Wolff M. Pure subdural hematomas: a postmortem analysis of their form and bleeding points. *Neurosurgery* 2002;50:503–8; discussion 508–9.

38. Mathew P, Oluoch-Olunya DL, Condon BR, et al. Acute subdural haematoma in the conscious patient: outcome with initial non-operative management. *Acta Neurochir (Wien)* 1993;121:100–8.

39. Givner A, Gurney J, O'Connor D, et al. Reimaging in pediatric neurotrauma: factors associated with progression of intracranial injury. *J Pediatr Surg* 2002;37:381–5.

40. Oertel M, Kelly DF, McArthur D, et al. Progressive hemorrhage after head trauma: predictors and consequences of the evolving injury. *J Neurosurg* 2002;96:109–16. doi:10.3171/ jns.2002.96.1.0109

41. Bullock MR, Chesnut R, Ghajar J, et al. Surgical management of acute subdural hematomas. *Neurosurgery* 2006;58:S16–24; discussion i–iv.

42. Servadei F, Nasi MT, Cremonini AM, et al. Importance of a reliable admission Glasgow Coma Scale score for determining the need for evacuation of posttraumatic subdural hematomas: a prospective study of 65 patients. *J Trauma* 1998;44: 868–73.

43. Rescue ASDH. www.rescueasdh.org

44. dex-CSDH Trial. www.dexcsdh.org

45. Brennan PM, Kolias AG, Joannides AJ, et al. The management and outcome for patients with chronic subdural hematoma: a prospective, multicenter, observational cohort study in the United Kingdom. *J Neurosurg* 2017;127:732–9. doi:10.3171/ 2016.8.JNS16134

46. Mayer S, Rowland L. Head injury. In: *Merritt's Neurology.* Philadelphia: Lippincott Williams & Wilkins; 2000.

47. Labadie EL, Glover D. Physiopathogenesis of subdural hematomas. Part 1: Histological and biochemical comparisons of subcutaneous hematoma in rats with subdural hematoma in man. *J Neurosurg* 1976;45:382–92. doi:10.3171/jns.1976.45.4.0382

48. Yadav Y, Parihar V, Namdev H, et al. Chronic subdural hematoma. *Asian J Neurosurg* 2016;11:330. doi:10.4103/1793-5482.145102

49. Berghauser Pont LME, Dirven CMF, Dippel DWJ, et al. The role of corticosteroids in the management of chronic subdural hematoma: a systematic review. *Eur J Neurol* 2012;19:1397–403. doi:10.1111/j.1468-1331.2012.03768.x

50. Krupa M. Comparison of two surgical methods as to early results in chronic subdural hematoma. *Ann Acad Med Stetin* 2009;55:39–47.

51. Lega BC, Danish SF, Malhotra NR, et al. Choosing the best operation for chronic subdural hematoma: a decision analysis. *J Neurosurg* 2010;113:615–21. doi:10.3171/2009.9.JNS08825

52. Markwalder TM. Chronic subdural hematomas: a review. *J Neurosurg* 1981;54:637–45. doi:10.3171/jns.1981.54.5.0637

53. Chon K-H, Lee J-M, Koh E-J, et al. Independent predictors for recurrence of chronic subdural hematoma. *Acta Neurochir (Wien)* 2012;154:1541–8. doi:10.1007/s00701-012-1399-9

54. Santarius T, Qureshi HU, Sivakumaran R, et al. The role of external drains and peritoneal conduits in the treatment of recurrent chronic subdural hematoma. *World Neurosurg* 2010;73:747–50. doi:10.1016/j.wneu.2010.03.031

55. Oh H-J, Lee K-S, Shim J-J, et al. Postoperative course and recurrence of chronic subdural hematoma. *J Korean Neurosurg Soc* 2010;48:518–23. doi:10.3340/jkns.2010.48.6.518

56. Aoki N. Subdural tapping and irrigation for the treatment of chronic subdural hematoma in adults. *Neurosurgery* 1984;14:545–8.

57. Suzuki K, Sugita K, Akai T, et al. Treatment of chronic subdural hematoma by closed-system drainage without irrigation. *Surg Neurol* 1998;50:231–4.

58. Benzel EC, Bridges RM, Hadden TA, et al. The single burr hole technique for the evacuation of non-acute subdural hematomas. *J Trauma* 1994;36:190–4.

59. Santarius T, Kirkpatrick PJ, Ganesan D, et al. Use of drains versus no drains after burr-hole evacuation of chronic subdural haematoma: a randomised controlled trial. *Lancet Lond Engl* 2009;374:1067–73. doi:10.1016/S0140-6736(09)61115-6

60. Ishfaq A, Ahmed I, Bhatti SH. Effect of head positioning on outcome after burr hole craniostomy for chronic subdural haematoma. *J Coll Physicians Surg–Pak JCPSP* 2009;19:492–5. doi:08.2009/JCPSP.492495

61. Abouzari M, Rashidi A, Rezaii J, et al. The role of postoperative patient posture in the recurrence of traumatic chronic subdural hematoma after burr-hole surgery. *Neurosurgery* 2007;61:794–7; discussion 797. doi:10.1227/01.NEU.0000298908.94129.67

62. Yamaki T, Hirakawa K, Ueguchi T, et al. Chronological evaluation of acute traumatic intracerebral haematoma. *Acta Neurochir (Wien)* 1990;103:112–5.

63. Gentleman D, Nath F, Macpherson P. Diagnosis and management of delayed traumatic intracerebral haematomas. *Br J Neurosurg* 1989;3:367–72.

64. Sprick C, Bettag M, Bock WJ. Delayed traumatic intracranial hematomas–clinical study of seven years. *Neurosurg Rev* 1989;12 Suppl 1:228–30.

65. Kaufman HH, Moake JL, Olson JD, et al. Delayed and recurrent intracranial hematomas related to disseminated intravascular clotting and fibrinolysis in head injury. *Neurosurgery* 1980;7:445–9.

66. Durham SR, Liu KC, Selden NR. Utility of serial computed tomography imaging in pediatric patients with head trauma. *J Neurosurg* 2006;105:365–9. doi:10.3171/ped.2006.105.5.365

67. Tseng SH. Delayed traumatic intracerebral hemorrhage: a study of prognostic factors. *J Formos Med Assoc Taiwan Yi Zhi* 1992;91:585–9.

68. Gallbraith S, Teasdale G. Predicting the need for operation in the patient with an occult traumatic intracranial hematoma. *J Neurosurg* 1981;55:75–81. doi:10.3171/jns.1981.55.1.0075

69. Mathiesen T, Kakarieka A, Edner G. Traumatic intracerebral lesions without extracerebral haematoma in 218 patients. *Acta Neurochir (Wien)* 1995;137:155–63; discussion 163.

70. Bullock MR, Chesnut R, Ghajar J, et al. Surgical management of traumatic parenchymal lesions. *Neurosurgery* 2006;58:S25–46; discussion i–iv. doi:10.1227/01.NEU.0000210365.36914.E3

71. Bullock MR, Chesnut R, Ghajar J, et al. Surgical management of posterior fossa mass lesions. *Neurosurgery* 2006;58:S47–55; discussion i–iv. doi:10.1227/01.NEU.0000210366.36914.38

72. Rinkel GJ, van Gijn J, Wijdicks EF. Subarachnoid hemorrhage without detectable aneurysm. A review of the causes. *Stroke* 1993;24:1403–9.

73. Eisenberg HM, Gary HE, Aldrich EF, et al. Initial CT findings in 753 patients with severe head injury: a report from the NIH Traumatic Coma Data Bank. *J Neurosurg* 1990;73:688–98. doi:10.3171/jns.1990.73.5.0688

74. Holloway KL, Barnes T, Choi S, et al. Ventriculostomy infections: the effect of monitoring duration and catheter exchange in 584 patients. *J Neurosurg* 1996;85:419–24. doi:10.3171/jns.1996.85.3.0419

75. Bochicchio M, Latronico N, Zappa S, et al. Bedside burr hole for intracranial pressure monitoring performed by intensive care physicians: a 5-year experience. *Intensive Care Med* 1996;22:1070–4.

76. Hayashi M, Handa Y, Kobayashi H, et al. Plateau-wave phenomenon (I). Correlation between the appearance of plateau waves and CSF circulation in patients with intracranial hypertension. *Brain J Neurol* 1991;114 (Pt 6):2681–91.

77. Cooper DJ, Rosenfeld JV, Murray L, et al. Decompressive craniectomy in diffuse traumatic brain injury. *N Engl J Med* 2011;364:1493–502. doi:10.1056/NEJMoa1102077

78. Hutchinson PJ, Kolias AG, Timofeev IS, et al. Trial of decompressive craniectomy for traumatic intracranial hypertension. *N Engl J Med* 2016;375:1119–30. doi:10.1056/NEJMoa1605215

79. Jourdan C, Convert J, Mottolese C, et al. Evaluation of the clinical benefit of decompression hemicraniectomy in intracranial hypertension not controlled by medical treatment. *Neurochirurgie* 1993;39:304–10.

80. Jennett B, Miller JD. Infection after depressed fracture of skull. Implications for management of nonmissile injuries. *J Neurosurg* 1972;36:333–9. doi:10.3171/jns.1972.36.3.0333

81. Yokota H, Eguchi T, Nobayashi M, et al. Persistent intracranial hypertension caused by superior sagittal sinus stenosis following depressed skull fracture: case report and review of the literature. *J Neurosurg* 2006;104:849–52. doi:10.3171/jns.2006.104.5.849

82. Fuentes S, Metellus P, Levrier O, et al. Depressed skull fracture overlying the superior sagittal sinus causing benign intracranial hypertension: description of two cases and review of the literature. *Br J Neurosurg* 2005;19:438–42. doi:10.1080/02688690500390193

83. Heary RF, Hunt CD, Krieger AJ, et al. Nonsurgical treatment of compound depressed skull fractures. *J Trauma* 1993;35:441–7.

Chapter 18

Craniofacial Trauma
Injury Patterns and Management

Kathrin J. Whitehouse and Paul McArdle

Introduction

The complexity of management of the patient with a severe craniofacial injury demands multidisciplinary care to deal with neurosurgical, maxillofacial, otolaryngological and ophthalmic problems. These teams should be available in all Major Trauma Centres. A dedicated craniofacial service with multiprofessional teamworking ensures that the long-term issues of neurorehabilitation, psychiatric support and support of the family are met as well as the early challenges of airway threat, resuscitation, head injury and fracture management. Inadequate investigation, planning and management results in missed or inadequately treated injuries; and the increased risk of late complications including poor functional and aesthetic results as well as the need for potentially sub-optimal rescue revision procedures.

Early Management

Craniofacial injuries challenge the surgical team at all stages in their management. The severity of these injuries superimposed on the background of systemic trauma demand a methodical systematic approach to diagnosis and management such as that embodied within the principles of ATLS.[1] At presentation, the airway compromise associated with massive facial bleeding must be suspected and treated as part of the primary survey. Definitive airway management and haemorrhage control minimise the risk of secondary brain injury at a time when autoregulatory control of brain perfusion may be compromised.

Airway Management

The concept of a shared airway must be followed for craniofacial cases with an understanding of surgical and anaesthetic needs. In the early post-injury phase careful ventilatory management is required to optimise CO_2 and hence intracranial pressure, and combined with judicious fluid management, may be used to reduce brain swelling. Early placement of a definitive airway is required in those with compromise; or potential for later compromise secondary to swelling, foreign bodies, bleeding into the airway or deteriorating consciousness.

Later, intraoperatively, restoration of occlusion may require intermaxillary fixation. A tracheostomy may facilitate post-operative airway management by reducing dead space and allowing early weaning of the patient, whilst retaining a definitive airway and facilitating earlier neurosurgical assessment. Alternatively, where long-term neurosurgical sequelae are not anticipated, submental or nasal intubation may be performed.[2] Submental intubation is a low-risk procedure, is quick to perform and may be reversed immediately at the conclusion of the surgical procedure with minimal risks. Nasal intubation may be considered when central comminuted midface trauma is not a concern. It should however be performed under direct observation by an experienced anaesthetist in the presence of anterior skull base comminution.

The establishment of a correct occlusal relationship between the upper and lower jaws is essential to long-term achievement of masticatory function and, in cases of severe midfacial trauma, is a key step in achieving a base from which to rebuild the midface. In the cases where there is a complete dentition, oral intubation will not be possible and alternative methods of establishing the intraoperative airway should be used. Where the dentition is incomplete, it may be possible to pass an armoured tube between or behind the remaining teeth. If an extended period of recovery is likely, then tracheostomy may be the preferred option to facilitate postoperative management of the respiratory tract.

Cervical Spine Stabilisation and Circulatory Control

After high-energy injuries, a combination of facial fractures and reduced Glasgow Coma Score (GCS) is associated with an increased prevalence of cervical spine injury, therefore inline triple immobilisation should be maintained until this is excluded or treated.[3,4] Cervical spine immobilisation complicates an already difficult intubation and demands high levels of anaesthetic expertise along with the facility to be able to provide an immediate emergency surgical airway, if needed, at short notice. In recent years improvements associated with video-assisted airway visualisation have led to a decreased requirement for the surgical airway, reducing patient morbidity; however, prevertebral swelling secondary to vertebral fracture and profuse upper airway haemorrhage may still require emergency surgical airway provision. A skilled multidisciplinary trauma team should therefore be available 24 hours a day in specialist trauma centres as part of a receiving team for such complex cases.

Hypotension is a common finding in severe head injury, occurring in 34% of patients. Each pre-hospital 10 point increase in systolic pressure, is associated with a linear decrease in the adjusted odds of death of 18.8% (i.e. each 10 mmHg interval from 119 to 40 mmHg).[5,6] Although exsanguination is uncommon as a result of facial injury, intractable bleeding may occur. Usually early fracture reduction along with the placement of anterior and posterior nasal packs is the key to arresting life-threatening haemorrhage. Rarely, endovascular treatment may be required to control intractable oronasal bleeding, as haemorrhage associated with fractures involving the skull base may be poorly controlled by ligation of the external carotid system owing to retrograde flow from the internal carotid and vertebrobasilar systems.[7] Only once the patient is adequately stabilised, can full craniofacial assessment, as part of the secondary survey, be undertaken to identify and assess the injuries sustained.

Craniofacial Assessment

The complete assessment of a craniofacial injury requires examination of the head and neck, hard and soft tissues, cranial nerve examination and assessment of orbital injury, supplemented by radiological evaluation. Although the GCS will have been evaluated in the primary survey, neurological observations should continue during the period of potential deterioration. Intracranial pressure monitoring may be deemed necessary.

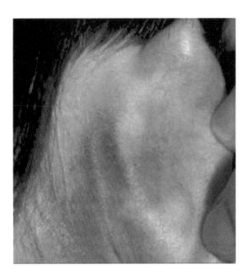

Figure 18.1 Battle's sign. Post-auricular bruising, without direct trauma to this region, is diagnostic of a basal skull fracture.

Signs of skull base fractures classically include periorbital ecchymosis, haemotympanum, CSF rhinorrhoea, otorrhoea and Battle's sign (Figure 18.1). In addition, fractures of the temporal bone may result in hearing loss and facial nerve palsy, whilst fractures of the cribriform plate may result in loss of olfaction. Various syndromes exist as a result of orbital trauma, including superior orbital fissure syndrome, traumatic optic nerve lesions, traumatic mydriasis, carotico-cavernous fistula, retrobulbar haemorrhage, traumatic retinal angiopathy and cavernous sinus thrombosis. Visual acuity should be checked with a Snellen chart. Eye movement should be assessed and diplopia excluded. Visual fields should be checked to confrontation and resting globe position documented. Periorbital oedema may make examination difficult, but this should only encourage a more rigorous inspection as loss of vision may otherwise go unnoticed. Clear protocols and team training are required to ensure such processes take place if visual loss is to be prevented in some cases, particularly in those patients taking anticoagulant medications. In cases of doubt formal ophthalmological opinion, measurement of intra-ocular pressures and slit lamp examination may be necessary.

When examining the scalp, it is easy to miss lacerations covered by congealed blood matted within the hair. The environment in which the trauma occurred should be taken into consideration when cleaning and assessing – one should be wary of glass fragments, tar, dirt and other potentially dangerous contaminants/debris. Careful debridement and suturing will help prevent infection and necrosis of skin margins particularly with occipital lacerations. Complex flap reconstruction is only required when large areas of tissue loss are present. Tissue glue for scalp closure is rarely successful and may promote infection. If partial thickness losses occur, these are often best dressed and left to heal. Subsequent serial excision, if required, will help deal with any areas of traumatic alopecia.

The facial soft tissues should be assessed. Lacerations should be dealt with as quickly as possible. Unlike other anatomical areas, it is not necessary to leave open contaminated lacerations due to robust blood supply, so layered closure is usually all that is required. If lacerations are complex and require general anaesthesia to enable closure, then these may be lightly tacked, photographed and dressed with betadine soaked packs until definitive surgery. Lacerations crossing vital structures demand special attention including those of the eyelids, overlying the facial nerve and overlying the parotid duct. It should be documented that facial sutures should be removed at 5 days, as in complex cases these are often easy to forget, leaving poor scars. We recommend a narrow (6/0) gauge non-absorbable non-braided suture placed with loop magnification to optimise the outcome Particular care should be taken to accurately juxtapose cuts that cross the vermillion border. Do not shave the eyebrow to suture cuts that cross it.

Fractures of the nasoethmoidal area may result in telecanthus and will require careful reconstruction with adequate surgical exposure if long-term poor facial aesthetics are to be avoided secondary to blunting of the lid margins. Associated nasal fractures should be documented as these are easy to miss in complex facial trauma and may lead to poor postoperative nasal airflow if neglected. Plain films are of no value in their assessment. Anterior rhinoscopy should be performed to rule out a septal haematoma and examine for septal deviation. A septal haematoma usually causes nasal obstruction and is seen as a red soft tissue swelling extending from the septum. It may be bilateral and in such cases requires drainage to prevent septal necrosis. A basic clinical assessment of hearing is made, and otoscopy should be performed to examine for haemotympanum, tympanic membrane perforation and CSF leak.

Facial fractures may be indicated by step deformity. In particular, the orbital rims, zygomaticofacial suture and maxilla should be palpated. Anaesthesia of the infraorbital distribution may indicate a fracture of the zygoma or midface. A direct blow to the nerve may also result in altered sensation secondary to neuropraxia, without a fracture. Similar injuries may also affect the supratrochlear and supra-orbital distributions. Movement at the level of the nasofrontal area on manipulation of the maxilla is indicative of a high Le Fort fracture.

Orotracheal intubation and the presence of a cervical collar make facial fracture assessment difficult, as occlusion cannot be checked. However, careful examination for lacerations within the gingivae, steps in the dentition and the presence of a sublingual haematoma may indicate the presence of an undetected mandibular fracture which may have been missed on the initial radiological evaluation, as CT cuts are frequently not continued low enough to include the mandible. Displaced fractures of the central midface above the maxillary alveolus disturb occlusion, resulting in an altered bite. As displaced bony fragments move posteriorly down the incline of the cranial base, so the posterior teeth occlude resulting in an anterior open bite.

Imaging in Craniofacial Injury

Craniofacial injuries are usually best assessed with high-resolution CT with coronal and sagittal reconstructions, to provide important information regarding the skull base and orbits. Fine cuts facilitate assessment of the likely sites for dural tears in the presence of CSF leaks. Three-dimensional reformatting is helpful for communication with patients and relatives, facilitates teaching and may help identify orientation and size of specific bone fragments such as the mandibular condyles and those carrying the medial canthal ligament (Figure 18.2). Contrast is not usually required unless intracranial vascular injuries are suspected. In these cases, CT or MR angiography may help.

Classification of Craniofacial Fractures

Throughout time, there have been multiple different classification systems developed, for example recently the Maxillofacial Injury Severity Score (MFISS), which assigns weights in

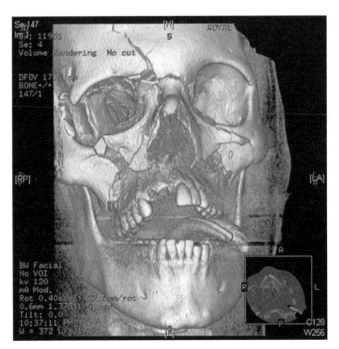

Figure 18.2 Complex craniofacial trauma. Note the frontal bone fracture in the vicinity of the frontal air sinus. In addition, there is evidence of complex mid- and lateral- facial trauma characterised by nasoethmoid fractures, bilateral maxillary fractures and fractures of the right orbit. The airway has been secured, reflecting a systematic approach to the management of the patient.

three categories – malocclusion, limited mouth opening and facial deformity; and Facial Fracture Severity Score (FFSS) which assigns numbers to different areas of the face depending on the fracture pattern.

Le Fort's famous classification[8] described three levels of fracture, and Wassmund[9] described four subtypes. We shall concentrate on the Le Fort classification here. Le Fort II and III fractures may involve the skull base, and result in CSF leak in about 30% of cases, usually from the cribriform plate.[10] Approximately 60% of midfacial injuries fall into the Le Fort categories.[11]

However, with comminuted facial injuries that occur in high-energy trauma, these simple low-energy-impact categories no longer suffice. With improvements in the reconstruction of facial form and function careful anatomic descriptions are best used to detail the reconstructive procedures that will be required. These may usefully be divided into central, centrolateral and lateral midfacial fractures; or a combination (see Table 18.1 and Figure 18.3).

Injuries involving the orbit, zygomatico-orbital complex, mid face, nasoethmoidal areas, maxilla and mandible each require specific treatment and deserve individual assessment as well as a combined assessment of the overall injury pattern that will determine likely long-term complications if inadequately managed.

Central Craniofacial Fractures

These injuries can occur following even low-energy trauma, including a simple nasal fracture. In more complex injuries with craniofacial disassociation the pterygoid muscles pull the mobile midface dorsally and caudally, resulting in occlusal disturbance. The palate may fracture antero-posteriorly along the midline suture, and unrepaired may result in an oronasal fistula as well as a poor occlusion. Manufacture of a palatal splint may help stabilise

Table 18.1 Central, centrolateral and lateral fracture subtypes and their relationship to the Le Fort classification

	Central	Centrolateral	Lateral
Le Fort	I – horizontal maxillary fracture separating teeth from upper face	III – craniofacial disjunction, through pterygoid plates, through the zygoma and lateral orbit to the nasofrontal suture	
	II – pyramidal, with fracture extending from the pterygoid plates across the infraorbital rims and up to the nasofrontal junction		
Other	Naso-ethmoidal, naso-maxillary	Naso-orbital-ethmoidal	Zygoma and lateral orbit

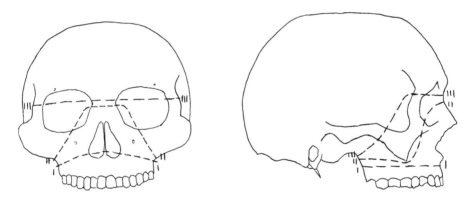

Figure 18.3 Fracture patterns in the Le Fort Classification. Note that Wassmund II fractures are equivalent to Le Fort II and Wassmund IV are equivalent to Le Fort III.

such fractures, allowing adequate fracture reduction as well as protecting the healing palate and encouraging mucosalisation. Impressions to create study models as part of the initial assessment are useful in creating such splints as well as aiding the manufacture of arch bars that will facilitate the re-establishment of an accurately reduced occlusion. Those fractures in the central frontobasal region communicate with the paranasal sinuses and so present an increased risk of ascending infection and meningitis in the presence of a dural tear. Fractures of the cribriform plate can be associated with CSF leak from dural tears around the olfactory nerves. Anosmia may result.

Centrolateral Craniofacial Fractures

The fracture line passes through the zygomatic arches, the lateral orbital wall and the frontal skull base. Combinations with other fracture lines and multiple fractures are possible. This causes cranio-facial disarticulation (basal, pyramidal or at the level of the skull base) and can be differentiated from unclassifiable fractures (comminuted fractures, fractures where there has been bone loss).

Lateral Craniofacial Fractures

Lateral craniofacial injuries involve the zygoma and lateral orbit. As they lie lateral to the sinuses, the risk of a persistent CSF leak is reduced, along with the risk of meningitis. Therefore, the need for the repair depends upon the extent of cosmetic deformity secondary to bony depression, and the ocular functional deficit due to changes in orbital volume affecting the orbital contents. Reconstruction is aimed at restoring the orbital volume and contour in the presence of displaced fractures of the orbital walls, and to optimise function. To achieve this, bone grafting may be required. The orbital rims provide important protection for the eyes whilst the thin bone of the orbital floor and medial wall collapse readily absorbing energy so protecting vital orbital structures. In the same way, crumpling of the mid-face may reduce the likelihood of brain injury, although the evidence for this concept in the literature is mixed.[12] In complex orbital and midfacial trauma, stereolithographic models and Computer Aided Design and Manufactured modelled implants (CADCAM) offer the possibility of perfect anatomical reconstruction, particularly helpful when complex anatomical structures are damaged. For instance, when the whole orbital floor is disrupted, computer-aided superimposition of the contralateral normal orbit overlaid against the injured orbit facilitates the construction of titanium or lightweight plastic implants which may be used to reproduce the original anatomical state. In the orbit this reduces long-term sequelae of enophthalmous and motility disorders and speeds reconstruction.

Aims of Reconstruction

The goal of reconstruction is to restore facial form whilst ensuring isolation and separation of the paranasal sinuses from the brain, by repair of the dura and the surrounding bone. Well-planned approaches to the craniofacial skeleton provide access for repair, whilst anticipating the need to minimise brain retraction through incisions that will heal aesthetically.

In both high- and low-energy trauma, rigid internal fixation using low-profile titanium plates stabilises fractures, restores anatomical form and provides the skeletal framework over which the soft tissues can be redraped. The historical problems of loss of facial height and projection that resulted from closed management of these fractures can now be avoided, along with the danger of airway compromise previously associated with wiring of the jaws. Precise replacement of small fragments allows restoration of volume and function in critical areas such as the orbit and enables the anatomical re-establishment of soft tissue form, for example at the medial canthus.

Surgical reconstruction aims to restore height, width and projection of the facial buttresses, which normally absorb and transmit forces from the jaws during eating. Reconstruction of the anterior maxillary buttress (from piriform rim to frontal process of the maxilla) and the zygomaticomaxillary buttress provide the basis for restoration of vertical height. Reconstruction of the zygomatic arch provides the guide to upper mid facial projection and width, providing it is remembered that the arch is essentially straight. If it is plated as a curved arch, the tendency is to reduce anterior projection and widen the face. Reconstruction of the mandible and frontal bone also determine facial width.

These reconstructed buttresses provide the base from which reassembly of the facial skeleton can take place. Surgical access includes the sublabial and bicoronal approaches; and the subciliary, transconjunctival and mid lid incisions to obtain access to the orbit. Using these in combination permits access to the whole of the facial skeleton without compromising long-term facial aesthetics.

Orbital Injuries

The characteristics of ocular injuries sustained relate to the trauma aetiology. One in five patients with midfacial fractures as a result of a motor vehicle collision, and one in ten patients with midfacial fractures secondary to assault, sustain severe ocular trauma.[13] In these cases pupillary responses, visual acuity, ocular motility and consequent diplopia should be documented and a formal ophthalmic opinion sought. Impaired visual acuity is the principal predictor of ocular injury. The presence of a blow-out fracture, comminuted zygomatic fractures, double vision and amnesia raise still further the likelihood of severe ocular trauma.[14] The symptoms of pain and proptosis in the presence of decreasing visual acuity, an enlarging pupil, ophthalmoplegia and tense soft tissues raise the likelihood of a retrobulbar haemorrhage, which is an ocular emergency. Immediate surgical decompression with cantholysis via a lateral canthotomy or a medial blepharoplasty may rescue sight, as otherwise central retinal artery ischaemia will result in blindness. In our experience, concomitant use of anticoagulation has resulted in a significant increase in the incidence of orbital compartment syndrome which may develop after CT assessment, requiring regular eye observation and early intervention in the presence of decreasing visual acuity and increasing intra-ocular pressures. Emergency temporisation may be achieved with the use of high-dose steroids, acetezolamide 500 mg IV followed by 125–250 mg IV 4–6 hourly and mannitol 20%, 2 g/kg IV over 2 hours until decompression is performed. Surgical decompression would normally be carried out under local anaesthesia, as timely intervention is critical to alleviate the intraorbital pressure rise responsible for this form of compartment syndrome.

Fine cut axial and coronal CT provides the necessary detail to guide diagnosis and reconstruction in orbital trauma. This also allows detailed assessment of the anterior skull base. Coronal reformats should be obtained when injury precludes standard examination. As the most common causes of reduced vision relate to potentially treatable pathologies such as retrobulbar haemorrhage, optic nerve compression presumably secondary to oedema and surgical emphysema, the importance of early,[15] and if necessary, repeated CT scanning is underlined.

Restitution of the orbital tissues aims to provide a fully reconstructed bony orbit with restoration of orbital volume and shape, ocular motility, soft tissue aesthetics, lacrimation and visual function. Early and accurate identification of the nature and extent of injuries, combined with careful surgery, will help prevent the late complications of enophthalmos and of restricted ocular motility with resultant diplopia. Further aspects of management of orbital injuries are outside the remit of this chapter.

Operative Considerations in Facial Fracture Management

Sequencing in Pan-facial Injury

In pan-facial injury with severe comminution, the loss of anatomical landmarks complicates reconstruction. As the reconstruction is of a curved structure, minor malpositioning of bone fragments in an area may be amplified and result in significant discrepancies elsewhere. Careful planning and sequencing will help reduce these problems.

Following clinical and radiographic assessment, the incisions required for access are planned. Three dimensional reconstructions can identify the size and position of bone fragments important for rebuilding the facial skeleton, and can be used to show patients and relatives the injuries and extent of reconstruction required. If possible, study models of the dentition should be made in the dentate patient prior to surgery. The occlusal relationship of the upper and lower teeth may then be used to help guide the positioning of the maxilla to the mandible. Construction of preformed arch bars saves time at surgery.

Using the principles described by Manson, reconstruction is planned dividing the face and cranium into units.[10] The upper and lower units of the face are artificially divided at the Le Fort I level. The sequence in which reconstruction takes place is planned carefully, determined by the nature of the injury and in particular by the non-injured areas, which provide the foundation and reference points from which the rebuilding starts. An example of such a sequence is given below:

- Radiological assessment
- Consent
- Secure the airway definitively for surgery (see above)
- Lower lid incisions
  The approach to the orbit should be made prior to the bicoronal approach as subsequent oedema may prevent accurate identification of the lower lid skin creases.
- Orbital floor exposure
  Although orbital floor exploration may take place at this stage, it will not usually be possible to reconstruct this area until the maxilla has been disimpacted and the orbital rim restored.
- Bicoronal flap
  A well-designed bicoronal incision provides excellent access, is hidden well back in the hair line, preserves the function of the facial nerve and allows a thick pericranial flap to be elevated from the site of the incision (if necessary) extending laterally along the upper margins of the temporalis attachment. Reflection down to, and preservation of, the supratrochlear and supraorbital vessels provide a vascularised flap that can cover a cranialised sinus and support a basal dural repair. If the incision to preserve the temporal branch of the facial nerve is extended to include the deep temporalis fascia, then the detached facial soft tissues can be re-suspended by reattachment of the temporalis fascia. Further soft tissue support may be provided by suspensory sutures attached to frontal bone plates.
- Exposure of orbits
  The superior aspect of the orbit may now be explored. It may be necessary to osteotomise the foramen surrounding the supra orbital vessels at the orbital rim to mobilise these vessels and allow access to the orbital roof. Access to the lateral wall is made easier once the zygomatic arch is exposed. Dissection in the orbit enables full exposure of the fractures and careful elevation of the temporalis muscle from the lateral orbital wall allows assessment of accurate fracture reduction. It also provides a site for burrhole placement that can be hidden underneath the muscle improving post-operative aesthetics.
- Exposure of zygomas as required.
  When the zygoma is comminuted, the whole of the arch should be exposed and disimpacted. This will facilitate mobilisation of the impacted maxilla.

- Frontal craniotomy
  Pre-plating of frontal fractures prior to craniotomy makes reconstruction much easier providing allowance is made for ability to place the pericranial flap into the anterior cranial fossa at the conclusion of the surgery. Burr holes can be hidden under temporalis.
- Maxillary disimpaction
  Once the zygomas are disimpacted, the maxilla is free for disimpaction. McMahon et al. recommend that this should be done with the anterior cranial fossa exposed when the anterior skull base is fractured.[16] Significant defects in the floor of the anterior fossa may be bone grafted including those of the orbital roof. Plates are not generally placed in the anterior fossa for fear of infection and the difficulty of later removal.
- Frontal sinus management
  The frontal sinus is cranialised or obliterated and sealed with an overlaid pericranial flap. This is discussed in further detail below.
- Orbital roof management
  The orbital roof may be explored subcranially or intracranially. Intracranial exploration is ideal as otherwise there is a risk of fractures tearing the dura. Fractures that extend posteriorly across the skull base may defy safe reduction, and mobilisation of the frontal area may have to be made via a frontobasal osteotomy to prevent injury.
- Dural repair
  The dura is repaired after manipulation of anterior fossa fractures is complete. An intradural repair may be required, particularly for low tears where access is limited by the constraints of brain retraction. Patches of pericranial flap may be inlaid over the defects and sealed with fibrin glue or dural sealants. The brain is then protected with dampened patties, whilst the next stages of repair take place, as the pericranial flap cannot be laid into place until the frontal, orbital and nasal reconstructions are complete.
- Frontonasal reconstruction
  A cantilevered split calvarial bone graft may be needed to restore frontonasal projection particularly in cases of gross nasal bone comminution. Early restitution prevents late contraction of the overlying soft tissue envelope.
- Medial orbital margin reconstruction and nasomaxillary reconstruction.
  The anterior nasoethmoidal area may now be reconstructed, ensuring that the nasal bridge width is kept narrow, as broadening may occur as a late consequence. Accurate placement of the medial canthal ligament can be challenging, and direct exposure may be necessary to enable identification. Painstaking overcorrection to position the ligament to the level of the anterior projection of the globe superiorly and medially is required, with medial transnasal wiring or plating, to secure the superior position of the canthus from solid bone in the glabellar region. If broadening of the intercanthal distance occurs, the resulting lid aesthetics are poor. Direct exposure of the canthal ligament may be required to enable its identification.
- Zygomatic disimpaction
  Fractures of the root of the zygoma should be identified and plated. If the temporalis insertion is released cranially and the muscle reflected down, it will allow access to the lateral wall of the orbit. Identification and reduction of the orbital process of the zygoma to the greater wing of the sphenoid at the lateral orbital wall is an excellent guide to the

accuracy of fracture reduction and is important in restoring the volume of the orbit. Failure to reduce a fracture at this site may result in enophthalmos.

- Zygomatic plating
  Fractures of the arch and root should be reduced and plated. Frequently, it is necessary to suspend the zygoma at the frontozygomatic suture with a wire or 1.0 mm plate to help support the zygoma whilst allowing it to be rotated as needed as the orbital rim repair is completed, and at a later stage when the zygomatic complex and maxilla are reunited. Once these manoeuvres are complete, it may be necessary to convert this to a weight-bearing plate to prevent relapse during the recovery period.
- Infra-orbital rim reconstruction and restitution of the medial orbit
  Lost orbital rim bone fragments displaced into the antrum are retrieved and plated into position. Exposure of the orbital floor will help avoid malpositioning of rim fragments that frequently over-rotate, lifting spurs of orbital floor bone into the orbit. Union across to the medial orbit now completes this horizontal buttress. Careful dissection of the infraorbital fissure will help reduce long-term loss of sensation in the infra orbital nerve distribution
- Grafting of the orbital walls
  Orbital shape and volume is restored with split calvarial bone grafts. These may be cantilevered off plates at the orbital rim. Post-operative closure of the periosteum over these plates makes them impalpable, improving cosmesis and reducing the risk of infection.
- Exposure of the mandibular condyles and reconstruction to height
  Lower facial height is determined by the occlusion and by the intact mandibular condyle. Where there are bilateral fractures, reconstruction will prevent loss of facial height and a resulting anterior open bite. High intracapsular fractures cannot be plated successfully, and when bilateral will create the need for intermaxillary fixation to be maintained postoperatively to try to prevent this occurrence.
- Mandibular reconstruction
  If the maxillary dentition is intact with no midline palatal split (present in about 8% of maxillary midfacial fractures) and no dentoalveolar fractures, then the mandible can be accurately reconstructed with temporary intermaxillary fixation to localise the fragments. If not, then the palatal split should first be plated or splinted and the mandible used as a guide for width. In cases with a midline mandibular split, careful assessment should be made at fracture reduction to avoid flaring of the mandibular rami.
- Maxillary plating at the Le Fort I level
  The upper and lower facial segments may now be reunited by plating of the vertical buttresses.
- Soft tissue resuspension
  Where dissection is not required across areas of the facial skeleton, then the soft tissues should be left attached to the periosteum. In all other areas, the periosteum should be resuspended with non-resorbable sutures.

Frontal Sinus Fracture Management

Frontal sinus fractures are reported to occur in 2%–12% of cranial fractures and 5% of facial fractures (Figure 18.4). One-third involves the anterior wall alone, whilst two-thirds of cases

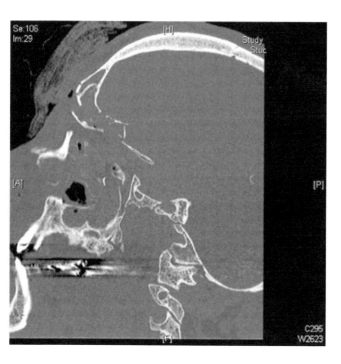

Figure 18.4 A sagittal reformat showing complex craniofacial trauma. The anterior cranial fossa floor has been fractured and appears to be in communication with the frontal air sinus.

involve a combination of fractures of the frontal recess and posterior, and anterior walls. Very rarely is the floor affected alone.[17] Up to one third have an associated CSF leak. Other complications of frontal sinus fractures include mucocoele, pyelocoele, brain abscess, frontal osteomyelitis and meningitis.

The management of the fractured frontal sinus is controversial. The following principles seem clear.

Undisplaced fractures of the anterior wall do not require correction. Gross comminution and depression of the anterior wall require correction to avoid aesthetic deformity. Overlying lacerations should be used only if extensive and when limited access is required for repair. The bicoronal incision is best for cosmesis, adequate visualisation of the fractures, and restoration of form, with debridement of the sinus if needed. The pericranial tissues are preserved if needed for repair. Multiple small fragments can be difficult to locate in the presence of severe comminution, when bone grafting with split calvarium may produce a more satisfactory end result. Fractures affecting the anterior wall alone should be rigidly fixed and the sinus mucosa left *in situ* if the frontonasal duct is not affected by the fracture. Plating of comminuted bone fragments held in place by sinus lining may be useful prior to removal of the anterior wall to allow accurate apposition of bone fragments. Early treatment with removal of fragments displaced into the frontal sinus will help prevent infection.[18]

Isolated *fractures of the posterior wall* require treatment when displaced by the thickness of the posterior wall or in the presence of CSF leak that persists despite conservative management. A frontal craniotomy facilitates access and exploration of the posterior wall, the frontal and the basal dura. Burr holes placed laterally under the temporalis reduce cosmetic deformity. A low bone flap provides access to the sinus and minimises brain retraction when the basal dura is explored, although difficulty may be experienced moving the saw across both tables of the sinus. Cranialisation is preferred over obliteration, as success is difficult unless the sinus is small, and there are high rates of infection with fat grafts and allografts.[19,20] However, if there is only moderate displacement of the fracture and no involvement of the nasofrontal duct, obliteration may be favoured as there is less brain retraction required.

To cranialise the frontal sinus, the posterior wall is removed, all sinus mucosa is removed, and the communication to the nasal cavity is sealed. Vascularised pericranial graft can be internalised and laid over the denuded sinus, perhaps using a dural sealant to reduce the risk of mucocoele formation. Obliteration of the frontal sinus involves removing the sinus mucosa and filling the sinus with fat, pericranium, or bone.

Management of fractures of the posterior wall, with associated CSF rhinorrhoea which stops within 7 days, presents an area of uncertainty. The arrest of the leak may be secondary to brain plugging the dural defect rather than spontaneous repair. The Mayo clinic reported a delayed onset of meningitis in 16% of patients, at an average of 6.5 years after a CSF leak lasting greater than 24 hours.[21] Eljamel and Foy describe a 7.5% CSF leak recurrence rate following spontaneous cessation, and a meningitis rate of 30.6% in those recurrences.[22] Communication between the brain and paranasal sinuses appears to place the patient at significant risk from ascending infection and supports the case for early intervention. Donald and Bernstein allude to the fact that sinus lining appears to invaginate the bone lining the sinus and that only by drilling out the sinus can it be rendered truly safe.[23] For this reason, cranialisation of the sinus and inlaying of a vascularised pericranial flap to separate the brain and obturation of the nasofrontal duct is the preferred option.

The evidence for intervention in management of fractures involving the frontonasal duct on the floor of the frontal sinus is difficult to interpret. Intubation of the duct may result in late problems with stenosis. Conservative management may leave the patient susceptible to mucocoele and pyelocoele formation, whilst obliteration may be difficult secondary to extensive pneumatisation. Preoperative imaging to determine the presence of a fracture involving the frontonasal duct is not always reliable.

Timing of Surgical Intervention

The timing of reconstruction in the presence of brain injury requires careful planning. Secondary injury could result from operating on patients with raised intracranial pressure (ICP); or hypotension from anaesthesia or surgical blood loss. Therefore, patients should be stable in terms of their ICP and cardiovascular parameters before aggressive intervention is considered. Retraction on vulnerable brain tissue may cause oedema and further brain injury. Facial swelling itself precludes early intervention, as the assessment of facial contour and the planning of incisions is difficult. Soft tissues may also be difficult to handle if oedematous. The definitive management of facial injuries may need to be deferred to allow the patient to stabilise. However, delay may compromise the final soft tissue, as healing and fibrosis may have commenced.

Another important consideration is that of airway management. Patients with facial swelling, or brain injury, may require prolonged intubation. The timing of surgery will need to be planned with extubation or tracheostomy in mind. Intermaxillary fixation may be required, necessitating either nasal intubation or tracheostomy. The logistics of multi-specialty operating, and availability of specialist kits and theatre space will also require co-ordination.

Cerebrospinal Fluid Leak

A CSF leak implies a dural tear and the possibility of ascending infection. Some opine that repair should be based on the extent of the associated fractures, accepting that dural tears are present in most cases when explored.

The first sign of CSF leak may be a tramline of CSF mixed with blood from the patient's nose. The glucose oxidase test strip test is unreliable and should not be used in diagnosis. Beta-2-transferrin analysis of a collected specimen has a sensitivity of 99% and specificity of 97%, but high levels of protein can confound any results. Beta-trace-protein is a less sensitive and less specific assay.[24]

High-resolution CT has a high sensitivity for identification of the site of CSF leak, with a fracture measuring over 3 mm in the anterior cranial fossa in the presence of pneumocephalus being highly suggestive of a CSF fistula, even if CSF leak is not clinically evident. MR cisternography, CT cisternography (requiring intrathecal radiopaque contrast), and intrathecal fluorescein with intraoperative visualisation are useful adjuncts for localisation of a CSF leak.[25]

The leak may be managed conservatively, depending on the location and the need for exploration of other injuries. Conservative management includes bed rest, head elevation, avoidance of coughing, sneezing and straining and the use of stool softeners/laxatives. Two to three days of conservative management has found to be effective in up to 68% of cases, improving to 85% after 7 days; however, the meningitis rate can be up to 11%.[26] If this fails, CSF diversion via lumbar drain or external ventricular drain can be attempted for up to 7 days, aiming to drain 5–10 ml/h. There is a risk of low-pressure headaches and meningitis with this therapy.

Meningitis occurs in around 5%–10% of those with CSF leak, with a mortality rate under 10%. *Streptococcus pneumoniae* is the most frequent causative organism. Meningitis can be treated with sensitivity-appropriate antibiotics, and, more definitively, surgical closure of the dural defect. A Cochrane review of prophylactic antibiotic usage in CSF leaks found no significant evidence that antibiotics reduce the risk of meningitis, nor improvement in mortality.[27] Prophylactic Pneumococcal Conjugate Vaccine (PCV) 13 may be beneficial, but as yet there are no randomised trials examining this.

In cases where a leak stops spontaneously, it may be due to necrotic brain tissue plugging the defect, and can result in delayed presentations with either recurrent meningitis (71%) or intermittent nasal discharge (30%); however, these delayed complications are rare.[28] Other symptoms of occult CSF leak include headaches, salty taste, or cerebral abscess.

There are some circumstances where surgery is indicated as the primary management. If there is a concomitant intracranial injury that requires operation, a culprit dural defect can be repaired at the same opportunity. CSF leaks with fractures with a defect over 1 cm in any dimension, or close to the midline are unlikely to heal with conservative management, and so may require operation. Associated encephalocoele or meningocoele may impede fracture closure and require operative reduction. Ideally, those that have had meningitis should have completed treatment for the meningitis and be clinically well before definitive closure.

Anterior cranial fossa leaks can be repaired by placing a graft via extradural endoscopic approach, with intraoperative localisation using fluorescein, if required. Alternative extracranial approaches include the bicoronal approach (which allows for assessment of the brain, and intradural repair), and the transpalpebral and transconjunctival transorbital approaches.

References

1. American College of Surgeons. *Advanced trauma life support manual*. Chicago: American College of Surgeons Committee on Trauma; 2004.

2. Hernandez Altemir F. The submental route for endotracheal intubation: a new technique. *J Maxillofac Surg*.1986;14 (1):64–65.

3. Williams J, Jehle D, Cottington E, Shufflebarger C. Head, facial, and clavicular trauma as a predictor of cervical-spine injury. *Ann Emerg Med* 1992;21(6):719–22.

4. Hills MW, Deane SA. Head injury and facial injury: is there an increased risk of cervical spine injury? *J Trauma* 1993;34 (4):549–53.

5. Vella MA. Acute management of traumatic brain injury. *Surg Clin N Am* 2017;95 (5):1015–30.

6. Spaite DW, Hu C, Bobrow BJ, et al. Mortality and prehospital blood pressure in patients with major traumatic brain injury: implications for the hypotension threshold. *JAMA Surg* 2017;152(4):360–8.

7. Komiyama M, Nishikawa M, Kan M, Shigemoto T, Kaji A. Endovascular treatment of intractable oronasal bleeding associated with severe craniofacial injury. *J Trauma* 1998;44(2):330–4.

8. Le Fort RL. Etude expérimentale sur les fractures de la mâchoire supérieure. *Rev Chir Paris* 1901;23:208–27.

9. Wassmund M. *Frakturen und Luxationen des Gesichtsschädels*. Meusser; 1927.

10. Manson PN. Maxillofacial injuries. *Emerg Med Clin North Am* 1984;2(4): 168–78.

11. Manson PN, Clarke N, Robertson B, et al. Subunit principles in midface fractures: the importance of sagittal buttresses, soft tissue reductions and sequencing treatment of segmental fractures. *Plastic Reconstruc Surg* 1999;103(4):1287–307.

12. Martin RC, Spain DA, Richardson JD. Do facial fractures protect the brain or are they a marker for severe head injury? *Am Surg* 2002;68(5):477–81.

13. al-Qurainy IA, Stassen LF, Dutton GN, Moos KF, el-Attar A. The characteristics of midfacial fractures and the association with ocular injury: a prospective study. *Br J Oral Maxillofac Surg* 1991;29(5): 291–301.

14. al-Qurainy IA, Titterington DM, Dutton GN, Stassen LF, Moos KF, el-Attar A. Midfacial fractures and the eye: the development of a system for detecting patients at risk of eye injury. *Br J Oral Maxillofac Surg* 1991;29(6):363–7.

15. Lee HJ, Jilani M, Frohman L, Baker S. CT of orbital trauma. *Emerg Radiol* 2004;10 (4):168–72.

16. McMahon JD, Koppel DA, Devlin M, Moos KF. Maxillary and panfacial fractures. In: Wardbooth P, Epply BL, Schmelzeizen R, eds. *Maxillofacial trauma and esthetic reconstruction*. Churchill Livingstone; 2003.

17. Wallis A, Donald PJ. Frontal sinus fractures: a review of 72 cases. *Laryngoscope* 1988;98:593–8.

18. Gruss JS, Pollock RA, Phillips JH, Antonyshyn O. Combined injuries to the cranium and face. *Br J Plastic Surg* 1999;42:385–98.

19. Wilson BC, Davidson B, Corey JP, Haydon RC 3rd. Comparison of complications following frontal sinus fractures managed with or without obliteration over ten years. *Laryngoscope* 1998;98(5):516–20.

20. Bell RB, Dierks EJ, Brar P, Potter JK, Potter BE. A protocol for the management of frontal sinus fractures emphasising sinus preservation. *J Oral Maxillofac Surg* 2007;65(5):825–39.

21. Friedman JA, Ebersold MJ, Quast LM. Post traumatic cerebrospinal fluid leakage. *World J Surg* 2001;25(8):1062–6.

22. Eljamel MS, Foy PM. Acute traumatic CSF fistulae: the risk of intracranial infection. *Br J Neurosurg* 1990;4(6):479–83.

23. Donald PJ, Bernstein L. Compound frontal sinus injuries with intracranial penetration. *Laryngoscope* 1978;88:225–32.

24. Warnecke A, Averbeck T, Wurster U, et al. Diagnostic relevance of beta2-transferrin for the detection of cerebrospinal fluid fistulas. *Arch Otolaryngol Head Neck Surg* 2004;130:1178–84.

25. Phang SY, Whitehouse KJ, Lee L, Khalil H, McArdle P, Whitfield PC. Management of CSF leak in base of skull fractures in adults. *Br J Neurosurg* 2016;30(6):596–604.

26. Mincy JE. Posttraumatic cerebrospinal fluid fistula of the frontal fossa. *J Trauma* 1966;6:618–22.

27. Ratilal BO, Costa J, Sampaio C, Pappamikail L. Antibiotic prophylaxis for preventing meningitis in patients with basilar skull fractures. *Cochrane Database Syst Rev* 2011;8:CD004884.

28. Scholsem M, Scholtes F, Collignon F, et al. Surgical management of anterior cranial base fractures with cerebrospinal fluid fistulae: a single institution experience. *Neurosurgery* 2008;62:463–9.

Chapter 19

Cranioplasty after Head Injury

Stephen Honeybul

Introduction

There continues to be considerable interest in the use of decompressive craniectomy following severe traumatic brain injury. The results of trials have confirmed the significant survival advantage; however, evidence that outcome is improved when compared with those patients who survive following medical management is less forthcoming.[1,2] This may be for a number of reasons not least of which is the morbidity associated with the initial decompressive craniectomy and the subsequent cranioplasty. If use of the procedure is to continue, ongoing research is required to clarify issues regarding optimal surgical timing and surgical technique, the most appropriate reconstructive materials and minimisation of surgical complications.

Surgical Timing

Once the patient recovers from the initial injury and the cerebral swelling has subsided, a cranioplasty is required order to restore cosmesis and protection, improve cerebral hydrodynamics and in certain cases improve neurological function.

The optimal timing of cranioplasty has not been clearly established; however, for many years it was suggested that the procedure should be delayed for a number of months to reduce the risk of infection. More recently this practice has been called into question as it has been clearly demonstrated that early cranioplasty can be safely performed.[3]

In view of these findings it would seem logical to replace the bone flap as soon as clinically possible to avoid the need for prolonged use of protective head-gear which is often uncomfortable and not particularly dignified. In addition, it is becoming increasingly apparent that there is a subgroup of patients who are particularly susceptible to the presence of a large skull defect and for these patients the cranioplasty may provide therapeutic benefit.

Neurological Susceptibility due to a Large Skull Defect

In 1939 Grant and Norcross coined the term 'syndrome of the trephine' to describe the symptoms of headache, vertigo, tinnitus, fatigue, insomnia, memory disturbance, seizures, mood swings and behavioural disturbance that was observed in some individuals with a large skull defect.[4] Subsequently many terms have been introduced that revolve around a common theme, including post-traumatic syndrome,[5] syndrome of the sinking scalp flap[6] and motor trephined syndrome.[7] The classical descriptions are of an initial period of improvement after the decompressive surgery followed by a period of neurological deterioration. The diagnosis is confirmed when the symptoms resolve or improve following replacement of the bone flap. Until recently these conditions were described as being relatively uncommon; however, it is becoming evident that certain patients are particularly susceptible to having large skull defects. Clinical presentation can range from the classical description of a reversal of neurological deficits, to a more subtle but quantifiable improvement in neurocognitive function or merely just a failure to clinically improve. Indeed, given the variation in clinical signs exhibited it is often difficult to provide a specific diagnosis. For example; a patient may develop postural headaches and increasing lethargy and therefore are deemed to have 'Syndrome of the trephined', but they may also develop a focal deficit and are therefore given a diagnosis of 'motor trephined syndrome'. In view of this variation it may be simpler to use a blanket term such as Neurological Susceptibility to a Skull Defect' (NSSD) that applies to all clinical manifestations attributable to the absence of a bone flap.[8]

The underlying pathophysiology responsible for the various neurological manifestations has yet to be established; however, a number of theories have been proposed including; direct effects of atmospheric air on the brain, alterations in CSF hydrodynamics and changes in cerebral blood flow and metabolism. Overall the effect that the skull defect has on neurological function may not be due to a single pathophysiological mechanism, rather it may in fact be multifactorial. Indeed, support for this hypothesis would come from the wide variety of clinical manifestations reported.

The number of patients who have been reported to exhibit some degree of neurological dysfunction has been variable. Stiver found that amongst 55 patients who had had a decompressive hemicraniectomy, 10 patients (26%) developed a delayed monoparesis which was reversed following cranioplasty.[7] More recently, a prospective cohort study found a measurable improvement in some aspect of neurological function in 4 (16%) out of 25 patients who were assessed a few days before and after cranioplasty.[9]

Overall it would appear unequivocal that some patients are particularly susceptible to having a large skull defect and further studies will be required to determine the true incidence and those factors that predispose to this condition in order to minimise the impact that this can have on patient rehabilitation.

Choice of Materials

The material most commonly used for reconstruction has been the patient's own bone that has been stored in a refrigerated sterile container. This is because autologous bone is cheap, biocompatible, strong, radiolucent and has an ideal contour. However it has been demonstrated that use of autologous bone is associated with a high failure rate due to either infection or bony resorption.[10,11] When this occurs the original bone flap has to be discarded and an alloplastic material utilised. A number of these have been used and they all have their relative merits.

Titanium

Titanium has the advantage of being strong and biocompatible. Advances in computer assisted design and manufacturing allows the production of large custom-made prefabricated plates. Favourable long-term functional and aesthetic outcomes have been reported and it would seem to represent a viable alternative to autologous bone. One of the frequently cited disadvantages has been cost; however, a recent randomised controlled trial comparing primary titanium cranioplasty with autologous bone found that titanium was associated with better cosmetic and functional outcomes without increasing overall health care costs.[12]

Whilst ongoing use of autologous bone would appear reasonable, these findings would support the use of primary titanium cranioplasty especially in young patients in whom bone resorption has been shown to be a significant problem.[11]

Alternative Materials

Methylmethacrylate is an alternative material that has been used for many years. It is cheap, possesses good biomechanical properties and is relatively simple to use. However, its highly exothermic setting reaction can cause tissue injury and its failure to osseointegrate will always place it at a disadvantage when compared with titanium or hydroxyapatite. The need to mould the cement to an appropriate contour can be time consuming when restoring large or complicated defects; however, the introduction of computer-assisted design modelling has addressed this problem and very acceptable results can be achieved with relatively limited additional costs.[13]

Amongst the ceramics, hydroxyapatite is probably the most frequently used and because it is the principal component of bone it has the advantage of being biocompatible and osteoconductive.[14] It is most suitable for the repair of relatively small defects; however, it can be combined with miniplates in order to repair more extensive deficits.[15] Despite good biocompatibility, hydroxyapatite can sometimes provoke a significant inflammatory reaction which may limit use in certain cases.[16] A final consideration is the significant cost especially when using customised prostheses and despite numerous reports of their use in craniofacial reconstruction, significant advantages over and above acrylics and titanium remain to be demonstrated. Finally, there are a number of promising experimental materials including carbon fibre,[17] PEEK,[18] bone growth factors[19] and stem cells.[20] Currently these materials are in the development phase and in most cases their initial use may be limited to relatively small defects. They will also have to prove their worth in the clinical setting when there are currently many suitable materials already available.

Surgical Techniques

In most neurosurgical centres cranioplasty procedures are viewed as straightforward surgical procedures that are delegated to relatively junior staff. However, the results of the aforementioned randomised controlled trial may require this practice to be reconsidered.[21] Patients were randomised to receive either their autologous bone that had been stored in a refrigerator or a primary titanium cranioplasty. To limit possible confounding due to differences in surgical technique and surgical expertise within and between treatment arms all surgical procedures were performed by the senior author. A standardised technique was used in which there was strict adherence to aseptic technique. In doing so the infection rate was reduced from approximately 9% in the period prior to the trial, to 0%. In view of these finding it may be necessary to consider involving more senior staff in the surgical management of these cases.

Management of Temporal Muscle

Management of the temporal muscle during cranioplasty can be problematic for a number of reasons (Figure 19.1). Firstly, the muscle often becomes damaged when it is detached from the temporal bone during the initial craniectomy procedure. The dissection is often performed using monopolar coagulation in order to minimise blood loss; however, this can damage the vascular supply from the anterior and posterior deep temporal arteries and

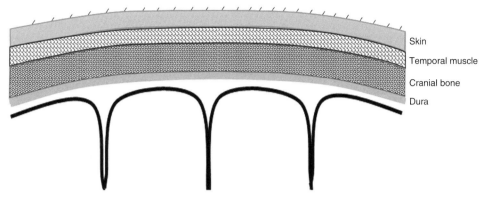

Figure 19.1 Schematic representation of normal skull anatomy. Skin and galea overlying temporal muscle, bone, dura and cerebral cortex.

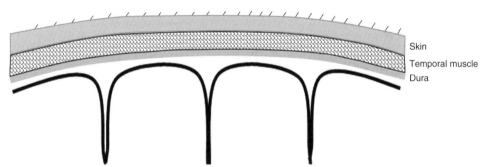

Figure 19.2 Following decompressive craniectomy, the temporalis muscle becomes adherent to the underlying dura.

innervation from the masseteric and middle temporal nerves. This can lead to loss of muscle bulk due to a combination of fibre retraction and atrophy.

Following the decompressive procedure the muscle is often left lying over the exposed dura (Figure 19.2) and in cases where a duroplasty has been performed, the dura substitute. This often leads to further scarring and muscle retraction and during the subsequent cranioplasty the absence of a clear dissection plane can lead to a considerable amount of raw muscle exposure. This in turn can increase the risk of postoperative haematoma formation which is a relatively common complication following cranioplasty.[22] Finally, there are functional and aesthetic problems that relate to muscle loss leading to masticatory difficulties and the unsatisfactory appearance due to temporal hollowing.

In an attempt to address these issues several methods have been described. In general they revolve around a common theme in which some sort of synthetic barrier is placed between the dura (and duroplasty) and the temporalis muscle at the time of closure following the initial decompressive procedure (Figures 19.3, 19.4 and 19.5). Examples include silicone, silicon elastomer, bovine pericardium, polytetrafluoroethylene and seprafilm.[23]

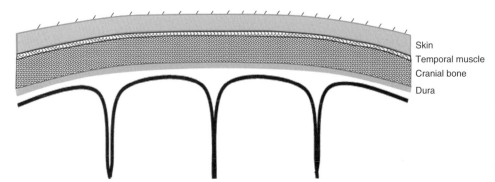

Figure 19.3 During the cranioplasty procedure, further dissection of the temporal muscle leads to atrophy of the muscle and subsequent temporal hollowing.

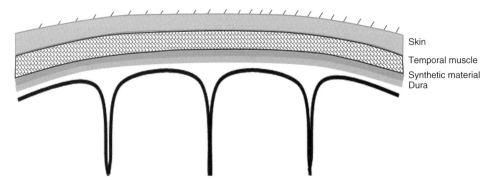

Figure 19.4 To prevent adhesions between the temporal muscle and the dura, a synthetic material can be placed over the dura, deep to the temporal muscle, at the time of closure following the initial surgical decompression.

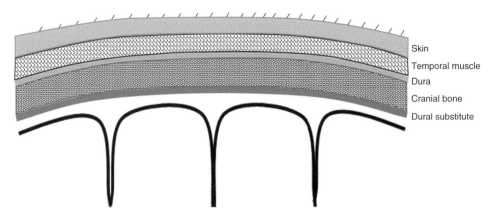

Figure 19.5 An alternative approach is to open the dura and leave it on a temporal muscle pedicle. The dural defect can be repaired with a proprietary dural substitute.

All of these methods would appear reasonable; however, this is not always possible and in many cases the temporal muscle becomes firmly adherent to the dura especially when a pericranial duroplasty has been performed. In order to avoid further damage to the temporal muscle an alternate approach would be to open the dura and reflect it laterally attached to the undersurface of the temporal muscle.[23] Once the dissection reaches the inferior aspect of the craniotomy the dura must be cut such that it remains attached to the temporal muscle and can then be reflected extracranially. When the cranioplasty is secured, the temporal muscle is sutured into its anatomical position with the dura attached to its inferior aspects.

It is not by any means suggested that this should represent a routine form of surgical reconstruction, especially if is found that there are cortical adhesions once the dura has been opened. In these circumstances the dura should be closed and the temporal muscle must either be dissected off the dura or remain attached with the cranioplasty placed over both structures. However, if there are no cortical adhesions reflecting the dura laterally provides a better cosmetic result and avoids further damage to the temporal muscle.

Complications of Cranioplasty

Overall it is clear that further work is required in order to determine the optimal surgical timing, reconstructive materials and surgical technique in order to maximise clinical benefit. However, it is also clear that there is a need to minimise morbidity due to surgical complications.

Sudden Death

In 2011, massive uncontrolled cerebral swelling leading to death following cranioplasty was reported in three young males who had survived following decompressive craniectomy for severe traumatic brain injury.[24] At the time this was thought to be a very rare event; however, since then there an increasing number of reports of this complication. Currently there has been 19 cases of this complication.[25]

Eight of these publications were isolated case reports; however, those that have been reported as part of a cohort study have reported a relatively high incidence. The initial three cases were from a cohort of 138 neurotrauma patient's cases operated on between 2004 and 2009 giving an incidence of 2.2%.[25] In 2014, Broughton reported two deaths amongst a cohort of 87 patients operated on between 2004 and 2011 giving an incidence of 2.3%.[26] Finally, Sviri has recently reported four deaths amongst a cohort of 57 patients operated on between 2005 and 2010 giving an incidence of 7%.[27]

The pathophysiology behind this exaggerated response to what should be a relatively benign surgical intervention has yet to be established. It has been suggested that it may relate to a failure in autoregulation such that the cerebral vasculature cannot respond adequately when the bone flap is replaced and there are rapid haemodynamic pressure changes. Whilst this has not been demonstrated, it would be difficult to attribute the massive and uncontrolled cerebral swelling to any other mechanism. However some sort of trigger or precipitating event would seem to be required and it has been suggested that either the application of a suction drain or a post-operative seizures may be responsible.[27]

If interest is maintained in the use of the decompressive craniectomy, close attention and wider reporting of this type of complication is required to focus attention on possible management strategies and to determine which patients are at most risk of this devastating complication

Postoperative Collections

The development of post-operative fluid collections can vary depending on site (subgaleal, extradural, subdural and intracerebral) and composition (acute, subacute and chronic haematoma/effusion). A number of studies have reported a relatively high incidence of these collections and whilst most can be treated conservatively a significant number required a return to theatre for surgical evacuation exposing the patient to further surgical morbidity.[22] It is not known why the rate of these collections is so high; however, it may relate to the degree of 'dead space' that often occurs when the brain has sunken in following resolution of the initial swelling. It may also relate to the amount of soft tissue scaring that is often encountered in re-do surgery especially when the temporalis muscle, must be dissected from the dura. The aforementioned technique whereby the dura is opened and reflected laterally, pedicled on the temporalis muscle may reduce the incidence of post-operative fluid collections; however, this remains to be established.

Infection

A higher than expected incidence of infection following cranioplasty has been reported for many years.[10] Although a clear explanation for this is unclear, it has been suggested that timing of cranioplasty may be an important factor and it has been suggested that the procedure should be delayed for a number of months in order to avoid the possibility of operating on a potentially contaminated wound. However more recent studies have failed to demonstrate any correlation between timing and infection.[3]

An alternative explanation may relate to surgical technique as was demonstrated by the aforementioned randomised controlled trial.[12] There is little doubt that the procedure is technically straightforward and in most institutions, it is performed by the relatively junior neurosurgical staff. However, the reopening of previous incisions, dissection of scarred tissue planes as well as the use of implants can lead to many instances where sterility may be compromised in inexperienced hands and this would seem to be confirmed by the results of cranioplasty trial.[22] In order to limit confounding factors, all procedures were performed by a single senior neurosurgeon in one series, using a standardised surgical technique with strict adherence to asepsis. This resulted in no primary infections in the 64 patients involved in the trial. The subsequent changes in management of cranioplasty procedure were such that there have been no cranioplasty infections in the 3 years following the trial within the two neurotrauma hospitals in Western Australia. Given these findings it may be necessary to place greater emphasis on basic surgical technique when these procedures are being performed.

Bone Resorption

The incidence of bone flap resorption following autologous cranioplasty has been reported to be between 3% and 31.6% in adults and up to 50% within the paediatric population.[10,28,29] This wide variation may reflect either biological variability or more likely be a reflection of the variability regarding the exact definition of significant bone resorption, methods of assessment and length of follow-up required.

In the aforementioned randomised controlled trial,[12] radiological assessments were performed at a standardised 12 month time point after cranioplasty, as previous studies have indicated that most resorption occurs within this time period.[28]

The bone flaps were adjudged a failure if there was resorption of bone through both the inner and outer table such that cranial protection was compromised. It must be acknowledged that there will always be some degree of subjectivity when making these types of assessment although for those bone flaps that were adjudged to be a complete failure, there was often little doubt. However, as noted by Stieglitz et al.,[30] many patients with significant resorption do not spontaneously report this occurrence and were unaware that this can be a potential problem. This highlights the need for long-term clinical and radiological surveillance, especially in young adults who may wish to return to a full working and recreational lifestyle. In these circumstances the protective role of the cranial vault requires careful consideration and the use of more robust reconstructive materials such as titanium may need to be considered as a primary restorative material.

Conclusions

If use of decompressive craniectomy in the management of severe traumatic brain injury continues, then further work will be needed to refine the technique of the constructive cranioplasty in order to minimise morbidity and provide patients with clinical benefit.

Recent studies have suggested that early surgical reconstruction can be safe and beneficial, but it has also demonstrated the need for strict adherence to aseptic technique. It is likely that autologous bone will continue to be used; however, given the choice of viable alternatives, further work will be required to assess their clinical efficacy and cost effectiveness. Finally it must be noted that whilst the procedure is technically straightforward, it has been associated with significant surgical complications which can have a significant impact on this group of previously injured and therefore vulnerable patients. Every effort must be made to minimise these complications in order to provide maximal clinical benefit.

References

1. Hutchinson PJ, Kolias AG, Timofeev IS, et al. Trial of decompressive craniectomy for traumatic intracranial hypertension. *N Engl J Med* 2016;375:1119–30.

2. Honeybul S. Decompressive craniectomy for severe traumatic brain injury reduces mortality but increases survival with severe disability. *Evid Based Med* 2017;22:61.

3. Honeybul S, Ho KM. Cranioplasty: morbidity and failure. *Br J Neurosurg* 2016;30:523–8.

4. Grant FC, Norcross NC. Repair of cranial defects by cranioplasty. *Ann Surg* 1939;110:488–512.

5. Granthan E, Landis H. Cranioplasty and the post traumatic syndrome. *J Neurosurg* 1947;5:19–22.

6. Yamaura A, Makino H. Neurological deficits in the presence of the sinking skin flap following decompressive craniectomy. *Neurol Med Chir (Tokyo)* 1977;17:43–53.

7. Stiver SI, Wintermark M, Manley GT. Reversible monoparesis following decompressive hemicraniectomy for traumatic brain injury. *J Neurosurg* 2008;109:245–54.

8. Honeybul S. Neurological susceptibility to a skull defect. *Surg Neurol Int* 2014;5:83.

9. Honeybul S, Janzen C, Kruger K, et al. The incidence of neurologic susceptibility to a skull defect. *World Neurosurg* 2016;86:147–52.

10. Matsuno A, Tanaka H, Iwamuro H, et al. Analyses of the factors influencing bone graft infection after delayed cranioplasty. *Acta Neurochir (Wien)* 2006;148:535–40.

11. Dünisch P, Walter J, Sakr Y, et al. Risk factors of aseptic bone resorption: a study after autologous bone flap reinsertion due to decompressive craniotomy. *J Neurosurg* 2013;118:1141–7.

12. Honeybul S, Morrison DA, Ho KM, et al. A randomized controlled trial comparing autologous cranioplasty with custom-made titanium cranioplasty. *J Neurosurg* 2017;126:81–90.

13. Hieu LC, Bohez E, Vander Sloten J, et al. Design and manufacturing of cranioplasty implants by 3-axis CNC milling. *Technol Health Care* 2002;10:413–23.

14. Costantino PD, Chaplin JM, Wolpoe ME, et al. Applications of fast-setting hydroxyapatite cement: cranioplasty. *Otolaryngol Head Neck Surg* 2000;123:409–12.

15. Durham SR, McComb JG, Levy ML. Correction of large (>25 cm(2)) cranial defects with 'reinforced' hydroxyapatite cement: technique and complications. *Neurosurgery* 2003;52:842–5.

16. Wong RK, Gandolfi BM, St-Hilaire H, et al. Complications of hydroxyapatite bone cement in secondary pediatric craniofacial reconstruction. *J Craniofac Surg* 2011;22:247–51.

17. Saringer W, Nöbauer-Huhmann I, Knosp E. Cranioplasty with individual carbon fibre reinforced polymer (CFRP) medical grade implants based on CAD/CAM technique. *Acta Neurochir (Wien)* 2002;144:1193–203.

18. Scolozzi P, Martinez A, Jaques B. Complex orbito-fronto-temporal reconstruction using computer-designed PEEK implant. *J Craniofac Surg* 2007;18:224–8.

19. Arnaud E. Advances in cranioplasty with osteoinductive biomaterials: summary of experimental studies and clinical prospects. *Childs Nerv Syst* 2000;16:659–68.

20. Morrison DA, Kop AM, Nilasaroya A, Sturm M, Shaw K, Honeybul S. Cranial reconstruction using allogeneic mesenchymal stromal cells: a phase 1 first-in-human trial. *J Tissue Eng Regen Med* 2017 [Epub ahead of print]

21. Joffe J, Harris M, Kahugu F, et al. A prospective study of computer-aided design and manufacture of titanium plate for cranioplasty and its clinical outcome. *Br J Neurosurg* 1999;13:576–80.

22. Gooch MR, Gin GE, Kenning TJ, et al. Complications of cranioplasty following decompressive craniectomy: analysis of 62 cases. *Neurosurg Focus* 2009;26:E9.

23. Honeybul S. Management of the temporal muscle during cranioplasty: technical note. *J Neurosurg Pediatr* 2016;17:701–4.

24. Honeybul S. Sudden death following cranioplasty: a complication of decompressive craniectomy for head injury. *Br J Neurosurg* 2011;25:343–5.

25. Honeybul S, Damodaran O, Lind CR, et al. Malignant cerebral swelling following cranioplasty. *J Clin Neurosci* 2016; 29:3–6.

26. Broughton E, Pobereskin L, Whitfield PC. Seven years of cranioplasty in aregional neurosurgical centre. *Br J Neurosurg* 2014;28:34–9.

27. Sviri GE. Massive cerebral swelling immediately after cranioplasty, a fatal and unpredictable complication: report of 4 cases. *J Neurosurg* 2015;123:1188–93.

28. Honeybul S, Ho KM. How 'successful' is calvarial reconstruction using frozen autologous bone? *Plast Reconstr Surg* 2012;130:1110–17.

29. Grant GA, Jolley M, Ellenbogen RG, et al. Failure of autologous bone-assisted cranioplasty following decompressive craniectomy in children and adolescents. *J Neurosurg* 2004;100(2Suppl Pediatrics):163–8.

30. Stieglitz LH, Fung C, Murek M, et al. What happens to the bone flap? Long-term outcome after reimplantation of cryoconserved bone flaps in a consecutive series of 92 patients. *Acta Neurochir (Wien)* 2015;157:275–80.

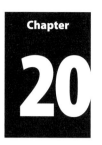

Chapter 20

Neurosurgical Complications of Head Injury

Ellie Edlmann and Peter C. Whitfield

Skull Base Fractures, Cerebrospinal Fluid Leaks and Pneumocephalus

A traumatic skull base fracture can breach the dura, leading to a communication, or fistula, from the intracranial cavity to the external environment. This leads to a risk of cerebrospinal fluid (CSF) leak in 10%–30% of patients, highest in fractures of the anterior cranial fossa.[1] CSF can subsequently leak from the nose (rhinorrhoea) or ear (otorrhoea). Many CSF leaks will seal spontaneously within 1–2 weeks with conservative management, but if CSF leakage is prolonged, then operative repair of the fistula is needed (see Chapter 18 for details on CSF leak diagnosis and management).

For anterior fossa leaks, surgical repair with a trans-nasal approach is commonly employed enabling an endoscopic extradural repair. Visualisation of the leakage has the best chance of success and is optimised by looking for discolouration of fluorescein soaked pledgets on contact with CSF. Soft tissues such as muscle, fat and fascia are commonly used to plug the defect and are usually supplanted with tissue glues and transient placement of a lumbar CSF drain to protect the repair. The success rate of such procedures exceeds 90% and has led to this being the treatment of choice.[2] Cranial approaches are generally only performed if a nasal approach has failed or if CSF is leaking through a fracture of the petrous temporal bone. A bicoronal approach is normally used for refractory anterior fossa CSF leaks, whilst a subtemporal approach, coupled with a mastoidectomy, provides good access to temporal bone fistulae. An intradural approach to the anterior fossa is more invasive than an extra-dural approach, but offers better prospects of success due to the ability to place an inlay graft. This should be done with careful placement of a graft (fascia or pericranium) across the contoured floor of the fractured anterior fossa (see Chapter 18 for management of frontal sinus fractures).

Rarely, a delayed CSF leak can occur some years after trauma. The pathogenesis of such a leak is uncertain, but the most common explanation is that following trauma, brain tissue plugged any dural breach and that changes over time have led to re-opening of the fistula.

Pneumocephalus

Pneumocephalus is air within the cranial cavity, and is commonly seen after trauma, particularly to the skull base. Small volumes of air are usually asymptomatic and self-resolve, but should alert the clinician to an underlying fracture and potential source of a CSF leak. Rarely, tension pneumocephalus can be develop if the anatomy of a fracture results in one-way flow of air.[3] This can cause headaches, agitation, seizures and neurological deterioration, necessitating urgent surgical aspiration of the air. If the volume of pneumocephalus is large but the patient is stable, then 30° head-up bed rest, high-flow oxygen (which encourages gas reabsorption into the blood stream) and surgical repair of any defect should be considered.

Meningitis Prophylaxis

Around 5%–10% of patients with a CSF leak are reported to develop meningitis, therefore the value of prophylactic antibiotics has been extensively debated.[1] Whilst some authors have shown a trend towards lower meningitis rates with antibiotic prophylaxis, it has not been concluded to significantly reduce the risk and therefore is not recommended as standard management.[4-6] Administration of Pneumococcal Conjugate Vaccine (PCV) 13 is common in the UK for patients with a CSF leak to minimise the risk of *Streptococcus pneumonia,* the most common causative organism for post-traumatic meningitis,[7] despite the evidence base for this being limited.

Growing Skull Fracture

If a young child (<3 years) sustains a skull fracture with an underlying dural tear, a growing skull fracture can develop. Clinicians should be aware of this rare complication. Growing skull fractures usually present weeks or months after the primary injury, although a small number of cases have presented years after trauma. From a pathological perspective, the brain herniates through the dural tear and keeps the fracture open, preventing healing of the bone. This brain may form a leptomeningeal cyst at the point of herniation. A craniotomy is required to expose the full extent of the dural tear. Dural repair must be achieved to prevent brain herniation. The bone flap is then replaced or reconstituted, to achieve maximal cover of the bone defect. The fracture will then usually heal.

Depressed Skull Fractures

Depressed skull fractures occur where comminuted bone fragments and scalp tissues have been forced inwards breaching the dura, usually due to high-impact forces at the point of contact with a sharp object. In penetrating trauma, the patient may have a deceptively normal level of consciousness, at least initially. However, vigilance is needed as compound (open) depressed skull fractures are associated with a high risk of seizures (up to 15%), intracranial infection (1.9%–10.6%) and mortality (1.4%–19%).[8] Whilst there are no controlled, prospective clinical trials on depressed skull fractures, there are some general principles in their management that can be followed (see Figure 20.1).

All obvious open wounds should be photographed and covered with a sterile dressing in the emergency department. The wound requires early debridement and dural repair to reduce the risk of developing intracranial infection. Where accessible, fragments of bone and contaminated material should be retrieved. Thorough irrigation of the wound with excision of devitalised tissues and primary closure of the scalp is recommended. Particular care must be exercised if a compound depressed fracture overlies the posterior two-thirds of the sagittal sinus or a transverse sinus. Elevation of bone fragments can lead to torrential bleeding, which may prove difficult to control. It is prudent to treat such fractures with wound toilet, cautious decontamination and closure of the scalp, avoiding removal of bone fragments where the risks outweigh the potential benefits.

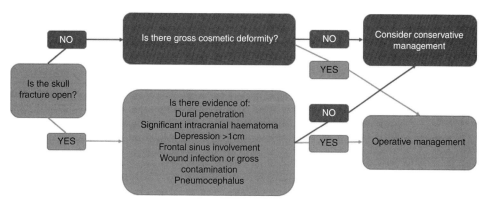

Figure 20.1 Principles of depressed skull fracture management.[8]

A closed depressed fracture does not require surgery except for cosmetic reasons and protection of the intracranial contents. This can be performed within the first week following surgery through a carefully planned, unobtrusive scalp incision.

Regarding antibiotic prophylaxis, the British Society for Antimicrobial Chemotherapy recommend a 5 day course of broad-spectrum (e.g. Co-amoxiclav or cefuroxime plus metronidazole) prophylactic antibiotic for penetrating craniocerebral injuries, although the evidence base is limited.[9]

Central Nervous System Infections Following TBI

Patients with severe TBI are at high risk of central nervous system (CNS) infection from penetrating injury, open fractures, CSF leaks and surgical incisions including EVDs and ICP monitors. Prolonged intensive-care stays also result in the development of systemic infections and colonisation with resistant organisms.

Surgical-Site Infections, Empyema and Abscess

Post-operative surgical site infections (SSIs) from craniotomy or craniectomy for TBI are a common source of infection. Wounds should be closely observed for erythema or discharge with prompt swabbing and treatment commencement if there is any concern. Superficial infections can be adequately treated with systemic antibiotics but there should be a low threshold to perform imaging to assess for evidence of deeper infection. Rarely a subdural empyema or cerebral abscess can form, particularly following penetrating head injuries and open skull fractures. The superficial wound may look acceptable in cases of deep infection, therefore a change in the clinical signs, such as a new seizure, is an indicator for further investigation. Contrast CT or diffusion MRI are the most appropriate investigations for suspected cranial SSI investigation. Distinguishing an empyema from a subdural hygroma/haematoma can be challenging and therefore the clinical picture should be carefully considered. Surgical treatment usually involves wound exploration and thorough irrigation, if deep infection is suspected then the subdural space should also be explored and the bone flap along with any dural substitute may need removal. For cerebral abscesses, marsupialisation or excision of the abscess may be appropriate if accessible; however, burr hole aspiration is commonly undertaken. Prolonged systemic antibiotics and regular post-operative surveillance CT/MR is necessary for at least 6–8 weeks to exclude abscess re-accumulation.

Meningitis/ Ventriculitis

Any trauma causing a dural breach, usually a basal skull fracture, can lead to a CSF leak exposing the patient to the risk of meningitis (see above). However, iatrogenic CSF drainage via an external ventricular drain (EVD) is a major potential source of infection. A recent UK prospective audit on 495 EVD catheters found an infection risk of 9.3%, with increased infection rates in catheters left *in situ* for more than 7 days or frequently sampled.[10] Maximum preventative strategies should be taken during EVD placement and vigilance for symptoms and signs of infection such as fever, photophobia, nuchal rigidity and altered level of consciousness is needed. Antibiotic and silver-impregnated catheters can be used instead of plain catheters, and a meta-analysis has suggested they reduce infection rate although the data are not conclusive.[11] Prophylactic systemic antibiotics should be avoided however, as they may increase the rate of resistant organisms.[12]

Early diagnosis and treatment by CSF sampling via lumbar puncture (if there is no contra-indicating mass lesion/swelling on CT) or EVD is essential. CSF microscopy and culture can identify the causative organism and guide antibiotic treatment, but may be negative if the patient has already been exposed to antibiotics. The commonest infecting organism in post-traumatic meningitis is *Streptococcus pneumoniae*, whilst EVD-related meningitis is more commonly gram-positive coagulase-negative staphylococci (35%), followed by staphylococcus aureus and (21%) enterococcus (10%).[10,11] Intravenous antibiotics with CNS penetration and appropriate sensitivity to the infecting organism should be administered early, in addition to intra-ventricular antibiotics if there is an EVD *in situ*. Ventriculitis offers a treatment challenge and has a high morbidity and mortality. Imaging can be useful to track progression, and signs such as enhancement of ventricular lining or ventricular loculation cause concern. Such findings may indicate the need for multiple EVD or shunt placements sometimes supplemented with endoscopic fenestration of loculated CSF collections.

Seizure Treatment and Prophylaxis

Seizures following a head injury, referred to as post-traumatic seizures (PTS), are a common occurrence and can be categorised as early (within 7 days) or late (after 7 days from injury).[13] If seizures are recurrent more than 7 days following injury, then this is usually classed as post-traumatic epilepsy (PTE). PTS can manifest as overt clinical seizures or sub-clinical seizures only detectable on EEG.

One population-based study on 4541 adults and children who survived TBI between 1935 and 1984 found around a 10% cumulative risk of PTE at 5 years.[14] Another report found a lower risk of only 5%, but also identified that early PTS were the biggest risk factor, increasing the likelihood of PTE fourfold.[15] The risk of epilepsy remains increased for more than 10 years following even mild TBI (see Table 20.1).[16] Recognised risk factors for developing PTS and PTE include subdural haematoma, contusions, penetrating injuries and depressed skull fractures with associated post-traumatic amnesia.[14,15,17,18]

In 1990 a landmark placebo-control trial of phenytoin in seizure control in severe TBI reported a 73% reduction in early seizures in patients on phenytoin compared with placebo,

Table 20.1 Risk of post-traumatic epilepsy following mild and severe TBI

	6 months post-TBI	3–5 years post-TBI	Over 10 years post-TBI
Mild TBI	5.46	1.99	1.51
Severe TBI	21.26	3.52	4.29

Note: Numbers represent the adjusted relative risk of epilepsy compared to patients with no history of TBI.[16]

although there was no effect on incidence of late seizures.[19] Amongst other research, this trial helped determine the 2016 Brain Trauma Foundation guidelines which recommend 1 week of phenytoin to prevent early PTS in severe TBI, where benefit is thought to outweigh complications.[13] This was supported by a Cochrane review in 2015, reporting that anti-epileptic drugs (AEDs) can be used to prevent early PTS, with the caveat that evidence is of low-quality and there is no associated impact on development of late seizures or mortality.[20] Therefore, in general many neurosurgeons give 1 week of AED prophylaxis in severe TBI patients to prevent PTS. However, choice of AED is drifting away from phenytoin and towards newer AEDs such as Levetiracetam. In Temkin's study, challenges were encountered in trying to achieve therapeutic phenytoin levels, whereas levetiracetam requires no level monitoring, has a lower side-effect profile and apparent equal efficacy.[21–26]

In addition to severe TBI, there are other circumstances when AED prophylaxis may also be beneficial. For example, moderate TBI with contusions infers a particularly high risk of early PTS, with one study reporting recurrent seizures in 85.7% of such patients even in the absence of craniotomy.[17] These patients were also at high risk of developing late PTS, with average onset of late seizures around 7 months and highest rates in patients who had an abnormal EEG on discharge.

As intensive care management of TBI becomes more sophisticated it may be possible to target AED prophylaxis more specifically at the patients who will benefit from it most. Continuous electroencephalogram (EEG) monitoring on 70 intensive care patients with severe TBI found 33% had convulsive or non-convulsive seizures at a mean of 3 days after injury.[27] EEG could also aid seizure prediction with 12 out of 18 patients having high-frequency bursts on EEG before developing seizures.

Overall, the issue of AED prophylaxis and prevention of seizures is important and further definitive studies are needed in this area. The long-term effects of seizures on patient quality of life should not be underestimated, with implications for independence and driving. All patients should be advised to stop driving and inform the DVLA following PTS, and specific guidelines on restrictions are in place depending on the severity of head injury and the timing and number of seizures.

Chronic Subdural Haematoma

Chronic subdural haematoma (CSDH) commonly complicates mild TBI in the elderly, with a mean patient age of 77 years.[28] The initial trauma may not even be recalled and the mean time interval from trauma to symptom presentation is 7–8 weeks. The pathophysiology is complex, but despite early theories on bleeding from bridging veins, it appears more likely that trauma splits open the dural space and initiates an inflammatory response.[29] The inflammatory cells and markers are then responsible for forming new membranes which contain immature, leaky blood vessels that allow chronic bleeding and fluid exudation. Patients with a conservatively managed acute subdural haematoma, are also at risk of progressing on to an expanding CSDH and should be carefully monitored for symptom progression. In such cases repeat imaging should be performed at 10–14 days to detect evolution of a CSDH.

Symptom onset in CSDH is often gradual and can be varied, including gait disturbance, cognitive decline, focal deficit, headache and eventually drowsiness or coma.[28] The mainstay of treatment is surgical drainage with burr holes or mini-craniotomy, although there is increasing interest in using medical treatments, such as steroids. These can be used as an adjunct to surgery in preventing CSDH recurrence, or can lead to complete CSDH resolution as a stand-alone therapy.[30] There are currently two ongoing randomised trials to assess the efficacy of steroid treatment in CSDH.[31,32]

Hydrocephalus

Post-traumatic hydrocephalus has an incidence ranging from 0.7% to 45% of patients.[33] CSF diversion with an EVD may be undertaken acutely to prevent or treat acute obstructive hydrocephalus secondary to traumatic intraventricular haemorrhage (tIVH). Alternatively, an EVD may be placed as a therapeutic manoeuvre in the management of refractory raised ICP. In some cases, this leads to shunt-dependency requiring permanent shunting. One study on 71 severe TBI patients found that 22.5% required permanent drainage with a CSF shunt before discharge from hospital.[33] A multivariate analysis identified craniotomy within 48 hours of admission and culture-positive CSF as risk factors leading to permanent shunting.

Patients with significant tIVH have a higher risk of EVD blockage/failure and therefore interest has grown in utilising intraventricular thrombolytic agents such as recombinant-tissue plasminogen activator (r-TPA) to help dissolve clot. However, trial results have shown that r-TPA has no impact on long-term shunt dependency in patients with spontaneous IVH.[34] Therefore, it is unlikely to have an impact on shunt dependency in TBI patients and caution should be used in this patient group due to the co-existence of other potentially haemorrhagic injuries.

Communicating hydrocephalus can develop weeks to months following TBI. This is due to chronic failure of CSF absorption, likely secondary to haemorrhage at the time of the initial injury. Symptoms commonly include gradual decline in mobility and cognition. CSF dynamic studies have been used to identify post-traumatic hydrocephalus in 20% of TBI patients, and can also identify those who are most likely to benefit from shunt treatment.[35]

Cranial Nerve Trauma

Any of the cranial nerves (CN) can be injured following head injury and a recent review found 9.1% of TBI patients (312 out of 3417) had a single or multiple CN injury.[36] This is commonly associated with other injuries such as brain contusions (74%), complicated fractures (70%) and epidural haematomas (62%).[36] A full list of CN injuries, their location, type and clinical relevance can be seen in Table 20.2.

Vascular Complications

Traumatic vertebral artery injury (TVAI) has been reported in up to 20% of head injury patients and is likely to be even higher in those with associated cervical injury.[43] This incidence has increased with more frequent and sophisticated imaging techniques, but only

Table 20.2 Cranial nerve injury incidence, location and clinical relevance

Cranial nerve	Incidence	Location of injury	Clinical relevance
I	1.9%–61% in patients with severe TBI[36,37]	Anterior cranial fossa fracture.	No specific treatments. Observe carefully for associated CSF leak. Anosmia following severe injury rarely recovers but hyposmia from mild or severe injury often spontaneously improves.[37]
II	0.5%–5%[38]	Orbital injury causing direct optic nerve compression, contusion or transection.	Deteriorating visual acuity. Surgical decompression should be considered in patients with visual deterioration in whom visual evoked potentials are still present and is particularly successful in children.[38]
III, IV V and VI	2.3%[36]	Orbital fractures and sphenoid fractures around the superior orbital fissure.[39] Distal CN V branches can be injured by craniofacial fractures	III, IV, VI = Diplopia due to ophthalmoplegia CN III – ptosis, mydriasis and ophthalmoplegia with good rates of recovery. Steroids and superior orbital fissure decompression can be considered if bony compression present.[39] CN V – facial numbness in relevant distribution[40–42]

approximately 20% of patients with unilateral TVAI are symptomatic. Those that are symptomatic usually experience symptoms of posterior circulation infarction, and presentation can be delayed up to 3–6 months due to the time taken to develop pseudoaneurysms, stenosis or arterio-venous fistula.

CT angiography allows rapid and accurate diagnosis of TVAI without the risks of invasive digital subtraction angiography, although MRA and duplex USS are also utilised.[43]

Most TVAI cases are managed with anti-platelet therapy (50%) or observation alone (31%), due to the low risk of neurological sequaelae.[44] Anticoagulation and endovascular techniques such as stenting are reserved for symptomatic, high-grade lesions.[43]

Arteriovenous fistulae can also result following traumatic head injury and most commonly occur in the cavernous segment of the carotid artery, producing a caroticocavernous fistula (CCF). This presents with pulsatile proptosis, congestion of the scleral vessels and an obvious bruit. CCFs are treated with endovascular coiling, allowing successful occlusion of the fistula in most cases (80%), and subsequent clinical improvement.[45]

Traumatic intracranial aneurysms are rare, accounting for less than 1% of all cerebral aneurysms, and are most commonly found in the supraclinoid segment of the carotid artery and along the anterior carotid artery and its branches.[46] Blunt or penetrating trauma can cause damage to vessel wall and most commonly results in false aneurysm formation, although true aneurysms can also occur if only the intima is injured. Aneurysmal haemorrhage normally occurs within 3 weeks of trauma and carries a 50% mortality.[46] To overcome this, aggressive surgical or interventional management of traumatic aneurysms is advocated. Increased utility of vascular imaging protocols as part of cranial trauma scanning identifies such lesions earlier, allowing prompt treatment.

Sport Concussion and Post-traumatic Encephalopathy

Concussion is a complex pathophysiological process affecting the brain, induced by traumatic forces. Sportsmen are at a particular risk of concussive injury. Concussion typically results in short-lived impairment of neurological function and is associated with normal neuro-imaging studies. The pathological substrate is unknown. Not all patients with concussion have a history of 'loss of consciousness'. Concussion may be categorised as simple or complex. The former resolves without complication in 7–10 days. Complex concussion is associated with persistent symptoms and prolonged cognitive impairment. It also includes athletes who experience motor convulsive posturing at the time of impact or suffer multiple concussive episodes over time, often with decreasing impact force. Neuropsychological assessment may prove invaluable in evaluating and managing these cases.[47]

The Sports Concussion Assessment Tool (SCAT) is widely used to enable medical personnel and athletes to recognise the features of concussion. These include confusion, amnesia, loss of consciousness, headache, balance impairment, dizziness, vomiting, feeling 'stunned', visual symptoms, tinnitus and irritability. Simple cognitive questions (e.g. list the months backwards, starting with any month other than January or December; recall five nouns; digit recall) help assess whether a sports person is concussed. These tests are more reliable than assessing orientation in time, place and person.[47]

It has long been reported that a patient with a history of recent concussion can sustain severe life-threatening cerebral oedema if a second injury occurs soon after trauma.[48] To prevent this rare 'second impact syndrome', most sporting authorities implement a period of non-participation after a first injury. The International Rugby Board states that 'a player who has suffered concussion shall not participate in any match or training session for a minimum period of 3 weeks from the time of the injury, and may then only do so when symptom-free and declared fit, after proper medical examination. Such declaration must be recorded in a written report prepared by the person who carried out the medical examination of the player'. The return to play should follow a stepwise progression with an initial period of cognitive and physical rest. This is followed by resumption of non-contact exercise, sports training and then game participation. For cases with complex concussion, the rehabilitation period will be longer.

Sports potentially involving repeated head injury such as boxing, football, American football and wrestling can result in long-term neuropathological sequelae termed chronic traumatic encephalopathy (CTE).[49] This has also been termed 'punch drunk syndrome' or 'dementia pugilistica' and is a neurodegenerative disorder that results in cognitive, psychiatric and motor symptoms, usually in later life once the patient has retired from their sport.[49-51] Post-mortem and imaging studies have shown structural changes that appear to correlate with clinical reports. These changes include cerebral atrophy; degeneration of midline or paramedian structures including the fornix, thalamus, hypothalamus, corpus callosum and substantia nigra; cerebellar degeneration with Purkinje cell loss; haemosiderin staining and cortical gliosis; and β-amyloid plaque formation.[52,53] The British Medical Association has voiced concern about the risks associated with boxing, despite a systematic review that reports the harmful effects are small and of doubtful significance.[54,55] There are no clear diagnostic criteria for CTE and much debate about the severity of injury required to cause it; further research is needed in this area to clarify the true cause and incidence.

References

1. Phang SY, Whitehouse K, Lee L, Khalil H, McArdle P, Whitfield PC. Management of CSF leak in base of skull fractures in adults. *Br J Neurosurg* 2016;30(6):596–604.

2. Hegazy HM, Carrau RL, Snyderman CH, Kassam A, Zweig J. Transnasal endoscopic repair of cerebrospinal fluid rhinorrhoea: a meta-analysis. *Laryngoscopy* 2000;110:1166–72.

3. Solomiichuk VO, Lebed VO, Drizhdoz KI. Posttraumatic delayed subdural tension pneumocephalus. *Surg Neurol Int* 2013;4:37.

4. Eljamel MS. Antibiotic prophylaxis in unrepaired CSF fistulae. *Br J Neurosurg* 1993;7(5):501–5.

5. Neurosurgery Working Party of the British Society for Antimicrobial Chemotherapy. Antimicrobial prophylaxis in neurosurgery and after head injury: infection. *The Lancet* 1994;344(8936):1547–51.

6. Ratilal BO, Costa J, Pappamikali L, Sampaio C. Antibiotic prophylaxis for preventing meningitis in patients with basilar skull fractures. *Cochrane Database Syst Rev* 2015;28(4):CD004884.

7. Hedberg AL, Pauksens K, Enblad P, et al. Pneumococcal polysaccharide vaccination administered early after neurotrauma or neurosurgery. *Vaccine* 2017;35(6):909–15.

8. Bullock MR, Chesnut R, Ghaiar J, et al. Surgical management of depressed cranial fractures. *Neurosurgery* 2006;58(3 Suppl): S56–60.

9. Bayston R, de Louvois J, Brown EM, Johnston RA, Lees P, Pople IK. Use of antibiotics in penetrating craniocerebral injuries 'Infection in Neurosurgery' Working Party of British Society for Antimicrobial Chemotherapy. *Lancet* 2000;355:1813–17.

10. Jamjoom AAB, Joannides AJ, Poon MT, et al. Prospective, multicentre study of external ventricular drainage-related infections in the UK and Ireland. *J Neurol Neurosurg Psychiatry* 2018;89(2):120–6.

11. Cui Z, Wang B, Zhong Z, et al. Impact of antibiotic- and silver-impregnated external ventricular drains on the risk of infections: a systematic review and meta-analysis. *Am J Infect Control* 2015;43(7):e23–32.

12. Sonabend AM, Korenfield Y, Crisman C, Badjatia N, Mayer SA, Connolly ES Jr. Prevention of ventriculostomy-related infections with prophylactic antibiotics and antibiotic-coated external ventricular drains: a systematic review. *Neurosurgery* 2011;68(4):996–1005.

13. Carney N, Totten AM, O'Reilly C, et al. Guidelines for the management of severe traumatic brain injury, fourth edition. *Neurosurgery* 2017;80(1):6–15.

14. Annegers JF, Hauser A, Coan SP, Rocca WA. A population-based study of seizures after traumatic brain injuries. *N Engl J Med* 1998;338(1):20–4.

15. Jennett WB. Predicting epilepsy after blunt head injury. *Br Med J* 1965;1 (5444):1215–16.

16. Christensen J, Pedersen MG, Pdersen CB, Sidenius P, Olsen J, Vestergaard M. Long-term risk of epilepsy after traumatic brain injury in children and young adults. *Lancet* 2009;373(9669):1105–10.

17. De Reuck J. Risk factors for late onset seizures related to cerebral contusions in adults with a moderate traumatic brain injury. *Clin Neurol Neurosurg* 2011:113 (6):469–71.

18. Englander J, Bushnik T, Duong TT, et al. Analyzing risk factors for late post-traumatic seizures. *Arch Phys Med Rehabil* 2003;84:365–73.

19. Temkin NR, Dikmen SS, Wilensky AJ, Keihm J, Chabal S, Winn HR. A randomized, double-blind study of phenytoin for the prevention of

post-traumatic seizures. *N Engl J Med* 1990;323(8):497–502.

20. Thompson K, Pohlmann-Eden B, Campbell LA, Abel H. Pharmacological treatments for preventing epilepsy following traumatic head injury. *Cochrane Database Syst Rev* 2015;8:CD009900.

21. Temkin NH, Dikmen SS, Anderson GD, et al. Valproate therapy for prevention of posttraumatic seizures: a randomized trial. *J Neurosurg* 1999; 91(4):593–600.

22. Fuller KL, Wang YY, Cook MJ, Murphy MA, D'Souza WJ. Tolerability, safety and side effects of levetiracetam versus phenytoin in intravenous and total prophylactic regimen among craniotomy patients: a prospective randomized study. *Epilepsia.* 2013;54(1):45–57.

23. Jones KE, Puccio AM, Harshaman KJ, et al. Levetiracetam versus phenytoin for seizure prophylaxis in severe traumatic brain injury. *Neurosurg Focus* 2008;25(4):E3.

24. Zafar SN, Khan AA, Ghauri AA, Shamim MS. Phenytoin versus Leviteracetam for seizure prophylaxis after brain injury – a meta analysis. *BMC Neurol* 2012;12:30.

25. Lim DA, Tarapore P, Chang E, et al. Safety and feasibility of switching from phenytoin to levetiracetam monotherapy for glioma-related seizure control following craniotomy: a randomized phase II pilot study. *J Neurooncol* 2009;93(3): 349–54.

26. Szaflarski JP, Sangha KS, Lindsell CJ, Shutter LA. Prospective, randomized, single blinded comparative trial of intravenous levetiracetam versus phenytoin for seizure prophylaxis. *Neurocrit Care* 2010;12(2):165–72.

27. Ronne-Engstrom E, Winkler T. Continuous EEG monitoring in patients with traumatic brain injury reveals a high incidence of epileptiform activity. *Acta Neurol Scand* 2006;114(1):47–53.

28. Santarius T, Kirkpatrick PJ, Ganesan D, et al. Use of drains versus no drains after burr-hole evacuation of chronic subdural haematoma: a randomised controlled trial. *Lancet* 2009;374(9695):1067–73.

29. Edlmann E, Girogi-Coll S, Whitfield PC, Carpenter KLH, Hutchinson PJ. Pathophysiology of chronic subdural haematoma: inflammation, angiogenesis and implications for pharmacotherapy. *J Neuroinflammation* 2017;14(1):108.

30. Berghauser Pont LM, Dirven CM, Dippel DW, Verweij BH, Dammers R. The role of corticosteroids in the management of chronic subdural hematoma: a systematic review. *Eur J Neurol* 2012;19 (11):1397–403.

31. Emich S, Richling B, McCoy MR, et al. The efficacy of dexamethasone on reduction in the reoperation rate of chronic subdural haematoma – the DRESH study: straightforward study protocol for a randomized controlled trial. *Trials.* 2014;15(1):6.

32. Dex-CSDH.org. www.dexcsdh.org

33. Bauer DF, McGwin G Jr, Melton SM, George RL, Markert JM. Risk factors for conversion to permanent ventricular shunt in patients receiving therapeutic ventriculostomy for traumatic brain injury. *Neurosurgery* 2001;68(1):85–8.

34. Murthy SB, Awad I, Aldrich F, et al. Permanent CSF shunting after intraventricular hemorrhage in the CLEAR III trial. *Neurology* 2017;89(4):355–62.

35. Marmarou A, Foda MA, Bandho K, et al. Posttraumatic ventriculomegaly: hydrocephalus or atrophy? A new approach for diagnosis using CSF dynamics. *J Neurosurg* 1996;85(6):1026–35.

36. Jin H, Wang S, Hou L, et al. Clinical treatment of traumatic brain injury complicated by cranial nerve injury. *Injury* 2010;41(9):918–23.

37. Schofield PW, Moore TM, Gardner A. Traumatic brain injury and olfaction: a systematic review. *Front Neurol* 2014;5:5.

38. He Z, Li Q, Yuan J, et al. Evaluation of transcranial surgical decompression of the optic canal as a treatment option for traumatic optic neuropathy. *Clin Neurol Neurosurg* 2015;134:130–5.

39. Lin C, Dong Y, Lv L, Yu M, Hou L. Clinical features and functional recovery of

traumatic isolated oculomotor nerve palsy in mild head injury with sphenoid fracture. *J Neurosurg* 2013;118(2):364–9.

40. Brodie HA, Thompson TC. Management of complications from 820 temporal bone fractures. *Am J Otol* 1997;18(2):188–97.

41. Darrouzet V, Duclos JY, Liguoro D, Truilhe Y, De Bonfils C, Bebear JP. Management of facial paralysis resulting from temporal bone fractures: our experience in 115 cases. *Otolaryngol Head Neck Surg* 2001; 125(1):77–84.

42. Finsterer J, Grisold W. Disorders of the lower cranial nerves. *J Neurosci Rural Pract* 2015;6(3):377–91.

43. deSouza RM, Crocker MJ, Haliasos N, Rennie A, Saxena A. Blunt traumatic vertebral artery injury: a clinical review. *Eur Spine J* 2011;20(9):1405–16.

44. Alterman DM, Heidel RE, Daley BJ, et al. Contemporary outcomes of vertebral artery injury. *J Vasc Surg* 2013;57(3):741–6.

45. Joshi DK, Singh DD, Garg DD, Singh DH, Tandon DM. Assessment of clinical improvement in patients undergoing endovascular coiling in traumatic carotid cavernous fistulas. *Clin Neurol Neurosurg* 2016;149:46–54.

46. Larson PS, Reisner A, Morassutti DJ, Abdulhadi B, Harpring JE. Traumatic intracranial aneurysms. *Neurosurg Focus* 2000;8(1):e4.

47. McCrory P, Johnston K, Meeuwisse W, et al. Summary and agreement statement of the 2nd International conference on concussion in sport, Prague 2004. *Clin J Sport Med* 2005;15:48–57.

48. Saunders RL, Harbaugh RE. The second impact in catastrophic contact-sports head trauma. *JAMA* 1984;252(4):538–9.

49. Gavett BE, Stern RA, McKee AC. Chronic traumatic encephalopathy: a potential late effect of sport-related concussive and subconcussive head trauma. *Clin Sports Med* 2011;30(1):179–88.

50. Martland HS. Punch drunk. *JAMA* 1928;9a:1103–7.

51. Millspaugh JA. Dementia pugilistica. *US Naval Bull* 1937;35:297–302.

52. Corsellis JAN. Boxing and the brain. *Br Med J* 1989;298:105–9.

53. Roberts AH. *Brain damage in boxers: a study of the prevalence of traumatic encephalopathy among ex-professional boxers.* London: Pitman; 1969.

54. Loosemore M, Knowles CH, Whyte GP. Amateur boxing and risk of chronic traumatic brain injury: systematic review of observational studies. *Br Med J* 2007;335:809–12.

55. McCrory P. Boxing and the risk of chronic brain injury. *Br Med J* 2007;335:781–2.

Paediatric Head Injury Management

Greg James

Introduction

Fundamentally, the management of children who have sustained traumatic brain injuries (TBI) follows the same paradigm as management in adults – primary surgery to remove mass lesions and prevention of secondary injury with high-quality intensive care. However, there are some important nuances, particularly in infants and smaller children, which the practitioner should be aware of. Increasingly (particularly in the UK, following the introduction of the 'safe and sustainable' concept of centralised services[1]), children with TBI are managed by subspecialist paediatric neurosurgeons. However, all neurosurgeons at some point are likely to be asked to look after (or at least triage) a child with a TBI, and this chapter will hopefully lay out the necessary information to aid in such a situation.

It is important to note at this point that the field of TBI management is underpinned by an increasing evidence base, thanks to several high-quality studies (e.g. RESCUE ICP[2]). Whilst some of these studies include children and young people, the focus is generally on adults. There is a paucity of so-called Level 1 evidence for management of TBI in the paediatric population, and recommendations are based on application of principles from adult practice, expert opinion and relatively small case series in children and infants. Hopefully this situation will improve in the coming years – but for now, the practitioner should bear this in mind when weighing the evidence.

Epidemiology

The overall incidence of paediatric TBI remains high, with a recent meta-analysis finding a range from between 47 (Sweden) and 280 (Australia) per 100 000.[3,4] Clearly, precise numbers will depend somewhat on definition,[5,6] but it is estimated 7000 children die from TBI in the USA every year.[7] Indeed, TBI has been described as a silent epidemic.[8] Of the 1.4 million people who attend an Emergency Department in the UK with a head injury each year, between a third and half will be children or young people under the age of 15.[9]

Most studies divide TBI into three strata of severity based on Glasgow Coma Scale (GCS): mild ($\geq$13), moderate (9–12) and severe ($\leq$8). Mild TBI remains by far the most common presentation to Emergency Departments, with at least 80% of TBI being classified as mild in most series.[3]

Generally, other than in the infant age group (<2 years), boys are more at risk, with a risk ratio for incidence at around 1.8:1 in the global meta-analysis.[3] In addition to the well-documented increase in incidence, mortality from TBI is higher in boys – 4.3% versus 1.8% in one series.[10] In regards to age, there appears to be a 'bimodal' pattern of presentation in most series,[11–13] with a median age of 6.8[3] but peaks below 3 years and around 15 years.

There is also an increased incidence (and severity) of TBI in black compared to white Americans,[14] and some evidence of increased incidence in poorer socio-economic groups.[15]

In terms of the aetiology of TBI, worldwide the most common causes of injury are motor vehicle accidents (MVA), followed by falls, non-accidental injury/assault and sporting accidents.[3] This profile is somewhat age dependent, with non-accidental injury being common in the under 2-year-old group (perhaps as many as 25%–30%[9]), falls more prevalent in intermediate age children (2–15), and MVA and assault more often seen in older teenagers (>15 years).[4,16]

Assessment

Appropriate assessment of a child presenting with a head injury will depend on age of the child and severity of injury.

For children presenting in coma or with so-called polytrauma, most institutions will follow the American Trauma Life Support guidelines or a derivative thereof.[17] After stabilisation of the 'ABC' of airway, breathing and circulation, the priority in this situation is early CT of the brain and cervical spine to identify injuries requiring immediate surgical attention. In a comatose or intubated child, clinical examination of the pupils and external examination of the head and neck for lacerations, penetrating injuries or bruising suggestive of skull fracture ('Battle's sign' and 'panda eyes') are important. Unilateral or bilateral fixed pupillary dilatation is an ominous sign and expeditious surgical treatment is likely to be required.

For those children not in coma at the time of presentation (the majority), a more detailed neurological assessment should be undertaken. It is important that practitioners are familiar with the Paediatric Glasgow Coma Scale (Table 21.1)[18] as the adult form cannot be applied to young and pre-verbal children. Generally, the aim of this assessment is to decide whether or not to subject the child to a CT scan. The advantage of an early CT scan is obvious – a normal scan reassures families and staff and allows early discharge without a prolonged period of inpatient observation (although of course a normal CT scan does not obviate the potential for later issues and appropriate, ideally written, advice should be given to the family). However, CT scanning in children carries a non-negligible risk of malignancy,[19] and therefore a degree of judgement and 'gate-keeping' is required. Attempts have therefore been made to develop paradigms to aid clinical decision-making based on evidence.[20,21] In the UK, the National Institute for Clinical Evidence (NICE) has issued specific recommendations regarding this question.[9] Readers are directed to the full guideline for complete information, but a short summary follows.

Table 21.1 The paediatric Glasgow Coma Scale

Best eye opening	Best verbal response	Best motor response
1 – none	1 – none	1 – none
2 – to pain	2 – occasional moans/whimpers	2 – extends to pain
3 – to command	3 – inappropriate crying	3 – flexes to pain
4 – spontaneous	4 – less than normal/irritable crying	4 – localises to pain
	5 – normal	5 – obeys command

For children who have sustained a head injury and have any **one** of the following risk factors, perform a CT head scan within 1 hour:

- Suspicion of non-accidental injury.
- Post-traumatic seizure but no history of epilepsy.
- On initial emergency department assessment, GCS less than 14, or for children under 1 year GCS (paediatric) less than 15.
- At 2 hours after the injury, GCS less than 15.
- Suspected open or depressed skull fracture or tense fontanelle.
- Any sign of basal skull fracture (haemotympanum, 'panda' eyes, cerebrospinal fluid leakage from the ear or nose, Battle's sign).
- Focal neurological deficit.
- For children under 1 year, presence of bruise, swelling or laceration of more than 5 cm on the head.

For children who have sustained a head injury and have **more than one** of the following risk factors (and none of those in the list above), perform a CT head scan within 1 hour:

- Loss of consciousness lasting more than 5 min (witnessed).
- Abnormal drowsiness.
- Three or more discrete episodes of vomiting.
- Dangerous mechanism of injury (high-speed road traffic accident either as pedestrian, cyclist or vehicle occupant, fall from a height of greater than 3 m, high-speed injury from a projectile or other object).
- Amnesia (anterograde or retrograde) lasting more than 5 min.

For those children who have only one of the risk factors listed in the second list, a period of observation is undertaken, and a CT scan performed if they continue to vomit or develop other symptoms.

In addition to this assessment, a full history and examination is undertaken, checking for salient points such as bleeding risks due to blood dyscrasias or pharmacological agents. Assessment of paediatric TBI must always contain a safeguarding consideration.[22] Each institution (and country) has its own rules and protocols regarding child safeguarding and it is mandatory for all practitioners to be familiar with them. A full discussion of safeguarding considerations in children is beyond the scope of this chapter, the 'bottom line' is to err on the side of safety: if non-accidental injury is suspected (however remote the suspicion), the paediatrician or nurse responsible for child safeguarding should be contacted and the case discussed. Many UK institutions now have protocols in place – for example mandatory safeguarding investigation for all TBI in children under 1 year of age.

Surgical Considerations

Extradural Haematoma

Extradural haematoma (EDH) appears to be more common in children than adults as a proportion of TBI.[23] The management is similar – most neurosurgeons will operate and extirpate an EDH in a symptomatic patient – the surgery is straightforward, with low morbidity and will usually permit early discharge from hospital.[24] However, reports exist of successful conservative management of EDH in children, even of relatively large

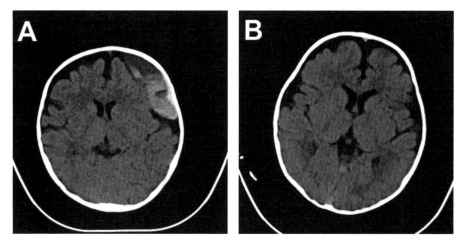

Figure 21.1 Conservative management of extradural haematoma in a child. A 10-month-old infant presented with irritability and vomiting. He had been born with a trache-oesophageal fistula, and his central line had caused a deep vein thrombosis for which he was anticoagulated on subcutaneous low-molecular weight heparin. (a) His CT scan showed a sizable left frontal EDH with mass effect. By the time of transfer to the neurosurgical unit, he was asymptomatic and neurologically normal. Craniotomy was offered but the family wished to avoid surgery due to complications of previous (non-neurosurgical) operations. The anticoagulation was discontinued. He was monitored in neurosurgical high-dependency unit for 1 week and remained asymptomatic throughout. He was discharged home. (b) A 1 month post-presentation CT demonstrated complete resolution of the EDH. He remains well at 1 year post-presentation.

EDH.[25–27] One study suggests children with no neurological deficit and a EDH volume of <15 ml on initial scan are good candidates for conservative treatment.[28] Conservative management requires close clinical observation and follow-up scanning, and may have a role in selected larger volume supratentorial cases (Figure 21.1). Conversely, due to restricted space in the posterior fossa, surgical evacuation is recommended for infratentorial EDH in children,[29] although this is a much less common anatomical location.

Overall outcomes from EDH in children (operated or conservatively managed) are good, with low levels of mortality and neurological morbidity.[24,30–33] Generally, if appropriately managed in the acute period, long-term sequelae are uncommon. One interesting phenomenon, not reported in adults, is the rare risk of calcification of an EDH causing skull deformity or mass effect.[34]

Subdural Haematoma

Whilst EDH is more prevalent in children when compared to adults, the converse is true in subdural haematoma (SDH).[35,36] Acute SDH (ASDH) is most usually seen after a high-energy injury such as a high-speed MVA and is, by definition, associated with an underlying brain injury. Polytrauma is common in these patients and ATLS guidelines should be followed to ensure optimisation of systemic factors such as oxygenation and tissue perfusion along with management of the ASDH.[17] Similar to adults, surgical treatment involves evacuation of the haematoma, with or without decompressive craniectomy,[37,38] followed by (in most cases) transfer to an Intensive Care Unit (ICU) for sedation and intracranial pressure (ICP) monitoring to manage the associated brain swelling.

One facet of SDH in children to warrant further discussion is the management of 'chronic' SDH seen in association with non-accidental injury. Classically, these are young infants (<1 year) presenting with irritability, macrocrania and symptoms of intracranial hypertension. There is often a vague or inconsistent history of one of more minor head injuries. Clinical assessment may detect retinal haemorrhages and long-bone fractures.[39] Imaging (CT or MRI) demonstrates subdural collections appearing to contain blood of mixed ages (often chronic).[40,41] Whilst these collections appear (both radiologically and macroscopically at operation) similar to the classic chronic SDH seen commonly in the elderly population, they have a high recurrence risk and appear to be better thought of, from a practical perspective, as a form of 'external hydrocephalus'. This is presumably due to disruption of the arachnoid membrane allowing CSF egress into the subdural space.[42] In our institution, we approach these SDH in a step-wise manner. Small SDH may be managed conservatively, but in the presence of symptoms and/or an increasing head circumference we recommend treatment. Initially, the subdurals can be tapped via a transfontanelle needle. This procedure can be carried out on the ward using local anaesthesia and relatively large volumes (50 ml) can be obtained. It is important to monitor the infant during and after the procedure as they can become systemically volume depleted when a large volume is taken. Sometimes, one or two large transfontanelle aspirates can be enough to treat these collections successfully. If the infant is requiring regular aspirates, a more definitive procedure can be undertaken in theatre. Burr hole washout, with or without a period of external drainage of the subdural space can be undertaken.[43] For those infants in which the collections re-accumulate despite surgical washout, and for those with very large bilateral collections, the definitive treatment is insertion of a subduro-peritoneal shunt (Figure 21.2). Whilst this is almost always successful in treating the mass effect of the collections, it requires long-term follow-up and maintenance. We have experience of children becoming 'shunt-dependent' even following complete radiological resolution of the collections.

Intraventricular Haemorrhage

Isolated intraventricular haemorrhage (IVH) following trauma is rare but reported – forming perhaps around 1% of TBI presentations in children.[44] It is more commonly seen in association with other haemorrhage, such as SDH or intracerebral contusions.[45] Traumatic IVH appears generally associated with poor overall outcomes, including a high risk of diffuse axonal injury,[45–47] although some better outcomes have been reported in selected cases.[48] Management of traumatic IVH includes close monitoring – clinically, ICP, and radiologically – for the risk of developing hydrocephalus. If hydrocephalus develops, the treatment of choice is insertion of an external ventricular drain. A rare cause of traumatic IVH, but one that should be entertained, is a cerebrovascular injury. In Figure 21.3 we demonstrate a case of a traumatic posterior inferior cerebellar artery pseudoaneurysm causing IVH. Both endovascular treatment of the pseudoaneurysm and permanent CSF shunting were required.

Skull Fractures

Linear skull vault fractures are relatively common in infancy and the vast majority can be managed conservatively.[49–52] The classic presentation is a small infant (<1 year) presenting after a fall with a swelling of the scalp and mild irritability. Neurological deficit or obtundation is rare, although vomiting may be a feature. Traditional thick-cut transverse

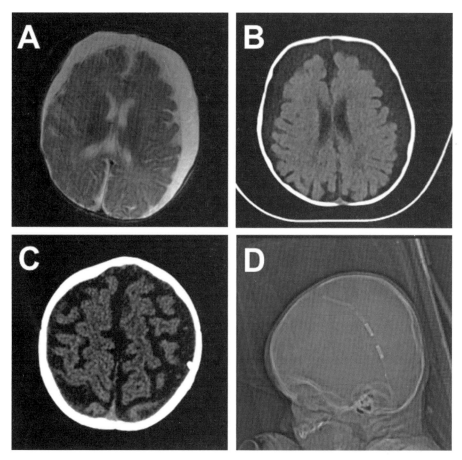

Figure 21.2 Non-accidental injury. This 3-month-old infant presented with irritability, macrocrania and a bulging fontanelle. The family gave an inconsistent history of a fall during a train journey some weeks prior. (a) MRI scan demonstrated large bilateral subdurals. (b) Initially, these were managed with repeated transfontanelle aspirations, but the collections persisted. (c, d) Therefore a subduro-peritoneal shunt was inserted, with resolution of the collections (the catheter can be seen in the left parietal region). Note the atrophy of the brain. The child's parents were investigated and prosecuted. The child is progressing well with an adopted family.

CT may miss linear fractures in the plane of the sections and 3D reconstructions are increasingly used – this technique has been demonstrated to have a greater sensitivity.[53,54] If there is a closed fracture, no underlying brain injury and the child is neurologically well, it is safe to discharge after a period of observation.[52,55] Open fractures (fractures with an overlying laceration) need appropriate wound toilet and closure, ideally by a neurosurgeon. Watertight dural closure should be achieved, if there has been a laceration. Our practice is to clean and replace any fracture fragments to avoid cranial gaps. Evidence suggests this method is safe.[56]

One phenomenon exclusively seen in the paediatric population is a growing skull fracture (GSF), sometimes called a traumatic leptomeningeal cyst.[57–59] GSF is a rare disease, seen only following head injury (1) in an infant with an open fontanelle and a rapidly growing head and (2) with skull fracture with an underlying dural injury. Essentially,

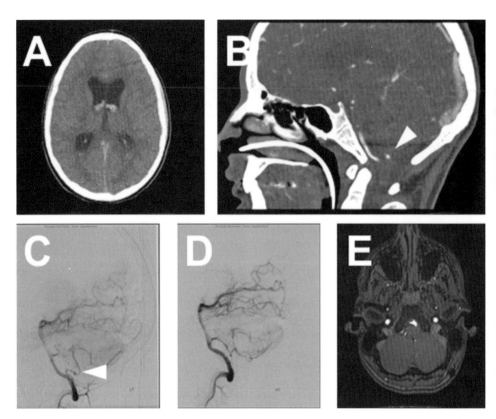

Figure 21.3 Traumatic neurovascular injury. This 13-year-old boy was involved in an altercation at school and was punched to the ground. He was initially lucid but became combative and was sedated and intubated. (a) His initial CT demonstrated predominantly intraventricular haemorrhage. (b) Because of the distribution of the blood, a CT angiogram was performed demonstrating a vascular lesion in the posterior fossa. (c) Catheter angiography confirmed a PICA pseudoaneurysm, (d) which was treated with coiling. (e) He required a VP shunt but has made a good recovery with no further bleeding, aneurysm recurrence or shunt revisions at 3 year follow-up.

pulsations of the growing brain gradually 'herniate' intracranial contents through the fracture, eroding the skull bone and chronically enlarging the defect (hence 'growing'). There is an associated leptomeningeal cyst, which itself can cause mass effect or seizures. As the name suggests, if left untreated it can result in a very significant defect. Children (usually 1–2 years old) present with a painless soft subcutaneous swelling on the head, sometimes associated with seizures or neurological deficit, following trauma (which may be comparatively minor) some weeks or months hitherto. Management involves repair of the dura and reconstructive cranioplasty, usually using autologous bone (Figure 21.4).

Decompressive Craniotomy and Craniectomy

Few topics in neurosurgery generate more controversy than the role of decompressive craniectomy (DC) in refractory intracranial hypertension following head injury, and children are not excepted from this disagreement.[60,61] Proponents of DC point to evidence from studies suggesting that early surgery can reduce ICP and increase survival,[2,62] whilst

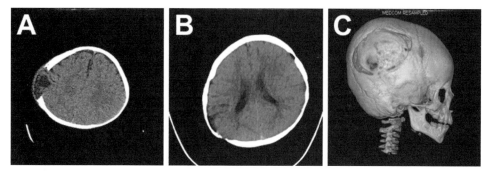

Figure 21.4 Growing skull fracture. This 18-month-old girl presented with a growing soft swelling under the scalp in the right parietal region. Her mother gave a history of her being struck by a suitcase on a train at age 6 months in India. Medical attention was appropriately sought, but no imaging was performed at that time. (a) CT at presentation to our unit demonstrated a growing skull fracture with erosion of the parietal bone and an underlying leptomeningeal cyst. (b, c) Surgical repair was undertaken with repair of the dural breach and split bone cranioplasty. Note resolution of the cyst on post-operative images. Four years later, she is neurologically normal, the cranial repair is stable and she has been discharged from the neurosurgery department.

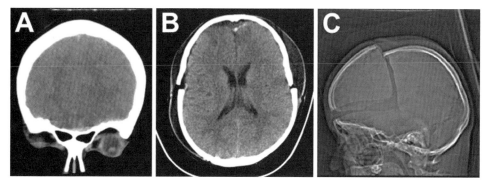

Figure 21.5 Decompressive craniotomy. This 9-year-old boy was struck by a car at 30 mph. He was intubated and ventilated at scene. (a) CT scan demonstrated bi-frontobasal contusions and loss of CSF sulcation. An ICP monitor was inserted and his pressure was high and refractory to medical treatment. Therefore, a decompressive craniotomy was undertaken with an expansion duraplasty. (b, c) The bone was left 'floating' to allow for expansion. At 5 years he has made a good recovery and not required cranioplasty.

detractors claim that increased survival is at the cost of a larger burden of surviving patients with severe neurological impairment, and significant operative morbidity.[63] Similar arguments are made on both sides in paediatric practice, and the evidence base to support such arguments is even more limited. A recent review of the literature regarding DC in children found a number of case series with overall similar outcomes to those reported in the adult literature.[61] Our institutional experience has been that children seem to have more neurological capacity for recovery than adults, and that we certainly utilise DC in children with uncontrolled ICP following a closed TBI (excepting those with prolonged fixed pupils or clinical or radiological evidence of non-survivable brain stem injury). From a technical perspective we have moved away from formal craniectomy and instead undertake an expansion duraplasty and leave the bone flap 'floating' (Figure 21.5). This can avoid the need for secondary cranioplasty surgery, and, anecdotally, appears to reduce symptoms of the so-called syndrome of the trephined. In children where a complete craniectomy is mandated (e.g. in very severe brain swelling or infection), we advocate early cranioplasty (within 3–4 weeks if possible), again to avoid flap sinkage, dural scarring and symptomatic intracranial hypotension.

Intensive Care Management

Intracranial Pressure Monitoring

Despite a recent, controversial, randomised controlled trial concluding that ICP monitoring does not improve outcome in TBI,[64] ICU care with invasive ICP monitoring remains the cornerstone of severe TBI management in the developed world. The practicalities of ICP monitoring in children is very similar to adults – intraparenchymal or intraventricular transducers can be used, inserted either in the operating room or in the ICU, and connected to an appropriate monitor to record a continuous trace. The open anterior fontanelle of small infants allows clinical examination by palpation to estimate ICP, and indeed devices have been developed to measure ICP non-invasively in these patients.[65,66] However, it is our preference to use invasive intraparenchymal monitoring for severe TBI even in small infants.

Normal values for ICP are not available for children. Although intuitively one might think that ICP is lower in children than in adults, available data do not support this,[67] and most experts recommend following similar protocols in adults as in children – that is avoiding ICPs of >20 mmHg for prolonged periods.[61]

Increasingly, there is a realisation that ICP alone is a limited indicator of intracranial physiology and outcome. Derived, multimodal variables such as PRx (the relationship between mean arterial blood pressure and ICP) can give more nuanced information about cerebral autoregulation and may guide intervention in a more useful manner. Whilst PRx was developed in adults initially, there is now evidence that it has a role in paediatric TBI.[68–70] A recent study demonstrated that both cerebral perfusion pressure (CPP) and PRx were better predictors of outcome in children with severe TBI than ICP alone.[71] We believe that there is an increasing role for multimodality monitoring in ICU management of these patients.

Osmotic Agents

Osmotic agents – primarily mannitol and hypertonic saline – are commonly used to temporarily alleviate intracranial hypertension in children with severe TBI, for example to 'buy time' for transfer from a local general hospital to a neurosciences centre. Currently, there is no evidence to suggest superiority of one over the other in paediatric practice, with both effecting a drop in ICP of around 10 mmHg following bolus administration.[72] Because there is no evidence than one agent is better than another, our current advice to referring units who need to administer a hyperosmotic agent prior to transfer is to simply use whichever one they are more familiar with.

Anticonvulsants

The use of prophylactic anticonvulsants for children with severe TBI remains controversial, with a recent study demonstrating a wide heterogeneity in practice across different paediatric neurosurgical centres[73] – in the USA, around 80% of children with severe TBI receive prophylaxis. The use of routine prophylaxis for mild and moderate TBI has been generally discontinued.[74]

The rationale for the routine use of anticonvulsants in children with severe TBI is that post-traumatic seizures are relatively common in this group[75] and that seizures are associated with worse clinical outcomes.[76] The main arguments against their routine use are related to the adverse event rate – around 75%–80% of children on anticonvulsant medication will suffer at least minor side effects.[77]

As well as the choice of whether to start anticonvulsants at all, if the clinician decides to institute treatment they must select an appropriate agent. Traditionally, this has been phenytoin – a reliable and familiar agent, albeit with a significant side effect profile. Recently, levetiracetam has been advocated as a potentially advantageous alternative[78]; however, a Cochrane systematic review failed to demonstrate superiority of any novel agent over phenytoin in this patient group.[79]

Hypothermia

Interest has persisted in the use of induced therapeutic hypothermia for traumatic brain injury, due to a plausible basic science mechanism and evidence from animal models.[80] Attempts to reproduce these results in clinical trials have been disappointing, such as the large Phase III trial published in 2001.[81] However, subgroup analysis of that trial suggested that the benefit was increased in the younger age groups studied – leading to the 'Cool Kids' randomised controlled trial examining the role of hypothermia in children with severe TBI. 77 patients were randomised to cooling (32°–33°C) or normothermia (36.5°–37.5°C). The trial was terminated early due to futility – no difference was detected between the two trial groups in terms of overall survival or poor outcome.[82] Therefore, routine use of cooling in children with severe TBI is not recommended.

Other Medical Management

Generally, recommendations for general ICU management of children with severe TBI follow those used in current adult practice. Our prime aim is to maintain 'normal' physiology such as arterial blood pressure, carbon dioxide tension and adequate oxygenation. Manoeuvres such as hyperventilation are reserved for acute episodes of intracranial hypertension as bridging measures, before, for example transfer to the CT scanner or operating room. A recent study found significant heterogeneity for ICU medical management of children with severe TBI[83] – presumably reflecting the absence of a consistent evidence base in this field.

Outcomes after TBI in Children

The needs of children who have suffered TBI do not end when they leave the operating room, intensive care unit or neurosurgical ward. It is increasingly recognised that even 'minor' TBI can have significant neuropsychological sequelae. In addition, children after TBI may suffer from epilepsy, hydrocephalus and endocrinopathies. Finally, an important question for many children and families is if and when they can return to sporting activity.

Neuropsychological Outcomes

Overall, a child's outcome from TBI is predicted by the severity of the presentation. For mild TBI, neuropsychological performance, evaluated at 6 months and 30 months post-injury, was equivalent to age-matched controls in the majority of domains. However long-term deficits were noted in verbal fluency and memory even in this group.[84] Ongoing research (such as the Brains Ahead! study) aims to elucidate both the patterns of deficit after mild TBI, as well as exploring possible treatments.[85]

For children with moderate and severe TBI, the outlook is notably worse.[86] Children who suffer these injuries are much more likely to suffer educational difficulties[87] and require intensive rehabilitation.[88] Memory, mood and concentration deficits are commonly seen,[89] with more severely affected children suffering problems with language, motor skills and planning. Overall, the incidence and severity of post-TBI cognitive and neurological deficits in children is similar to that seen caused by cerebral palsy.[90]

Post-traumatic Hydrocephalus

Post-traumatic hydrocephalus, as in adults, is a rare phenomenon but has been reported in children[91,92] – with an incidence of around 1% or less. The presence of a decompressive craniectomy appears to be a risk factor.[93,94]

Post-traumatic Epilepsy

Children are prone to developing seizures after head injury. Even in mild TBI, a large study found that 4% of children had at least one post-traumatic seizure, with 2% going on to develop intractable epilepsy.[95] The incidence of post-traumatic seizures rises to 25% in severe TBI, with risk factors including young age at injury, non-accidental aetiology and presence of subdural haematoma in a study of more than 2000 patients.[96]

Endocrine Dysfunction

It is increasingly recognised that children may suffer pituitary insufficiency after head injury, although it appears to be rarer than in adult TBI. A study of adult TBI found a prevalence of hypopituitarism of up to 50% in severe TBI,[97] whereas in children no cases of permanent hypopituitarism were detected in 198 TBI cases, although a low rate of individual hormone deficiencies and precocious puberty was detected.[98] However, a number of case reports and series have described pituitary dysfunction and stunting of growth in children[99] and endocrine referral should be considered in children presenting with relevant symptoms or failure to thrive after TBI. There is a general paucity of research in this important area, and several commentators have suggested the need for more definitive evidence.[100]

Return to Sporting Activity

Sport-related TBI is common, with an estimated 11 000 presentations per annum in the USA.[101] A common question from parents and children is related of timing of return to sporting activity – particularly in cases of impact sports such as rugby and American football – after concussion. A recent consensus statement from the American Academy of Sports Medicine[102] gives the following advice:

- Concussion symptoms should be resolved before returning to exercise.
- A return-to-play progression involves a gradual, step-wise increase in physical demands, sports-specific activities, and the risk for contact.

- If symptoms occur with activity, the progression should be halted and restarted at the preceding symptom-free step.
- Return to practice/play after concussion should occur only with medical clearance from a licensed health care provider trained in the evaluation and management of concussion.

As the long-term effects of sport-related concussion are increasingly recognised, neurosurgeons are likely to be asked for opinions regarding return to sports for children who have suffered TBI. In the absence of evidence, following published expert guidelines is recommended, as is deferring to the advice of specialist sports physicians.

Conclusion

TBI remains a common and potentially devastating disease in the paediatric population. Whilst, in the main, management is similar to TBI in adults, there are particular nuances of practice in children with head injury that need to be appreciated for optimal outcome. Whilst paediatric neurosurgical practice is likely to be further centralised in future, all neurosurgeons need to be familiar with managing TBI in children in emergent situations.

References

1. Mitchell P. Future UK paediatric neurosurgery. *Br J Neurosurg* 2010;24 (1):3–4; discussion 5–7.

2. Hutchinson PJ, Kolias AG, Timofeev IS, Corteen EA, Czosnyka M, Timothy J, et al. Trial of decompressive craniectomy for traumatic intracranial hypertension. *N Engl J Med* 2016;375(12):1119–30.

3. Dewan MC, Mummareddy N, Wellons JC3, Bonfield CM. Epidemiology of global pediatric traumatic brain injury: qualitative review. *World Neurosurg* 2016;91:497–509.

4. Thurman DJ. The epidemiology of traumatic brain injury in children and youths: a review of research since 1990. *J Child Neurol* 2016;31(1):20–7.

5. Menon DK, Schwab K, Wright DW, Maas AI, Demographics and Clinical Assessment Working Group of the International and Interagency Initiative toward Common Data Elements for Research on Traumatic Brain Injury and Psychological Health. Position statement: definition of traumatic brain injury. *Arch Phys Med Rehabil* 2010;91(11): 1637–40.

6. Savitsky B, Givon A, Rozenfeld M, Radomislensky I, Peleg K. Traumatic brain injury: it is all about definition. *Brain Injury* 2016;30(10):1194–200.

7. Langlois JA, Rutland-Brown W, Wald MM. The epidemiology and impact of traumatic brain injury: a brief overview. *J Head Trauma Rehabil* 2006;21(5):375–8.

8. Langlois JA, Marr A, Mitchko J, Johnson RL. Tracking the silent epidemic and educating the public: CDC's traumatic brain injury-associated activities under the TBI Act of 1996 and the Children's Health Act of 2000. *J Head Trauma Rehabil* 2005;20(3):196–204.

9. NICE. Head injury: assessment and early management. NICE Guideline; 2014.

10. Collins NC, Molcho M, Carney P, McEvoy L, Geoghegan L, Phillips JP, et al. Are boys and girls that different? An analysis of traumatic brain injury in children. *Emerg Med J* 2013;30(8):675–8.

11. Schneier AJ, Shields BJ, Hostetler SG, Xiang H, Smith GA. Incidence of pediatric traumatic brain injury and associated hospital resource utilization in the United States. *Pediatrics* 2006;118(2):483–92.

12. Amaranath JE, Ramanan M, Reagh J, Saekang E, Prasad N, Chaseling R, et al. Epidemiology of traumatic head injury from a major paediatric trauma centre in New South Wales, Australia. *ANZ J Surg* 2014;84(6):424–8.

13. Majdan M, Mauritz W, Rusnak M, Brazinova A, Rehorcikova V, Leitgeb J.

Long-term trends and patterns of fatal traumatic brain injuries in the pediatric and adolescent population of Austria in 1980–2012: analysis of 33 years. *J Neurotrauma* 2014;31(11):1046–55.

14. Langlois JA, Rutland-Brown W, Thomas KE. The incidence of traumatic brain injury among children in the United States: differences by race. *J Head Trauma Rehabil* 2005;20(3):229–38.

15. Parslow RC, Morris KP, Tasker RC, Forsyth RJ, Hawley CA, UK Paediatric Traumatic Brain Injury Study Steering Group, et al. Epidemiology of traumatic brain injury in children receiving intensive care in the UK. *Arch Dis Child* 2005;90 (11):1182–7.

16. Langlois JA, Kegler SR, Butler JA, Gotsch KE, Johnson RL, Reichard AA, et al. Traumatic brain injury-related hospital discharges: results from a 14-state surveillance system, 1997. *MMWR Surveill Summ* 2003;52(4):1–20.

17. *Advanced Trauma Life Support Manual*, 10th edn. American College of Surgeons, Chicago. 2018

18. Morray JP, Tyler DC, Jones TK, Stuntz JT, Lemire RJ. Coma scale for use in brain-injured children. *Crit Care Med* 1984;12(12):1018–20.

19. Pearce MS, Salotti JA, Little MP, McHugh K, Lee C, Kim KP, et al. Radiation exposure from CT scans in childhood and subsequent risk of leukaemia and brain tumours: a retrospective cohort study. *Lancet* 2012;380(9840):499–505.

20. Kuppermann N, Holmes JF, Dayan PS, Hoyle JDJ, Atabaki SM, Holubkov R, et al. Identification of children at very low risk of clinically-important brain injuries after head trauma: a prospective cohort study. *Lancet* 2009;374(9696):1160–70.

21. Dayan PS, Holmes JF, Atabaki S, Hoyle JJ, Tunik MG, Lichenstein R, et al. Association of traumatic brain injuries with vomiting in children with blunt head trauma. *Ann Emerg Med* 2014;63(6):657–65.

22. Payne FL, Fernandez DN, Jenner L, Paul SP. Recognition and nursing management of abusive head trauma in children. *Br J Nurs* 2017;26(17):974–81.

23. Godano U, Serracchioli A, Servadei F, Donati R, Piazza G. Intracranial lesions of surgical interest in minor head injuries in paediatric patients. *Childs Nerv Syst* 1992;8 (3):136–8.

24. Enicker B, Louw H, Madiba T. Acute extradural haematomas in children: A single neurosurgery unit's 12-year experience. *S Afr J Surg* 2016;54(4):28–33.

25. Khan MB, Riaz M, Javed G. Conservative management of significant supratentorial epidural hematomas in pediatric patients. *Childs Nerv Syst* 2014;30(7):1249–53.

26. Champagne P-O, He KX, Mercier C, Weil AG, Crevier L. Conservative management of large traumatic supratentorial epidural hematoma in the pediatric population. *Pediatr Neurosurg* 2017;52(3):168–72.

27. Skadorwa T, Zyganska E, Eibl M, Ciszek B. Distinct strategies in the treatment of epidural hematoma in children: clinical considerations. *Pediatr Neurosurg* 2013;49 (3):166–71.

28. Flaherty BF, Moore HE, Riva-Cambrin J, Bratton SL. Pediatric patients with traumatic epidural hematoma at low risk for deterioration and need for surgical treatment. *J Pediatr Surg* 2017;52(2):334–9.

29. Sencer A, Aras Y, Akcakaya MO, Goker B, Kiris T, Canbolat AT. Posterior fossa epidural hematomas in children: clinical experience with 40 cases. *J Neurosurg Pediatr* 2012;9(2):139–43.

30. Chowdhury SNK, Islam KMT, Mahmood E, Hossain SKS. Extradural haematoma in children: surgical experiences and prospective analysis of 170 cases. *Turk Neurosurg* 2012;22(1):39–43.

31. Teichert JH, Rosales PRJ, Lopes PB, Eneas LV, da Rocha TS. Extradural hematoma in children: case series of 33 patients. *Pediatr Neurosurg* 2012;48 (4):216–20.

32. Santos dos AL, Plese JP, Ciquini Junior O, Shu EB, Manreza LA, Marino Junior R.

Extradural hematomas in children. *Pediatr Neurosurg* 1994;21(1):50–4.

33. Nath PC, Mishra SS, Das S, Deo RC. Supratentorial extradural hematoma in children: An institutional clinical experience of 65 cases. *J Pediatr Neurosci* 2015;10(2):114–18.

34. Claiborne JR, Hoge MK, Wood BC, Couture DE, David LR. Extradural ossification following epidural hematoma in children: a rare but significant entity. *J Craniofacial Surg* 2015;26(5):1500–3.

35. Berney J, Favier J, Froidevaux AC. Paediatric head trauma: influence of age and sex. I. Epidemiology. *Childs Nerv Syst* 1994;10(8):509–16.

36. Berney J, Froidevaux AC, Favier J. Paediatric head trauma: influence of age and sex II. Biomechanical and anatomo-clinical correlations. *Childs Nerv Syst* 1994;10(8):517–23.

37. Kolias AG, Adams H, Timofeev I, Czosnyka M, Corteen EA, Pickard JD, et al. Decompressive craniectomy following traumatic brain injury: developing the evidence base. *Br J Neurosurg* 2016;30(2):246–50.

38. Kolias AG, Scotton WJ, Belli A, King AT, Brennan PM, Bulters DO, et al. Surgical management of acute subdural haematomas: current practice patterns in the United Kingdom and the Republic of Ireland. *Br J Neurosurg* 2013;27(3):330–3.

39. Fitzpatrick S, Leach P. Neurosurgical aspects of abusive head trauma management in children: a review for the training neurosurgeon. *Br J Neurosurg* 2019;33(1):47–50.

40. Sieswerda-Hoogendoorn T, Robben SGF, Karst WA, Moesker FM, van Aalderen WM, Lameris JS, et al. Abusive head trauma: differentiation between impact and non-impact cases based on neuroimaging findings and skeletal surveys. *Eur J Radiol* 2014;83(3):584–8.

41. Amagasa S, Matsui H, Tsuji S, Uematsu S, Moriya T, Kinoshita K. Characteristics distinguishing abusive head trauma from accidental head trauma in infants with traumatic intracranial hemorrhage in Japan. *Acute Med Surg* 2018;5(3):265–71.

42. Wright JN. CNS injuries in abusive head trauma. *AJR Am J Roentgenol* 2017;208(5):991–1001.

43. Melo JRT, Di Rocco F, Bourgeois M, Puget S, Blauwblomme T, Sainte-Rose C, et al. Surgical options for treatment of traumatic subdural hematomas in children younger than 2 years of age. *J Neurosurg Pediatr* 2014;13(4):456–61.

44. Lichenstein R, Glass TF, Quayle KS, Wootton-Gorges SL, Wisner DH, Miskin M, et al. Presentations and outcomes of children with intraventricular hemorrhages after blunt head trauma. *Arch Pediatr Adolesc Med* 2012;166(8):725–31.

45. Mata-Mbemba D, Mugikura S, Nakagawa A, Murata T, Kato Y, Tatewaki Y, et al. Intraventricular hemorrhage on initial computed tomography as marker of diffuse axonal injury after traumatic brain injury. *J Neurotrauma* 2015;32(5):359–65.

46. Muller H, Brock M. Primary intraventricular traumatic hemorrhage. *Surg Neurol* 1987;27(4):398–402.

47. Atzema C, Mower WR, Hoffman JR, Holmes JF, Killian AJ, Wolfson AB. Prevalence and prognosis of traumatic intraventricular hemorrhage in patients with blunt head trauma. *J Trauma* 2006;60(5):1010–7; discussion 1017.

48. Is M, Gezen F, Akgul M, Dosoglu M. Traumatic intraventricular hemorrhage with a good prognosis. *Turk Neurosurg* 2011;21(1):107–9.

49. Merhar SL, Kline-Fath BM, Nathan AT, Melton KR, Bierbrauer KS. Identification and management of neonatal skull fractures. *J Perinatol* 2016;36(8):640–2.

50. Powell EC, Atabaki SM, Wootton-Gorges S, Wisner D, Mahajan P, Glass T, et al. Isolated linear skull fractures in children with blunt head trauma. *Pediatrics* 2015;135(4):e851–7.

51. Mannix R, Monuteaux MC, Schutzman SA, Meehan WP, Nigrovic LE, Neuman MI. Isolated skull fractures: trends in

management in US pediatric emergency departments. *Ann Emerg Med* 2013;62 (4):327–31.

52. Arrey EN, Kerr ML, Fletcher S, Cox CSJ, Sandberg DI. Linear nondisplaced skull fractures in children: who should be observed or admitted? *J Neurosurg Pediatr* 2015;16(6):703–8.

53. Cho SM, Kim HG, Yoon SH, Chang KH, Park MS, Park Y-H, et al. Reappraisal of neonatal greenstick skull fractures caused by birth injuries: comparison of 3-dimensional reconstructed computed tomography and simple skull radiographs. *World Neurosurg* 2018;109:e305–12.

54. Orman G, Wagner MW, Seeburg D, Zamora CA, Oshmyansky A, Tekes A, et al. Pediatric skull fracture diagnosis: should 3D CT reconstructions be added as routine imaging? *J Neurosurg Pediatr* 2015;16 (4):426–31.

55. White IK, Pestereva E, Shaikh KA, Fulkerson DH. Transfer of children with isolated linear skull fractures: is it worth the cost? *J Neurosurg Pediatr* 2016;17 (5):602–6.

56. AbdelFatah MA. Management of bone fragments in nonmissile compound depressed skull fractures. *Acta Neurochir* 2016;158(12):2341–5.

57. Singh I, Rohilla S, Siddiqui SA, Kumar P. Growing skull fractures: guidelines for early diagnosis and surgical management. *Childs Nerv Syst* 2016;32(6):1117–22.

58. Vezina N, Al-Halabi B, Shash H, Dudley RR, Gilardino MS. A review of techniques used in the management of growing skull fractures. *J Craniofacial Surg* 2017;28(3):604–9.

59. Prasad GL, Gupta DK, Mahapatra AK, Borkar SA, Sharma BS. Surgical results of growing skull fractures in children: a single centre study of 43 cases. *Childs Nerv Syst* 2015;31(2):269–77.

60. Pechmann A, Anastasopoulos C, Korinthenberg R, van Velthoven-Wurster V, Kirschner J. Decompressive craniectomy after severe traumatic brain injury in children: complications and outcome. *Neuropediatrics* 2015;46(1):5–12.

61. Young AMH, Kolias AG, Hutchinson PJ. Decompressive craniectomy for traumatic intracranial hypertension: application in children. *Childs Nerv Syst* 2017;33 (10):1745–50.

62. Cooper DJ, Rosenfeld JV, Murray L, Arabi YM, Davies AR, D'Urso P, et al. Decompressive craniectomy in diffuse traumatic brain injury. *N Engl J Med* 2011;364(16):1493–502.

63. Honeybul S, Ho KM, Lind CRP, Gillett GR. The future of decompressive craniectomy for diffuse traumatic brain injury. *J Neurotrauma* 2011;28(10):2199–200.

64. Chesnut RM, Temkin N, Carney N, Dikmen S, Rondina C, Videtta W, et al. A trial of intracranial-pressure monitoring in traumatic brain injury. *N Engl J Med* 2012;367(26):2471–81.

65. Behmanesh B, Setzer M, Noack A, Bartels M, Quick-Weller J, Seifert V, et al. Noninvasive epicutaneous transfontanelle intracranial pressure monitoring in children under the age of 1 year: a novel technique. *J Neurosurg Pediatr* 2016;18 (3):372–6.

66. Behmanesh B, Bartels M, Gessler F, Filmann N, Seifert V, Setzer M, et al. Noninvasive transfontanelle monitoring of the intracerebral pressure in comparison with an invasive intradural intracranial pressure device: a prospective study. *Oper Neurosurg (Hagerstown)* 2017;13 (5):609–13.

67. Magnéli S, Howells T, Saiepour D, Nowinski D, Enblad P, Nilsson P. Telemetric intracranial pressure monitoring: a noninvasive method to follow up children with complex craniosynostoses: a case report. *Childs Nerv Syst* 2016;32(7):1311–5.

68. Ducharme-Crevier L. Cerebrovascular pressure reactivity in children with TBI. *Pediatr Neurol Briefs* 2015;29(10):77.

69. Hockel K, Diedler J, Neunhoeffer F, Heimberg E, Nagel C, Schuhmann MU. Time spent with impaired autoregulation is linked with outcome in severe infant/paediatric traumatic brain injury. *Acta Neurochir* 2017;159(11):2053–61.

70. Nagel C, Diedler J, Gerbig I, Heimberg E, Schuhmann MU, Hockel K. State of cerebrovascular autoregulation correlates with outcome in severe infant/pediatric traumatic brain injury. *Acta Neurochir Suppl* 2016;122:239–44.

71. Young AMH, Donnelly J, Czosnyka M, Jalloh I, Liu X, Aries MJ, et al. Continuous multimodality monitoring in children after traumatic brain injury-preliminary experience. *PLoS One* 2016;11(3):e0148817.

72. Roumeliotis N, Dong C, Pettersen G, Crevier L, Emeriaud G. Hyperosmolar therapy in pediatric traumatic brain injury: a retrospective study. *Childs Nerv Syst* 2016;32(12):2363–8.

73. Ostahowski PJ, Kannan N, Wainwright MS, Qiu Q, Mink RB, Groner JI, et al. Variation in seizure prophylaxis in severe pediatric traumatic brain injury. *J Neurosurg Pediatr* 2016;18 (4):499–506.

74. Tanaka T, Litofsky NS. Anti-epileptic drugs in pediatric traumatic brain injury. *Expert Rev Neurotherapeut* 2016;16 (10):1229–34.

75. Arndt DH, Lerner JT, Matsumoto JH, Madikians A, Yudovin S, Valino H, et al. Subclinical early posttraumatic seizures detected by continuous EEG monitoring in a consecutive pediatric cohort. *Epilepsia* 2013;54(10):1780–8.

76. Vespa PM, Miller C, McArthur D, Eliseo M, Etchepare M, Hirt D, et al. Nonconvulsive electrographic seizures after traumatic brain injury result in a delayed, prolonged increase in intracranial pressure and metabolic crisis. *Crit Care Med* 2007;35(12):2830–6.

77. Egunsola O, Choonara I, Sammons HM, Whitehouse WP. Safety of antiepileptic drugs in children and young people: a prospective cohort study. *Seizure* 2018;56:20–5.

78. Pearl PL, McCarter R, McGavin CL, Yu Y, Sandoval F, Trzcinski S, et al. Results of phase II levetiracetam trial following acute head injury in children at risk for posttraumatic epilepsy. *Epilepsia* 2013;54 (9):e135–7.

79. Thompson K, Pohlmann-Eden B, Campbell LA, Abel H. Pharmacological treatments for preventing epilepsy following traumatic head injury. *Cochrane Database Syst Rev* 2015;26(8):CD009900.

80. Clark RS, Kochanek PM, Marion DW, Schiding JK, White M, Palmer AM, et al. Mild posttraumatic hypothermia reduces mortality after severe controlled cortical impact in rats. *J Cereb Blood Flow Metab* 1996;16(2):253–61.

81. Clifton GL, Miller ER, Choi SC, Levin HS, McCauley S, Smith KR, et al. Lack of effect of induction of hypothermia after acute brain injury. *N Engl J Med* 2001;344 (8):556–63.

82. Adelson PD, Wisniewski SR, Beca J, Brown SD, Bell M, Muizelaar JP, et al. Comparison of hypothermia and normothermia after severe traumatic brain injury in children (Cool Kids): a phase 3, randomised controlled trial. *Lancet Neurol* 2013;12(6):546–53.

83. Bell MJ, Adelson PD, Hutchison JS, Kochanek PM, Tasker RC, Vavilala MS, et al. Differences in medical therapy goals for children with severe traumatic brain injury-an international study. *Pediatr Crit Care Med* 2013;14(8):811–8.

84. Anderson V, Catroppa C, Morse S, Haritou F, Rosenfeld J. Outcome from mild head injury in young children: a prospective study. *J Clin Exp Neuropsychol* 2001;23(6):705–17.

85. Renaud MI, Lambregts SAM, de Kloet AJ, Catsman-Berrevoets CE, van de Port IGL, van Heugten CM. Activities and participation of children and adolescents after mild traumatic brain injury and the effectiveness of an early intervention (Brains Ahead!): study protocol for a cohort study with a nested randomised controlled trial. *Trials* 2016;17(1):236.

86. Popernack ML, Gray N, Reuter-Rice K. Moderate-to-severe traumatic brain injury in children: complications and rehabilitation strategies. *J Pediatr Health Care* 2015;29(3):e1–7.

87. Prasad MR, Swank PR, Ewing-Cobbs L. Long-term school outcomes of children and

adolescents with traumatic brain injury. *J Head Trauma Rehabil* 2017;32(1):E24–E32.

88. Hayes L, Shaw S, Pearce MS, Forsyth RJ. Requirements for and current provision of rehabilitation services for children after severe acquired brain injury in the UK: a population-based study. *Arch Dis Child* 2017;102(9):813–20.

89. Babikian T, Merkley T, Savage RC, Giza CC, Levin H. Chronic aspects of pediatric traumatic brain injury: review of the literature. *J Neurotrauma* 2015;32 (23):1849–60.

90. Hayes L, Shaw S, Pearce MS, Forsyth RJ. Requirements for and current provision of rehabilitation services for children after severe acquired brain injury in the UK: a population-based study. *Arch Dis Child* 2017;102(9):813–20.

91. Gupta SK, Sharma T. Acute post-traumatic hydrocephalus in an infant due to aqueductal obstruction by a blood clot: a case report. *Childs Nerv Syst* 2009;25 (3):373–6.

92. Licata C, Cristofori L, Gambin R, Vivenza C, Turazzi S. Post-traumatic hydrocephalus. *J Neurosurg Sci* 2001;45(3):141–9.

93. Phuenpathom N, Ratanalert S, Saeheng S, Sripairojkul B. Post-traumatic hydrocephalus: experience in 17 consecutive cases. *J Med Assoc Thai* 1999;82(1):46–53.

94. Vadivelu S, Rekate HL, Esernio-Jenssen D, Mittler MA, Schneider SJ. Hydrocephalus associated with childhood nonaccidental head trauma. *Neurosurg Focus* 2016;41(5):E8.

95. Keret A, Bennett-Back O, Rosenthal G, Gilboa T, Shweiki M, Shoshan Y, et al.

Posttraumatic epilepsy: long-term follow-up of children with mild traumatic brain injury. *J Neurosurg Pediatr* 2017;20 (1):64–70.

96. Bennett KS, DeWitt PE, Harlaar N, Bennett TD. Seizures in children with severe traumatic brain injury. *Pediatr Crit Care Med* 2017;18(1):54–63.

97. Schneider HJ, Schneider M, Saller B, Petersenn S, Uhr M, Husemann B, et al. Prevalence of anterior pituitary insufficiency 3 and 12 months after traumatic brain injury. *Eur J Endocrinol* 2006;154(2):259–65.

98. Heather NL, Jefferies C, Hofman PL, Derraik JGB, Brennan C, Kelly P, et al. Permanent hypopituitarism is rare after structural traumatic brain injury in early childhood. *J Clin Endocrinol Metab* 2012;97(2):599–604.

99. Richmond E, Rogol AD. Traumatic brain injury: endocrine consequences in children and adults. *Endocrine* 2014;45(1):3–8.

100. Casano-Sancho P. Pituitary dysfunction after traumatic brain injury: are there definitive data in children? *Arch Dis Child* 2017;102(6):572–7.

101. Yue JK, Winkler EA, Burke JF, Chan AK, Dhall SS, Berger MS, et al. Pediatric sports-related traumatic brain injury in United States trauma centers. *Neurosurg Focus* 2016;40(4):E3.

102. Harmon KG, Drezner J, Gammons M, Guskiewicz K, Halstead M, Herring S, et al. American Medical Society for Sports Medicine position statement: concussion in sport. *Clin J Sport Med* 2013;23: 1–18.

Chapter 22

Assessment of Cognition and Capacity

Maggie Whyte and Fiona Summers

Introduction

The cognitive consequences of traumatic brain injury are wide ranging in severity and presentation. Early assessment of cognition can give indication of severity of injury, prognosis, can guide communication with the patient and inform rehabilitation. At later stages in recovery, cognitive assessment, as part of a wider evaluation, can be used to identify neuroanatomical areas of injury, quantify areas of cognitive deficit and discriminate between influences on cognitive functioning (e.g. primary impact of the brain injury, psychological disturbance, impact of other physical factors such as pain or fatigue). Cognitive assessment can also assist in predicting recovery and the likely future impact on daily living skills, inform adjustments that may need to be made to rehabilitation programmes and measure change as the patient recovers and responds to rehabilitation. Where cognition is impaired, decision-making may be affected and therefore clinician's are often required to consider cognition in assessment of capacity. In early stages of recovery this most likely relates to medical treatment however as recovery progresses, may relate to other welfare or financial matters. The following chapter outlines the cognitive consequences of traumatic brain injury, considerations for cognitive assessment and assessment of capacity with reference to the process of neuropsychological assessment.

Assessing Cognitive Functioning in the Acute Inpatient Environment

A detailed and comprehensive assessment of the patient's cognitive functioning is generally conducted in the post-acute rehabilitation environment by a neuropsychologist. However, on occasion, a request might be made to assess a patient's cognitive abilities whilst they are receiving acute medical treatment.[1] Even if the patient is in Post-Traumatic Amnesia (PTA) it may be possible to conduct brief cognitive assessments. Although fluctuations in the patient's level of consciousness during the acute period of recovery may devalue the results of any such assessment, Bishop et al. report that, when undertaken, the results and recommendations made in the neuropsychological report often have a significant bearing on the patient's placement at discharge.[1]

Furthermore, documenting the patient's cognitive strengths and weaknesses at the acute stage of recovery will be helpful when it comes to planning a rehabilitation programme. The neuropsychologist can make recommendations to other health professionals about ways of modifying their therapeutic approach in order to provide the patient with the optimum environment in which to realise their rehabilitation potential. Regular multidisciplinary consultation and review is helpful in assessing the potential benefits and disadvantages of a particular intervention. This process of review also allows alternative interventions to be considered according to the patient's changing presentation and stage of recovery. Bearing in mind factors such as aetiology and diagnosis, the results of any assessment conducted in the acute stage of the patient's recovery can be used to draw conclusions about likely prognosis which can influence future management decisions.[2]

Process of Neuropsychological Assessment

The process of neuropsychological assessment involves the complex integration of information gathered about the patient and their difficulties from medical notes, interview with the patient and others, observation and formal assessment. Pre-morbid factors influencing cognition in the person's medical, psychiatric, developmental, educational and occupational history are considered. The history of the injury and subsequent recovery, including measures of PTA and GCS, can give an initial impression of severity of injury. Consultation with the family may reveal important information about pre-morbid personality, abilities and lifestyle, and comments by family and staff on their observations of the patient's behaviour and abilities can usefully inform assessment. The neuropsychologist may also spend a period of time observing the patient particularly those with challenging behaviour and/or a severe TBI. The neuropsychologist will observe the patient during the interview and formal assessment in order to gather information on the presentation of difficulties, for example insight, processing speed or those which may influence performance on formal assessment including anxiety, motivation and secondary gain. Hodges provides a useful chapter on history taking including tips on physical examination.[3]

Formal cognitive assessment covers the main domains of cognitive functioning however the focus and choice of assessment is likely to vary, depending on the presentation of the patient and the impression of likely difficulties. Pre-morbid functioning is also tested and assessment results interpreted in view of this. The neuropsychologist will be aware of the limitations of the tests which are used, including information on the development of the assessments, the validity and reliability. Following assessment, the neuropsychologist draws the information together to construct a formulation identifying which aspects of the patient's presentation are as a result of the primary consequences of the brain injury, which are secondary consequences and which are a result of other influences, pre-morbid or co-existing.

There is much evidence to support the validity of neuropsychological assessment in predicting functional outcome after TBI and return to work.[4,5] Neuropsychological assessment has been shown to be a reliable diagnostic and prognostic indicator when compared with neuroimaging.[6,7] However, there is general agreement about the utility of using a combination of neuro-imaging and neuropsychological assessment when answering diagnostic or other clinical questions.

Cognitive Functioning

Impairments in cognitive functioning as a result of brain injury can be diffuse or focal depending on the nature of the injury. Diffuse brain injury, affecting many, although rarely all, areas of cognition, is common following closed brain injuries involving rapid acceleration or deceleration. Focal impairments in cognition are common following penetrating traumatic brain injuries. The type and extent of any impairment is influenced by the site, size and depth of any lesion. Whilst diffuse brain injury affects many aspects of cognition, focal deficits can also have a significant deleterious effect upon day-to-day functioning and quality of life. Areas of cognitive impairment commonly reported in the literature following brain injury include memory, attention, processing speed, executive functioning, perception and language.

Memory

Impairment in memory functioning is the most common complaint following brain injury and is associated with medial temporal lobes, the diencephalon, the basal forebrain nuclei and retrosplenial cortex. There are many different types of memory functioning. *Working memory* involves the temporary storage and manipulation of a limited amount of information for a short period of time and is often confused with term 'short-term memory'. Short-term memory is an outdated concept but still often used by clinicians. *Long-term memory* is subdivided into two broad areas: explicit (declarative) memory and implicit memory. Explicit memory involves the process of actively remembering, such as studying for an examination, and includes *semantic memory*, a representation knowledge of facts and concepts; for example mathematical equations, words and their meanings as well as *episodic memory* which involves long-term storage of events and personal experiences. Implicit memory is the process of non-conscious remembering and includes *procedural memory* of motor and cognitive skills, such as driving or riding a bike, priming and classical conditioning.

The distinction between anterograde and retrograde amnesia is important in clinical settings. *Anterograde or post-traumatic amnesia (PTA)* refers to the inability, or limited ability, to learn new information and knowledge from the point at which injury has occurred, but after a period of coma, whereas *retrograde amnesia* refers to the inability to recall events preceding the onset of brain injury. Retrograde amnesia can range from a few seconds to decades and consequently can cause significant distress for the patient and family members. Anterograde amnesia can cause considerable problems with return to work, academic study and simply remembering to do something (*prospective memory*). An important concept in memory functioning is the distinction between the registration of information, encoding and retrieval. Patients need to be able to attend to information (be this verbal, visual or tactile) for this to be encoded and consolidated for it then to be retrieved when necessary. The distinction between free recall (uncued retrieval involving an active search process) and recognition (familiarity) is therefore important as impaired recall with intact recognition suggests deficits in retrieval rather than encoding. Impairments in both suggest deficits in the encoding of information.

Attention

Impairment in attention is also common following brain injury and is associated with multiple brain systems including the parietal cortex, the frontal cortex and limbic system structures. Although there are many different types of attention, the most common are focused/selective attention, sustained attention/vigilance, divided attention and alternating attention. Focused or selective attention, also commonly referred to as concentration, is the capacity to highlight important stimuli whilst suppressing awareness of competing distractions.[8] Sustained attention refers to the ability to maintain attention over an extended period of time, whilst divided attention involves the ability to respond to more than one task at a time for example talking on the telephone whilst writing. Alternating attention, also referred to as set shifting, involves the ability to move attentional focus from one task to another. It is important to acknowledge that attentional abilities have limited capacity and impairments in attention have significant effects on other areas of cognition, particularly memory and executive functioning.

Processing Speed

Processing speed, the rate at which mental activities are performed, is commonly impaired following brain damage. Patients often describe slow processing speed as feeling as if they are one step behind everyone else in conversations. Patients with slow processing speed commonly take longer to respond to questions displaying delayed reaction times, which are important to consider during clinical interview.

Executive Functioning

Executive functioning refers to a range of functions associated with the ability to establish behaviour patterns and ways of thinking and to introspect upon them. Impairments in executive functioning (often called dysexecutive syndrome) were initially thought to be related solely to damage to the frontal lobes; however, research now suggests wider network brain involvement, although the frontal lobes still remain important. Executive functioning encompasses a wide and varied range of behaviours, including planning and organising, problem solving and reasoning (required in decision-making and important when considering capacity), the ability to achieve goals effectively, control of impulsivity (when impaired can result in aggression, inappropriate behaviour and excitability), confabulation (unintentional production of a false memory), mental flexibility (when impaired can result in rigid inflexible thinking) and sequencing. Lack of concern, apathy and lack of insight are also associated with impaired executive functioning and cause considerable problems for families and in rehabilitation who will often describe this as a 'personality change'.

Perception

Perceptual processes, the elaborations and interpretations of neural signals which enable one to become aware of external stimulations, are associated with damage to the occipital and parietal lobes with some involvement of the temporal lobes and subcortical regions. Impaired perceptual processes include agnosias (the inability to recognise the meaning, identity and nature of sensory stimuli presented either by touch, sight or sound), neglect and visual inattention. This includes structural perception and semantic processing of faces (prosopagnosia).

Speech and Language

Language and communication disorders following brain injury are frequent and include dysphasia (the impairment of language function), dysarthria (the impairment of coordinated muscle activity), impairments in pragmatic communication and discourse, acquired dyslexia (impaired reading) and dysgraphia (impaired writing) and the secondary effect of other cognitive impairments such as executive functioning on communication.

ACE III,
http://dementia.ie/images/uploads/site-images/ACE-III_Administration_(UK).pdf
Free app available (following an 8 min tutorial) including instructions for administration and scoring:

MoCA,
www.mocatest.org.
Paper and App available; requires mandatory online training and certification with fee.

Figure 22.1 Online resources for bedside testing of cognitive functioning

Bedside Testing

Clinical neuropsychologists have in-depth expertise in assessing cognitive functioning; however, it is acknowledged that cognitive screening may usefully be conducted by other professionals. The most common and widely used assessment tool to screen for cognitive impairment is the Mini Mental Status Examination (MMSE).[9] However, this tool lacks the sensitivity required for detecting mild brain injury, focuses mainly on memory functioning and neglects executive functioning (critical for TBI), lacks the specificity to identify focal impairments and is no longer free to use. In addition, it is strongly influenced by age, education, ethnicity and socioeconomic status although can be useful for monitoring change over time particularly in patients with moderate and severe impairments. The Addenbrooke's Cognitive Examination–III (ACE-III) provides a more in-depth yet brief assessment, including aspects of executive functioning. Research shows that the ACE-III cognitive domains correlate significantly with standardised neuropsychological tests and shows high sensitivity and specificity.[10] The Montreal Cognitive Assessment (MoCA) is also widely used screening assessment covering several cognitive domains. Both the ACE-III and the MoCA are available online (Figure 22.1), in many languages and have alternative forms. Research comparing the ACE-III and MoCA show the ACE-III as having slightly higher diagnostic accuracy[11] however are generally comparable. The ACE-III takes 10–20 min to complete compared to 10 min for the MoCA. Hodges[3] provides a useful guide to conducting bedside examinations of cognitive performance.

Assessing Capacity in Clinical Practice

In this section aspects which are important to consider in assessing capacity are explored along with a practical approach to assessing capacity.

Definition of Capacity

Regulation of how decisions are made for those who do not have the capacity to make them for themselves are governed by the laws of the country. In the British Isles this includes the Mental Capacity Act (2005) (MCA) in England and Wales, the Adults with Incapacity (Scotland) Act 2000 (AwI), the Assisted Decision Making (Capacity) Act 2015 in Ireland and the Mental Capacity Act (Northern Ireland) 2016. Definitions of incapacity differ between these legal frameworks (Figure 22.2) and each act lays out a number of principles that must be adhered to when applying the act. The clinical aspects of assessing capacity however remain the same.

The requirement for assessment of capacity in a patient with TBI may be triggered by the need for a particular decision to be made about medical treatment, other welfare or financial

Mental Capacity Act (2005)
www.legislation.gov.uk/ukpga/2005/9/pdfs/ukpga_20050009_en.pdf

2 stage definition

1   Determine whether there exists a disturbance in the mind or brain. Can be permanent or temporary cannot be established merely by reference to age, appearance, a condition or behaviour that might lead to unjustified assumptions about capacity.
2   Determine if this impairment or disturbance results in an inability to make or communicate decisions. If he/she is unable to:

> understand the information relevant to the decision
> retain that information
> use or weigh that information as part of the process of making a decision
> communicate the decision

Adults with Incapacity (Scotland) Act 2000
www.legislation.gov.uk/asp/2000/4/pdfs/asp_20000004_en.pdf

'incapable' means incapable of –

(a) acting; or
(b) making decisions; or
(c) communicating decisions; or
(d) understanding decisions; or
(e) retaining the memory of decisions,

as mentioned in any provision of this Act, by reason of mental disorder or of inability to communicate because of physical disability; but a person shall not fall within this definition by reason only of a lack or deficiency in a faculty of communication if that lack or deficiency can be made good by human or mechanical aid (whether of an interpretative nature or otherwise).

Figure 22.2 Definition of capacity to make decisions.

matters. For example a wish to self-discharge against medical advice, requirement for more supported living situation, selling of a house. Where assessment of capacity is required, the principles and guidance of the relevant law must be considered. This can raise a number of questions such as who should assess capacity and which specific decision requires assessment. Considerations may need to be made about what action to take when capacity fluctuates, decisions are seemingly unwise, decisions are required to be made urgently and where patients have given an advance directive. The following section expands on these aspects to consider in assessing decision-making.

Who Assesses Capacity?
The professionals recognised in legislation as those who provide assessment of capacity differ between countries. Under the MCA judgements about capacity are usually made by those directly concerned with the individual at the time the decision is required. Day-to-day decisions such as which coat to wear when going outside or whether or not to have a shower, may be judged by a carer. Where a medical doctor or health care professional proposes treatment, they must assess the person's capacity to consent. For legal transactions capacity must be assessed by a lawyer or legal practitioner. Where decisions are of more consequence or where there is the possibility of dispute, this may trigger a formal hearing where independent professional assessment is required usually conducted by a psychiatrist,

clinical psychologist or clinical neuropsychologist, although this may be another health professional with relevant expertise.[12]

Under the AwI act, medical treatment of an adult with incapacity requires certification by a medical doctor. Where decisions relate to finances and welfare matters, application to the courts must be made with report from two medical doctors, one of whom must be approved for the purposes of section 22 of the 1984 Mental Health Act Scotland as having special experience in the diagnosis or treatment of mental disorder. At the time of going to press, proposals to review this process are in consultation.

Capacity to Make a Decision Is Specific to the Decision in Question

Decisions, and the potential consequences of decisions, vary in complexity and therefore the level of cognitive skill required to make a decision is specific to the particular decision. For example, decisions on day-to-day spending in a food budget may require less complex cognitive processes than those required to make a decision about purchasing a house, decisions about suitable clothing to wear for the weather are less complex than decisions about the level of care required to safely maintain a residential placement. Therefore, when assessing capacity the specific decision in question must be considered.

Fluctuating Capacity

Capacity may fluctuate due to medical condition, medication, psychological state, psychiatric condition or other influences. Assessment of capacity must be conducted when the person is judged to be at their most competent. Where a person's condition is likely to improve and they may gain sufficient capacity to make the decision in question, then the decision should be deferred until after treatment and/or recovery. In some cases it may not be possible to delay the decision for example where a person's health may deteriorate or they may be put at risk.

Unwise Decisions

A person, with no impairment in decision-making capacity, may make a different decision under the same, or similar conditions as another person. A person may make decisions that others regard as unwise. In assessing capacity, it is the capacity of the person making the decision, not the wisdom of the decision that is under scrutiny. One of the guiding principles of the MCA is that *'a person is not to be treated as unable to make a decision merely because he makes an unwise decision'* although guidance points out that decisions which involve risk of harm or exploitation or are out of character may inform capacity assessment. If a decision regarded as unwise is made by a person with TBI then this might raise concerns about the person's ability to make decisions and trigger assessment of capacity.

Advance Decisions

The regulations monitoring adherence to advance directives vary across legislation. Under the MCA, an advance decision is valid only if made when the person is over 18 years of age and where it is to cover a situation where life saving treatment is to be refused, it must be recorded in writing. It is only applicable for the treatment specified in the advanced decision and does not apply if any of the circumstances specified in the advance decision are absent or that there are reasonable grounds for believing that circumstances exist that the person making the advance decision did not anticipate. Dimond examines legal interpretation and practical implications of this and other aspects of the MCA.[13] Advance directives are not legally binding in Scotland; however, past and present wishes must be taken into account. At time of going to press, regulation around advance directives are being considered under proposals for reform of the AWI act. Advance decisions are based on a prediction of our preference in future scenarios. This may not accurately reflect our wishes should we experience the predicted situation. McMillan et al. present a case of a patient with extremely severe brain injury, where discontinuation of life sustaining treatment was being considered.[14] Prior to brain injury, the patient had given an advanced directive that should she become incapable and dependent on life support, she did not wish to live. Using minimal hand responses on a button to indicate 'yes' and 'no', the patient's consistent wish to live was demonstrated. Follow-up study 6 years after injury continued to show the patient had a consistent wish to live.[15] The authors of this study recommend consideration of neuropsychological assessment in all cases where withdrawal of treatment is being considered and cognitive ability is not certain.

Urgent Decisions

Urgent decisions may be required to be made on behalf of a person unable to consent, for the preservation of the life or the prevention of serious deterioration in medical condition. In these cases, the MCA recommends immediate action should be taken in the person's best interests.[12] The Mental Welfare Commission for Scotland outlines several principles that should be taken into account when people who lack capacity require urgent treatment.[16]

Neuropsychological Factors Affecting Decision-Making

As an individual makes a decision, the process is subject to a number of influences including current circumstances, personal preferences, previous experience and prediction of likely outcomes. Decision-making involves complex processing of information, ability to generate options and weigh up the pros and cons of potential decisions. Thus a number of neurop-sychological skills are applied when making a decision. The following section describes the main neuropsychological processes which affect decision-making, namely communication, memory, attention, executive functioning, insight and mood.

Communication

In order to make a decision, a person needs to have sufficient verbal comprehension to understand information about the decision and sufficient verbal expression to communica-tion their opinion. Comprehension and expression may be assisted by communication aids. Involving a speech and language therapist or clinical psychologist to assist with assessment of comprehension and expressive language abilities and to assist communication during the capacity assessment should be considered.

Memory

Legal definitions of capacity in the UK require that the patient be able to retain the memory of the decision. Provision has been made in guidance however for patients who may present with severely impaired memory function but have preservation of other cognitive abilities to a level that allows competent decision-making. The MCA states that even if a person is only able to retain information relevant to the decision for a short period, this does not prevent him from being regarded as unable to make a decision. The mental welfare commission for Scotland in guidance on consent to treatment suggest that the person must be able to retain information for long enough to make a decision.[16] Thus rather than evidencing the ability to remember the decision, the emphasis is on the consistency of the decision and evidence for a competent decision-making process.

Attention

In order to be able to process information for decision-making, a person needs to be able to receive it and hold it in their working memory. Impairment in attention can result in the patient having access to insufficient information to enable them to make a decision.

Executive Functioning

Executive functioning refers to a range of cognitive abilities that allow us to manage and regulate our thinking processes and behaviour. In making a decision, a person needs to be able to consider available options, predict a range of outcomes, generate pros and cons of these outcomes and evaluate these to come to a reasoned decision. This requires a number of executive functioning processes including the ability to think flexibly, adapt to changing circumstances, use information effectively in problem solving, applying reasoning where there are several options, inhibit impulses and devote sufficient time to decision-making, action an intended plan and use reasoning about a decision when confronted with the situation in which the decision has to be made. Patients with executive functioning problems can often give a good description of the decision in question and may be able to discuss different options and pros and cons of a decision however carrying out the intended plan, or applying this information when confronted with the actual situation can be impaired (Figure 22.3).

It is often not possible to engineer situations which test a person's practical decision-making abilities; however, it is important to gather information from those who have observed the persons practical skills and actions.

Insight

Lack of insight, that is impaired awareness or appreciation of impairment, is common following TBI. As a result, patients may have difficulties taking cognitive impairment or

---

Mr A was receiving inpatient rehabilitation for a moderate TBI sustained in a road traffic accident resulting in right sided haemorrhage which had required evacuation. Two months following injury he was due to be discharged home, where he lived on his own. OT had raised concerns about his ability to attend to safety in the kitchen and he had been discussing his keenness to get back to DIY tasks at home. Mr A experienced dizziness and left sided weakness. Neuropsychologist discussed the risks of undertaking DIY at home and Mr A explained he knew it wasn't safe for him to use ladders at the moment due to the risk of falling and that he would wait for medical advice before using ladders and other DIY equipment. Two hours after this discussion a member of care staff discovered Mr A half way up a ladder which had been left outside. Mr A claimed he had seen the ladder and the gutter needing cleared and wished to help. Mr A was able to discuss and recognise the risks however confronted with the situation his impaired self-monitoring and difficulty using information on-line caused him to follow the visual cues and his inclination to be helpful without considering the risks, even though these had been so recently and competently discussed.

Figure 22.3 Case example.

physical limitations into account when making decisions. If a person is unable to appreciate the extent of their impairment then they do not have accurate information on which to judge what they are able or not able to do. Thus their ability to make accurate judgement about how their difficulties impact on daily function and the level of support they may require may be impaired. Lack of awareness of cognitive or physical limitations may mean a person is not able to make informed decisions about level of risk in situations, does not take measures to protect themselves from potential risk or is not able to judge appropriate action in hazardous situations. People with reduced insight are also less likely to take advice to compensate for their difficulties as they do not believe that they need to make allowances of their difficulties. Insight should not be confused with psychological denial where a person experiencing brain injury and the possible consequences has consciously or unconsciously avoided processing information on the consequences of their TBI. In this case, time and/or formal therapeutic intervention may be required before capacity is assessed.

Emotional State

Emotional state can affect decision-making directly, that is perceptions and interpretations are altered by mood and can bias choices in decision-making. Mood disorders can also have a detrimental effect on cognitive functions such as attention, memory and mental flexibility and therefore can impair decision-making ability. Treatment for mood disorders should be considered prior to assessment of capacity and assessment, if possible, should be delayed to allow for treatment of any psychological disorder affecting capacity.

With all of the above neuropsychological functions, it is important to note that impairment in any one or combination of the above does not automatically equate to impairment in capacity. The role of the clinician assessing capacity is to establish if deficits in the above are present and if so, the extent of impact they have on the decision-making process for the specific decision in question.

Process of Assessing Capacity

Clarify the Question

It is important to consider the specific area of decision-making capacity which requires assessment. The cognitive capacity required to make specific decisions varies with the decision. That is, the ability to evaluate the weather and decide which coat is appropriate to put on varies in the cognitive abilities and level of ability required to make a decisions about financial investments. Thus if a person is judged to be incapable of a certain decision, this does not infer that they are incapable of making another decision. Having a clear statement of the decision in question is the first stage in assessment of the cognitive capacity to make that decision.

Gather Information

In order to be able to assess whether a patient is able to make a competent decision, the assessing clinician must have information about the decision to be made. For non-medical professionals this can mean familiarisation with the pros and cons of particular medical procedure, to the level that would be expected by a patient making that decision following discussion with a doctor. This can be helpful to the patient as seeking an explanation understood from a non-medical perspective allows the explanation of confusing medical terms and reduces assumptions of knowledge that may be made by even an experienced doctor.

Therapists who have observed the patient in practical situations can be good sources of information about the patient's abilities including awareness of risk, ability to adjust behaviour, ability to plan and organise a task, all of which give indications of cognitive abilities of the patient and therefore information about possible abilities affecting capacity. Families are also important sources of information being able to give information about pre-morbid abilities and approaches to decision-making and also current behaviour which might indicate cognitive impairment. Information from others observations can provide examples of behaviours or response in situations which may indicate insight or lack of insight, good or poor decision-making, reasoning that matches or does not match action and the impact of mood on decision-making.

Conditions for Assessment

Medical wards, due to noise and other distractions, may not provide the optimal environment for assessment of capacity; however, it is not always practically possible to provide the ideal environmental conditions. Difficulties inhibiting distraction or increased sensitivity to noise may interfere with the processes of decision-making, therefore where possible background noise should be minimal. Many patients become fatigued as the day progresses which can negatively impact on cognition therefore time of day of assessment should be selected to optimise patients functioning. Similarly the assessing clinician needs to be conscious of their own interactions with the patient and take account of potential cognitive or sensory problems. Adjustment of speed and volume of speech may be required. Questions or information may have to be repeated several times or written down. Communication aids or joint sessions with speech and language therapist may be required.

Interview

During interview, engagement with the patient, listening and validating their responses is important in order to assess their understanding and views on the decision to be made. It is important to establish the patient's awareness of the decision, ensure that the patient has the relevant information to make the decision and that the information has been explained at a level appropriate to the individual's ability to understand. Grisso and Applebaum developed the MacArthur Competency Assessment Tool for Treatment specifically to guide assessment of capacity to make medical decisions.[17] They provide a semi-structure interview format to assess patients understanding, appreciation, reasoning and expression of choice. They describe an interview approach involving disclosure of information to the patient, enquiry of the patients understanding of the information, probing using prompts to establish patients recall and understanding of any information omitted during enquiry and re-disclosure of information with re-enquiry for both understanding of disorder and of treatment.

Prior to interview it is useful to consider the information required. Figure 22.4 lists questions the clinician may wish to consider. This will depend on a number of factors including the specific decision in question, the pros, cons and risks involved in different outcomes of the decision, the psychological state of the patient and the cognitive abilities of the patient. Each question asked is likely to lead to additional enquiry to establish understanding and the thinking processes behind decisions making.

- Can the patient explain situation and the decision to be made?
- What is their opinion on the decision?
- Are they able to recognise how their decision may influence the situation?
- Do they know and understand the consequences of their decision for themselves and others?
- Can they generate and consider both the immediate and long-term consequences of the decision?
- Can they give pros and cons for their decision?
- Are they aware of any risks associated with the decision and, if so, can they generate ways of reducing risk?
- Is there consistency between their reasoning and the decision they express?
- Can they consider alternative decisions?
- Can they give pros and cons for alternative decisions?
- Are they subject to any undue influence from others?
- Are there religious or cultural beliefs that may influence decision?

Figure 22.4 Checklist for the clinician assessing capacity.

Cognitive Assessment and Capacity

Measures of cognition give information about cognitive abilities that may impact on capacity but do not measure capacity per se. The decision to be made, the options available and the likely outcomes are all specific to the individual's situation and therefore require different cognitive capacities. Decision-making capacity is subject not only to cognitive ability but the application of cognitive skills, which will interact with an individual's past experience, pre-morbid abilities, emotional state and ability to use residual cognitive functioning. Therefore there is no specific cognitive test that can take this into account and be reliably predictive of capacity in a given situation. Performance on cognitive tests, no matter how strong the reliability or validity of the test, does not translate to legal competency.[18] Nonetheless, cognitive assessment is a useful tool in combination with other sources of information and may add to evidence in capacity assessment.

Neuropsychological approach to assessing cognition considers the evidence for likely impairment in particular areas and test selection is based on the hypothesis under test. Thus if a patient has sustained a frontal injury, observations of behaviour are consistent with dysexecutive syndrome and decision-making ability has been questioned, measures of executive functioning would be appropriate.

As described above, executive functioning has a key role in decision-making allowing generation of options and evaluation of outcomes. Therefore it is always important to consider executive functioning in capacity assessment. Screening instruments such as the MMSE do not have the specificity required to draw conclusions on executive impairment. Even neuropsychological assessment with good specificity and reliability in assessing executive functioning can sometimes not identify impairment. It is well recognised that some patients with executive impairment can perform very well on standardised executive functioning measures but are unable to utilise their skills in everyday tasks.[18] Conversely patients may perform poorly in a testing situation but manage well in daily life and be capable of making many everyday decisions.

Measurement of cognitive capacities known to affect decision-making can provide useful evidence; however, clinicians must be aware of the limitations of assessment and consider results along with information from other sources such as responses in interview, information from others and practical examples of decision-making by the patient. Where evidence is difficult to interpret, neuropsychological opinion from a clinical neuropsychologist is advisable.

Facilitating Capacity and Enabling Decision-Making

Many of the cognitive factors involved in making decisions can be improved or supported through cognitive rehabilitation. For example, a patient who has impairment in attention may be taught to attend to information, a patient with memory problems may be encouraged to use external memory aids, organisation of information may facilitate capacity for a patient with executive functioning problems. Strategies to compensate for the cognitive deficits are individual to the patient, the decision and their deficits. A detailed assessment to identify cognitive strengths and weaknesses of the patient is important to assist with directing rehabilitation and facilitating capacity.

Decision-making processes may also be affected by psychological disorder. Thinking biases in those with anxiety and depression may impact on evaluation of information for a decision. For example, where thought processes are affected by depression, negative predictions about the future and the outcome of decisions are more likely. Psychological intervention can be specifically targeted at improving decision-making through increasing awareness of the impact of thinking biases.

Involving Others in the Clinical Judgement

Making a clinical judgement about capacity involves integrating information, or collecting evidence, from several sources. Both professionals and family members will have important insights, views and examples to contribute. Even where clinicians are experienced in assessing capacity, clinical judgements may vary.[19] Best practice, although not always practical, is to hold a multidisciplinary case conference to discuss the evidence for capacity so that the professional making the decision is as well informed as possible.

Summary

Legal statutes specify the definition, principles and process of representing patients who do not have capacity to make decisions. In clinical practice a number of factors must be considered when assessing capacity including the specific decision to be made, fluctuating capacity, advance decisions and the urgency of the decision. Neuropsychological functioning can influence decision-making ability and the areas of communication, memory, attention, executive functioning, insight and emotional state require consideration in assessment. The process of assessment of capacity involves the integration of evidence from several sources including professionals working with the patient, the family of the patient, background medical information, interview with the patient and formal cognitive assessment. Clinical judgement about capacity can be complex and consultation with the wider multidisciplinary team is advised.

A number of resources are available for guidance on assessing capacity and managing clinical situations where the patient may not have capacity (Figure 22.5).

Mental Welfare Commission for Scotland
www.mwcscot.org.uk/publications/good-practice-guides/

Adults with Incapacity (2000) Scotland guidance
www.scotland.gov.uk/justice/incapacity

Mental Capacity Act guidance
www.gov.uk/government/publications/mental-capacity-act-code-of-practice

British Medical Association guidance
www.bma.org.uk/advice/employment/ethics/mental-capacity/assessing-mental-capacity

General Medical Council guidance
www.gmc-uk.org/guidance/ethical_guidance/consent_guidance_index.asp

British Psychological Society Guidance
www.bps.org.uk/news-and-policy/what-makes-good-assessment-capacity

Figure 22.5 Resources providing guidance on the assessment of capacity and the management of a patient lacking capacity

References

1. Bishop LC, Temple RO, Tremont G, Westervelt HJ, Stern RA. Utility of the neuropsychological evaluation in an acute medical hospital. *Clin Neuropsychol* 2003;17(4):468–73.

2. Harvey, PD. Clinical applications of neuropsychological assessment. *Dialogues in Clinical Neuroscience* 2012;14(1):91–9.

3. Hodges J. *Cognitive assessment for clinicians.* 3rd edn. New York: Oxford University Press;2017.

4. Wood RLL, Rutterford NA. Demographic and cognitive predictors of long-term psychosocial outcome following traumatic brain injury. *J Int Neuropsychol Soc* 2006;12(3):350–8.

5. Studerus-Germann AM, Engel DC, Stienen MN, von Ow D, Hildebrandt G, Gautschi OP. Three versus seven days to return-to-work after mild traumatic brain injury: a randomized parallel-group trial with neuropsychological assessment. *Int J Neurosci* 2017;127(10):900–8.

6. Galton C, Erzinclioglu S, Sahakian BJ, Antoun N, Hodges JR. A comparison of the Addenbrooke's Cognitive Examination (ACE), conventional neuropsychological assessment, and simple MRI-based medial temporal lobe evaluation in the early diagnosis of Alzheimer's disease. *Cogn Behav Neurol* 2005;18(3):144–50.

7. Scheid R, Walther K, Guthke T, Preul C, von Cramon DY. Cognitive sequelae of diffuse axonal injury. *Arch Neurol* 2006;63(3):418–24.

8. Lezak MD, Howieson DB, Bigler ED, Tranel D. *Neuropsychological assessment.* 5th edn. New York:Oxford University Press;2012.

9. Folstein MF, Folstein SE, McHeugh PR. Mini-mental state: a practical method for grading the cognitive state of outpatients for the clinician. *J Psychiatric Res* 1975;12:189–98.

10. Noone P. Addenbrooke's Cognitive Examination–III. *Occupational Med* 2015;65:418–20.

11. Matías-Guiu JA, Valles-Salgado M, Rognoni T, Hamre-Gil F, Moreno-Ramos T, Matías-Guiu J. Comparative diagnostic accuracy of the ACE-III, MIS, MMSE, MoCA, and RUDAS for screening of Alzheimer disease. *Dement Geriatr Cogn Disord* 2017;43(5–6):237–46.

12. Mental Capacity Act. Code of Practice issued by the Lord Chancellor on 23 April

2007 in accordance with sections 42 and 43 of the Act; 2005.

13. Dimond B. *Legal aspects of mental capacity. a practical guide for health and social care professionals.* Malden, MA: Blackwell;2016.

14. McMillan TM. Neuropsychological assessment after extremely severe head injury in a case of life or death. *Brain Injury* 1996;11:483–90.

15. McMillan TM, Herbert C. Neuropsychological assessment of a potential 'euthanasia' case: a 5 year follow up. *Brain Injury* 2000;14:197–203.

16. Mental Welfare Commission for Scotland. *Right to treat: delivering physical heath care to people who lack capacity and refuse or resist treatment.* Mental Welfare Commission for Scotland; July 2011

17. Grisso T, Applebaum PS. *Assessing competence to consent to treatment.* New York:Oxford University Press;1998.

18. Herbert C.Assessment of capacity in clients with executive dysfunction. In Oddy M, Worthington A, eds. *The rehabilitation of executive disorders: a guide to theory and practice.* Oxford: Oxford University Press;2009.

19. Whyte M, Wilson M, Hamilton J, Primrose W, Summers F. Adults with Incapacity (Scotland) Act 2000: implications for clinical psychology. *Clin Psychol* 2003;**31**:5–8.

Chapter 23

Families

Effective Communication and Facilitating Adjustment

Fiona Summers, Helen M. K. Gooday, Maggie Whyte
and Camilla Herbert

When I was in a coma, my wife would sit all night by my bedside and then go to work in the morning. It was a 24 hour job for her.
Saul, patient with TBI.

Introduction

The role of the family in recovery from brain injury is of central importance. Family members provide emotional and practical support, advocate for the patient and assist in rehabilitation. The experience of observing a family member following a traumatic injury is extremely challenging and families can experience high levels of distress, anger, guilt and denial in the early post-traumatic phase. These features are followed, in the longer term, by increasing social isolation, depression and anxiety about the future[1–3] and can persist for many years after discharge from hospital. Cognitive and personality changes in the individual with the brain injury are reported as the main causes of family distress than other consequences. Understanding the process of family adjustment and engaging families in a meaningful away is critical for all staff at the acute, post-acute and community stages of brain injury recovery.

Definition of the Family

The definition of family has changed significantly over the years. As well as the traditional definition, families can consist of partners and step-children, other relatives and close friends. There may be significant conflict, for example between parents and ex-partners or between parents who have divorced or current partners and family members. This may be challenging if a patient is unable to communicate. The clinical team need to establish who is next of kin and if there is already a power of attorney or any other legal documentation in place, prior to the brain injury. This may require a direct conversation with family members to establish the most appropriate person, or persons, to communicate with and involve in rehabilitation goals.

Engaging with Families in the Acute Stage

A number of factors are important to consider when engaging with families including the particular circumstances around the injury and the emotional response of family members.

The circumstances which resulted in the brain injury may be distressing and should be managed with sensitively. If there was a fatality, for example in a RTA, the relationship of the deceased to the person with the brain injury needs to be considered and the sensitivity of the situation, for example police investigations, reaction of family members or others (e.g. blame, distress).

Family reactions to brain injury can vary considerably with displays of different behaviours associated with emotional distress such as uncontrollable weeping, shaking, shouting, verbal and physical aggression, dissociation, confusion, blaming, numbness, confrontation and grief. Different family members will react in different ways at different times which can sometimes be overwhelming for clinical staff. During this initial stage family members often find it difficult to make sense of anything they are told and will often not recall information discussed. This can lead to situations of frustration for staff when families report they were not told critical information. Injury-related factors and socio-demographic variables have consistently been found to be poor predictors of psychological adjustment of both the injured person and their relatives.[4,5]

The aim for any member of the team is to deliver bad news clearly, honestly and sensitively. Initially this may involve giving information about the severity of the brain injury and an explanation of the critical care process; however, throughout the acute and rehabilitation stages of recovery bad news may need to be conveyed to family members at any time regarding progress and care needs. Discussing prognosis is difficult; however, it is something families often ask at the acute stages of a brain injury. Families consistently feedback that information given at this stage was overly negative therefore it is important that clinicians manage this sensitively. Prognosis in brain injury is often very difficult to predict and giving concrete statements of outcome can jeopardise future trust in the team expertise. For example should a clinician erroneously state that a patient will never walk again, the family are less likely to believe the teams opinion on other outcomes, particularly negative predictions.

There are important considerations when giving bad news at any stage of the patient's recovery and treatment. The clinical team should have a quiet, well-lit, appropriately furnished room to discuss sensitive issues with family members. Communication needs to be regular, clear and honest; however, this can be challenging for a variety of reasons for example the amount and complexity of information and the emotional distress of family members. There should be consideration to who in the team discusses a particular issue and when. Whomever is meeting with the family needs to give enough time for questions and discussions, turning off bleeps and other distractions, if possible. Rushing a meeting may make the family feel that their family member is not important and that the clinician has other patients in more need. To establish a strong therapeutic relationship with the family the clinical team need to listen carefully to the needs of the family, watch for reactions (e.g. confusion or distress), respond appropriately and reflect back. Consideration should be given to body language, facial expressions and tone of voice. Clinicians should avoid jargon and, where thought beneficial, consider using illustrations. Helping the family contain their distress through normalisation (acknowledgement that this is distressing time) and containment (providing them the space to acknowledge and express their emotions within a safe environment) is important. Many families are resilient when confronted with traumatic situations and manage well, under the circumstances, when a good clinical team is able and skilful in providing the support the family need.

Communication and the Team

Communication between different members of the team is important and without it family members could lose trust in how the team operates. In particular is a need for good lines of communication between those setting up rehabilitation goals and those being asked to implement them, for example physiotherapists developing a hoisting programme and care staff using hoists. The team also need to be aware that family members will notice any conflict in the team and it is critically important that no member of the team contradicts or criticises another member in the presence of the family even when errors have been made. Family members will naturally gravitate to team members with whom they develop a strong relationship (due to personality or other factors) and this should be seen as positive, providing therapeutic boundaries are maintained. Any member of the team, when opportunity arises and families members seem receptive, should use opportunities to have helpful informal conversations. Sherer et al. found that higher levels of family discord were associated with poorer therapeutic relationships and larger discrepancies between family and clinician perceptions of patient functioning were associated with compliance in therapy activities.[6]

Managing Expectations

At the acute stages of recovery, and often beyond, family members initial concerns after the relief that their family member has survived, are largely focused on physical recovery. They are less aware, even if this has been discussed, about any cognitive, behavioural and personality changes until later. It is part of the team's responsibility to manage these expectations. The team need to accept that families are still in the process of adjustment and whilst these issues should be raised and discussed the team should not attempt to 'force' this adjustment process. Another area which can cause conflict is when family members feel the clinical team are being dismissive of responses the family think indicates improvement for example if the patient appears to be responding to being spoken to by moving eyes or fingers. Whilst the team is familiar with the difference between voluntary and involuntary movement family members may not be and their desire for improvement may bias interpretation of any movements as signs of meaningful recovery. The importance of having hope for recovery has been highlighted in previous studies and is identified as a vital part of this process.[7-9] Kuipers et al., in their study on the factors which contribute to engaging families following brain injury, found that the importance of hope for families was fundamental to positive outcomes.[10] The clinical team need to foster hope and manage these situations with sensitivity and compassion using phrases such as 'with rehabilitation we could, not we will, but we could get'. The alternative to hope is hopelessness which is not what the team should wish for families; however, managing expectations particularly at the rehabilitation stages is important. In addition the team also need to be aware that the family often spend considerably more time with the patient than the clinical team and their involvement in noticing change is important.

Engaging the Family in Patient Care

It is important for the team to give the family a role and practical suggestions for engaging in all stages of recovery which might include, at the initial stages, ensuring family members interact with the patient (talking, holding hands), encouraging family members to bring in music the patient enjoys, family photo albums and familiar items to decorate the room if appropriate and suggesting family members write a recovery journal. Family members could also be involved in facilitating and supporting any rehabilitation goals and are often keen on doing so. The team however need to be mindful of those family members who do not wish to be actively involved in rehabilitation, often through anxiety and fear. The team also needs to be sensitive to religious and cultural norms.

Keeping the family informed of any new developments helps build trust, facilitates the therapeutic relationship with the team and supports family adjustment.[11] Changes in treatment or the environment may be very significant for families, even if the team regard them as minor, for example a change of bed or room, introduction or removal of equipment. If these changes occur without the family being informed, this can impact on the families trust in the team. Discussion with the family about how and when they would like to be kept informed is important, for example would they wish to be contacted late at night, what is their preferred method of communication (e.g. text, telephone). It is also essential that any plans or actions discussed with the family are carried out, or where plans change, that the reasoning is clearly explained to the family. Bond et al. demonstrated that family members consistently expressed a need to know, the need for consistent information and the need for involvement to help them make sense of their experience.[12]

Cultural Issues

When communicating with the family, cultural and religious sensitivity should to be considered and respected.[13] Patients can come from a wide variety of religious and cultural backgrounds (which can be hard to distinguish) and understanding this will help the clinical team care and support a patient and their family but also prevent mistakes that can lead to a breakdown in relationships. The team should consider how to address people, which festivals and rituals are important for the family and patient to follow, dietary requirements and food preparation. The needs of the patient and family may vary and it is important to ask families which traditions they follow and, where possible, these should be accommodated. Local multicultural centres can provide more detailed information.

Providing Information to Families

In the early stages after brain injury, it has been demonstrated that the most highly rated needs are for clear explanations of the patient's medical condition, discussion of realistic expectations for recovery, truthfulness and reassurance from medical professionals.[14,15] Discussing the nature of TBI can help family members better understand and enable them to develop a realistic perception of the patient's abilities.

It is helpful to provide high-quality, accurate and up-to-date written information for example booklets provided by Headway charity. The appropriate stage of recovery for giving information should be considered and a record of written information given should be documented in the patient's clinical notes. It is also important that relatives are given an opportunity to speak to a clinician about the information that they have received, and to ask questions. There are a number of websites that families can be directed to (e.g. www.headway.org, www.brainandspine.org), to provide information about brain injury and local support services that may be available.

Engaging with Families in Rehabilitation

Your family, they are the foundation for your recovery.
Duncan, patient with TBI.

It is widely recommended that family members are actively engaged in the patient's rehabilitation journey because evidence suggests that this is associated with better outcomes for patients.[6,16,17] However, services vary in the way that they conceptualise and organise involvement with, and support for, family members and there are also wide variations in the resources available to facilitate these processes. Under some conditions, family-supported rehabilitation can achieve better outcomes than direct clinician-delivered rehabilitation.[18] It is likely that, if family members have engaged in the rehabilitation process and have learned skills and developed confidence prior to the patient being discharged, this will have a direct benefit to the patient. There is evidence to suggest that patients whose family members are engaged in their rehabilitation, through active participation or by establishing a working relationship with rehabilitation professionals, go on to have better outcomes than those who do not.[6,19]

Foster et al. noted that the ability of family members to fully engage in rehabilitation may be hindered by the barriers (logistical and psychological) they encounter.[16] They describe how rehabilitation services can facilitate family engagement through a person-centred approach using an eight-tiered model. This is done by explicit structuring of services to include the following: early engagement, meeting cultural needs, keeping families together, actively listening, active involvement, education, skills training and support for community integration.

The clinical team who are working with the patient may have to attempt to provide support and education to the family despite limited resources. The structure suggested by Forster et al. for their routine interventions with families can be used effectively (Figure 23.1).[16]

It is helpful to have an initial case conference approximately 3 weeks after admission to the rehab unit (unless the admission is likely to be shorter) when the clinical team are familiar with the patient and their family. A care manager should be involved at an early stage, if input in relation to housing or a care package is required. This will facilitate discharge planning and avoid unnecessary delays.

To enable the patient and family to have a shared understanding of the rehabilitation issues and challenges, it can be useful if the patient is present at the meeting. If this is not possible the patient may feel excluded from decisions about their future therefore arrangements should be made for the patient to attend for a brief summary at the end of the meeting or for a clinician or family member to feedback to the patient following the meeting. These options should be discussed with the patient and family prior to the meeting.

Case conferences should have formal minutes taken, with minutes given to the patient (if appropriate), next of kin, primary care team and care manager, if input from social services is required. These should be free from jargon, and written so that they can be understood by professionals and patients. Medical and other technical terms should be explained. It is helpful if family members can see a draft of the minutes to ensure that they are in agreement with them, before they are finalised.

It can be helpful for relatives to attend some therapy sessions, if the patient does not object, and if their presence is not a cause of distraction. Encouragement from family members can sometimes have an impact on the patient's motivation to participate in sessions, and their progress. It may also give the clinical team valuable information about family relationships, which can have a direct bearing on the discharge plan.

It is important for the clinical team to be aware of external resources which may provide support to the family including the local social work department and charitable

Early Engagement	• Staff meet with the patient, and if available family members prior to transfer from the acute neurosurgical ward to give information about the rehabilitation unit, answer questions and begin to establish relationships. Written information about the rehabilitation unit is given to families. • Families are invited to visit the rehab unit if time allows before transfer. • In complex cases and where relationships have been challenging a case conference is held to ensure information is shared and communication with the family is consistent. • Following transfer members of the MDT endeavour to meet with the patient and family as soon as possible to explain their roles and answer any questions.
Meeting cultural needs	• Professional translators are engaged if required • Dietary requirements are provided for. • Wards have contacts for local leaders of the main religions practiced in the area.
Keeping families together	• Visiting hours are throughout the day although not at night, unless there are exceptional circumstances. • Family members have access to a kitchen where they can heat food or prepare snacks.
Actively listening	• Family members are encouraged to ask questions about their loved one's care and progress and are encouraged to attend therapy sessions (as long as the patient gives permission and their presence does not cause distraction). • weekly relatives clinic is held to give family members as opportunity to discuss their relatives care with a consultant. Families are updated on weekly ward round if in attendance.
Active Involvement	• Family members are encouraged to take part in personal care, if they wish to do so (and if the patient is in agreement). • They are invited to bring in music, magazines, DVDs and other material which the patient can enjoy outside therapy sessions, and to share in these activities. • If it is safe for the patient to leave the ward, relatives are encouraged to start taking them out of the ward to provide stimulation, and to encourage social interaction, e.g. by going to the hospital cafe or out to the cinema.
Education	• During formal and informal meetings with relatives, education is given about the patient's brain injury by medical staff and the nursing and therapy team. • Some relatives are much more likely to approach ward staff on a regular basis to exchange information. For those who do not, it is clinicians are proactive, and make as effort to introduce themselves to relatives who are visiting, give an update on progress (following permission from the patient), and demonstrate concern for the wellbeing of family members.
Skills Training	• Prior to discharge, it is clarified to what extent family members will be involved in hands-on care (as this will depend on the preferences of the patient and family, but also on the availability of care and support which can be provided via social services). • family members, if appropriate, are given training in relation to bowel and bladder management, gastrostomy feeding, feeding of modified diets, positioning, manual handling and management of pain and discomfort. Family members may also need training in managing the neuro-behavioural sequelae of brain injury, and may need to learn how to manage poor motivation, irritability, anxiety and low mood in their relative.
Support for community re-integration	• Prior to discharge, patients are encouraged to spend increasing length of time at home, initially during the day, and subsequently "on pass" at weekends, to integrate them back into the family unit, and to determine whether there are any further needs for equipment, home adaptations or support that had not previously been envisaged.

Figure 23.1 The person-centred model of family engagement used by the post-acute neurorehabilitation unit, Woodend Hospital, NHS Grampian.

organisations such as Headway (www.headway.org.uk). Family members should also be given advice in relation to financial issues and claiming benefits, and this may be available via charities such as the Citizen's Advice Bureau (citizensadvice.org.uk). If possible, access to these external organisations should be facilitated for example by arranging for workers to visit the unit to meet with relatives. Advice and support for families is also available on-line, and is provided via a number of charities, such as Carers UK, Age UK (information and advice for people aged over 60) and the Carer's Trust.

Practical Management of Difficult Situations

Engaging with Dissatisfied Relatives

From time to time the team may have to manage dissatisfied relatives, often due to distress, frustration, lack of progress and concerns about intensity or quality of therapy and/or nursing or medical input. It may be helpful to have an early team meeting with family members, as soon as possible after dissatisfaction has being noted, to clarify the nature of the concerns. It is important for staff to be open minded, as relatives may have legitimate concerns about the medical treatment or rehabilitation programme. Ensuring that family members feel that they are being listened to is important as is providing clear explanations, for example where therapy is causing pain, discomfort or anxiety, providing explanations about the rationale behind therapy and the long-term impact of not persisting. It may be appropriate to offer a second opinion from a consultant or senior therapist from another team.

Managing Visitors Who Have Substance Misuse Problems or Bring in Illicit Substances

Problems can arise if family members or friends arrive in the ward under the influence of alcohol or illegal drugs, or bring them into hospital for patients.

If visitors are suspected of being under the influence of alcohol or drugs, a senior member of the team should meet with them immediately, clarify the situation, explain that visiting is not possible under these circumstances and request that they leave the ward. Repeated meetings may be necessary to reinforce this message, with a 'firm but fair' approach, and if necessary, visitors may need to be informed that they will be barred from visiting if their behaviour does not change.

Local policies will determine the appropriate action if visitors bring in alcohol or illegal drugs. The situation can become more complex if relatives are bringing in illicit substances that are beneficial for symptom relief in their relatives, such as cannabis, which some patients find helpful for muscle spasms. In this situation, ward staff may have mixed feelings about banning or confiscating such substances; however, in the UK, and in many other countries, the possession of even small amounts of such drugs is illegal. If patients have capacity to make decisions, and decide to use illegal substances when away from the hospital site, it may be possible to prevent this activity with a harm-reduction approach including open discussion about the possible consequences and alternative courses of action.

Dealing with Abusive or Aggressive Visitors

Workplace aggression, both physical and verbal, can have a major impact on clinicians, and has a significant economic cost. Early recognition and use of de-escalation strategies are important[34]; however, if problems persist, deployment of additional staff in the ward may be temporarily necessary, including security staff and, if necessary, police. Ward staff should have information about how to contact the local police.

Following Discharge from Hospital: Family Outcomes and Intervention

He still looks the same, it isn't until people who know him before have spent some time with him that they start to understand and it's not just that he has changed, he doesn't seem to know who I am anymore. He never asks how my day has been. He doesn't play with the children unless I ask him to. When we have visitors I'm constantly on edge, worried about what he might say.
Claire, wife of a patient with brain injury

Few families have experience of the cognitive, emotional, behavioural and social changes that can occur as a result of brain injury and therefore do not have a framework of understanding from which to approach challenges and solve problems. Social isolation and reduced intimacy in relationships following traumatic brain injury is common.[20] Many, but not all, studies suggest that spouses experience different levels of stress and burden in caring for a partner or adult child with traumatic brain injury.[21] There can be tensions within families, commonly between a spouse or a partner and the brain-injured person's parents. Some of these are long-standing but exposed or exacerbated by the brain injury. It is often the case that the parents live separately from the brain-injured person and do not fully appreciate the situation faced by the spouse/partner. Social networks may reduce for family care givers due to constraints on their ability to pursue their own social activities whilst managing care responsibilities. The impact of brain injury on the family may not be obvious to others and therefore others may be less likely to offer of assistance. A care giver who is striving to manage may regard asking for help as an indication that they are unable to cope. Dynamics in relationships may have changed, for example the person with a brain injury may have provided emotional support in the family; however, their capacity to do so may have diminished due to organic or psychological factors. Family care givers experience a wide range of emotions which are particular to their own circumstances and influenced by the neurobehavioural consequences of brain injury.[22] Anxiety is commonly experienced often associated with uncertainty about the future and stress with managing the care demands. Difficulties influencing or changing the situation can instigate feelings of helplessness. Lack of insight can be extremely stressful for the family care giver who is endeavouring to provide or arrange support and the person with brain injury is unable to appreciate the need and therefore resistant to assistance. Carers often identify feelings of guilt, secondary anger or frustration that they experience towards the person with brain injury.

Frequency of marital breakdown after brain injury identifies divorce rates comparable to the national figures for divorce in the USA 15%[23] and UK 17%.[24] The rate increased to 49% when marital separations and divorces were considered together. Reduced relationship satisfaction and general functioning has been documented in couples who stay together.[25]

Sexual problems are common following brain injury.[26,27] In a large survey of adults after brain injury[26] 10% of the sample reported increase in sexual drive but the more common changes reported was hyposexuality. Difficulties can arise directly as a result of hormonal changes (17%) or more commonly by physical dysfunction that affects physical mobility (31%) flexibility and spontaneity. There are other indirect physical consequences that can restrict intimacy such as pain, fatigue, reduced physical fitness[28] and the impact of changes in appearance on self confidence can limit peoples willingness to engage in relationships.[29] Within a couple either person's attempt to fix difficulties can paradoxically amplify the problem and part of the role of professionals can be to re-establish previous ways of coping and communication or develop new ways of coping.[30]

Most studies that assess the long-term impact on families focus on those who have struggled to adjust,[21] but there is some evidence to suggest that a significant proportion of families cope remarkably well[31] and more recent research has focused more on the systems dynamic rather than on individual coping.[30]

Impact on the children of a parent's brain injury remains an under-researched area. In a comparison study of 16 families with a parent with ABI and 16 matched controls[32] parents with TBI and their spouses were similar to their comparison group in many parenting skills, but parents with TBI reported less goal setting, less encouragement of skill development, less emphasis on obedience to rules and orderliness, less promotion of work values, less nurturing, and lower levels of active involvement with their children. No differences in the frequency of behavioural problems were found between children of parents with TBI and children of parents without TBI. There is also little research on the impact of ABI on siblings, one paper refers to siblings as 'the forgotten victims' and concluded that having a sibling with a TBI can result in profound and enduring negative and positive life changes for non-injured siblings and recommended that professionals need to attend to the needs of siblings for support and guidance.[33]

Family dynamics pre- and post-injury are often complex and family therapy is sometimes recommended, but it is important to adjust the nature of the therapy to compensate for possible cognitive difficulties, with greater use of logbooks, memory aids and visible reminders.[34] As well as the brain injury symptoms there may be the experience of trauma and this can interfere with the patterns of communication previously established between the injured person and their partner or friends. A programme of education, advice and problem-solving training can be very effective. Whilst there are few formal family education/training programmes available in the UK, these are more common in the USA.[35]

Summary

The family of a person who has a brain injury is of primary importance to their immediate and long-term recovery. The MDT working with the patient and family need to consider their approach to engagement with the family, the impact of communication between team members on the family, managing expectations and providing information, involvement in rehabilitation and how to manage challenging situations with family members.

References

1. Kreutzer JS, Serio C, Berquist S. Family needs after brain injury: a quantitative analysis. *J Head Trauma Rehabil* 1994;9(3):104–15.

2. Wallace CA, Bogner J, Corrigan JD, Clinchot D, Mysiw WJ, Fugate LP. Primary caregivers of persons with brain injury: life change 1 year after injury. *Brain Inj* 1998;12 (6):483–93.

3. Knight RG, Devereux RT, Godfrey HPD. Caring for a family member with a traumatic brain injury. *Brain Inj* 1998;12 (6):467–81.

4. Gervasio AH, Kreutzer JS. Kinship and family members' psychological distress after traumatic brain injury: a large sample study. *J Head Trauma Rehabil* 1997;12 (3):14–26.

5. Gillen R, Tennen H, Affleck G, Steinpreis R. Distress, depressive symptoms and depressive disorder among caregivers of patients with brain injury. *J Head Trauma Rehabil* 1998;13 (3):31–43.

6. Sherer M, Evans CC, Leverenz J, et al. Therapeutic alliance in post-acute brain injury rehabilitation: predictors of strength of alliance and impact of alliance on outcome. *Brain Injury* 2007;21(7):663–72.

7. Bright FAS, Kayes NM, McCann CM, McPherson KM. Understanding hope after stroke: a systematic review of the literature using concept analysis. *Topics Stroke Rehab* 2001;18(5):490–508.

8. Keenan A, Joseph L. The needs of family members of severe traumatic brain injured patients during critical and acute care: a qualitative study. *Can J Neurosci Nurs* 2010;32(3):25–35.

9. Lucas MR. What brain tumor patients and their families have taught me. *J Neurosci Nurs* 2013;45(3):171–5.

10. Kuipers P, Doig E, Kendall M, Turner B, Mitchell M, Fleming J. Hope:afurther dimension for engaging family members of people with ABI. *NeuroRehabilitation* 2014;35(3):475–80.

11. Gan C, Gargo J, Kreutzer JS, et al. Development and preliminary evaluation of a structured family system intervention for adolescents with brain injury and their families. *Brain Injury* 2010;24:651–63.

12. Bond A, Draeger C, Mandleco B, Donnelly M. Trauma: needs of family members of patients with severe traumatic brain injury: implications for evidence-based practice. *Crit Care Nurse* 2003;23(4):63–72.

13. Yeates G. Working with families in neuropsychological rehabilitation. In: Wilson B, Gracey F, Evans JJ, Bateman A, eds. *Neuropsychological rehabilitation:theory, models, therapy and outcome.* Cambridge: Cambridge University Press; 2009.

14. Mauss-Clum N, Ryan M. Brain injury and the family. *J Neurosurg Nurs* 1981;13 (40):165–9.

15. Kreutzer JS, Serio C, Berquist S. Family needs following brain injury: a quantitative analysis. *J Head Trauma Rehab* 1994;9 (3):104–15.

16. Foster AM, Armstrong J, Buckley A, et al. Encouraging family engagement in the rehabilitation process: a rehabilitation provider's development of support strategies for family members of people with traumatic brain injury. *Disability Rehab* 2012;34(22):1855–62.

17. Kreutzer JS, Stejskal TM, Ketchum JM, et al. A preliminary investigation of the brain injury family intervention: impact on family members. *Brain Injury* 2009;23:535–47.

18. Braga LW, Da Paz AC, Ylvisaker M. Direct clinician-delivered versus indirect family-supported rehabilitation of children with traumatic brain injury: a randomised controlled trial. *Brain Injury* 2005;19:819–31.

19. Chua KS, Ng YS, Yap SG, et al. A brief review of traumatic brain injury rehabilitation. *Ann Acad Med Singap* 2007;36:31–42.

20. Ponsford J, Sloan S, Snow P. *Traumatic brain injury rehabilitation for everyday adaptive living.* 2nd edn. New York: Psychology Press; 2013.

21. Oddy M,Herbert CM. Intervention with families following brain injury: evidence-based practice. *Neuropsychol Rehab* 2003;13(1–2):259–73.

22. Schönberger M, Ponsford J, Olver J, Ponsford M. A longitudinal study of family functioning after TBI and relatives' emotional status. *Neuropsychol Rehab* 2010;20(6):813–29.

23. Kreutzer J, Marwitz J, Hsu N, Williams K, Riddick A. Marital stability after brain injury: an investigation and analysis. *Neurorehabilitation* 2007;22:53–9.

24. Wood RL, Yurdakel LK. Change in relationship status following traumatic brain injury. *Brain Injury* 1997;11:491–502.

25. Burridge ACH. Spousal relationship satisfaction following acquired bring injury: the role of insight and

socio-emotional skill. *Neuropsychol Rehab* 2007;17:95–105.

26. Sander AM, Maestas KL, Nick TG, Pappadis MR, Hammond FM, Hanks RA, Ripley DL. Predictors of sexual functioning and satisfaction 1 yr following TBI. *J Head Trauma Rehab* 2013;28(3):186–94.

27. Ponsford J. Sexual changes associated with traumatic brain injury. *Neuropsychol Rehab* 2003;13:275.

28. Ponsford J, Downing M, Stolwky R, Taffe CJ. Factors associated with sexuality following TBI. *J Head Trauma Rehab* 2013:28(3):195–201.

29. Palmer S, Herbert CM. Friendships and intimacy: promoting the maintenance and development of relationships in residential neurorehabilitation. *NeuroRehabilitation* 2016:38:291–8.

30. Bowen C, Yeates G, Palmer S. *A relational approach to rehabilitation.* London: Karnac; 2010.

31. Perlesz A, Kinsella G, Crowe S. Impact of traumatic brain injury on the family: a critical review. *Rehabil Psychol* 1999;44 (1):6–35.

32. Uysal S, Hibbard MR, Robillard D, Pappadopulos E, Jaffe M. The effect of parental traumatic brain injury on parenting and child behaviour. *J Head Trauma Rehab* 1998;13(6):57–71.

33. Degeneffe CE, Olney MF. 'We are the forgotten victims': Perspectives of adult siblings of persons with traumatic brain injury. *Brain Injury* 2010;24(12): 1416–27.

34. Solomon CR, Scherzer BP. Some guidelines for family therapists working with the traumatically brain injured and their families. *Brain Injury* 1991;5(3):253–66.

35. Kreutzer J, Taylor L. *Brain injury family intervention: an implementation manual.* www.tbicommunity.org/resources/index .htm

Principles of Rehabilitation

Jonathan J. Evans

Introduction

Rehabilitation has been defined in many ways, but in the broadest sense is concerned with maximising quality of life after injury or illness.[1] More specifically, rehabilitation is about maximising the ability and opportunity of the person with brain injury to participate in those activities of daily living, work, education, leisure and relationships that are valued by that person. Wade discusses the importance of models of illness (and health) and highlights the value of the World Health Organization International Classification of Functioning, Disability and Health (ICF) as a framework for understanding the process of rehabilitation.[2] The ICF emphasises that health (or illness) and functioning can be considered at the level of (i) body structure (pathology), (ii) body function (impairment) and (iii) participation in activities. As a simple example, someone who has a brain injury with frontal and temporal lobe damage (the pathology) may have impaired memory functioning and so not be able to carry out activities that are essential for his/her job (e.g. remembering task instructions) and hence not be able to return to (participate in) work. The value of the ICF is that it reminds us that rehabilitation should ultimately be concerned with maximising participation in valued activities, within the limitations imposed by impairments of physical, cognitive or emotional functioning. Rehabilitation is not synonymous with *restoration* of normal functioning. To use another simple example, the person who, despite extensive physiotherapy, cannot walk as a result of hemiplegia, cannot go to the local shop in the usual way, but nevertheless with a wheelchair can complete the activity of shopping independently. The wheelchair compensates for physical impairment, allowing participation in activities of daily living.

Rehabilitation treatments or interventions can be applied at all levels of the ICF, with the nature and focus of the rehabilitation process changing over time. The first minutes, hours or days after the injury are concerned with minimising the level of secondary damage that would otherwise occur, and maximising the physical integrity of the brain. Rehabilitation is then concerned with restoring impaired physical or cognitive skills. Finally, as the extent of the permanent level of physical, cognitive and emotional impairment becomes clear, so rehabilitation interventions are aimed at enabling the person with brain injury to compensate for impairments or with modifying the environment to minimise demands on impaired functions.

Models of Service

Rehabilitation is a complex process because patients have different needs at different times. Furthermore, brain injury can result in a huge range of possible consequences, with outcome dependent upon many factors including the severity of brain injury, the specific areas of brain damage, along with factors such as pre-morbid intellectual ability, psychological coping style and levels of social support. Given the range of possible immediate and longer-term outcomes of brain injury, a range of services is required to meet the needs of patients at different times post-injury and with different levels of impairment. This is reflected in recent models of service provision (Figure 24.1).[3–5]

Ideally, patients should be transferred to rehabilitation facilities as soon as they are medically stable.[6] Failure to do so can result in inappropriate management, which may lead to physical and behavioural complications.[7] McMillan suggests that, for those people with acquired brain injury (ABI) admitted for more than 48 hours, an early management/rehabilitation ward is needed.[3] The functions of this ward are to monitor prolonged coma and recovery, provide a safe environment, prevent contractures and sores developing,

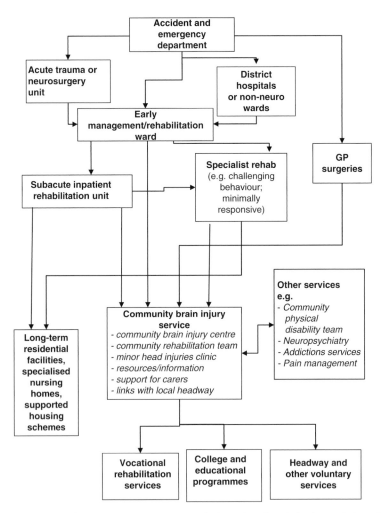

Figure 24.1 The Acquired Brain Injury Service Network. Reproduced with kind permission of the British Psychological Society.

maintain posture, offer active rehabilitation for those who are able, taking account of fatigue, and, as soon as appropriate, discharge to the next step in rehabilitation. Beyond this acute stage, several onward routes exist. Some patients will have physical disability and need to transfer to an environment with expertise in the management of physical disability. A small sub-group of patients require long-term coma care. These patients may remain in an unresponsive state for several months, or longer. They require specialised medical, nursing and therapy care in order to maintain their physical well-being. An important minority of patients develop challenging behaviour. Appropriate care in the acute stage of recovery can reduce the incidence of this, but the incidence of challenging behaviour increases rather than decreases following discharge from hospital.[7] Evidence has accumulated that appropriate management, intervention and environmental control can significantly reduce the severity of challenging behaviour and allow individuals to lead more independent lives. All brain injury services should be able to successfully manage mild and moderate degrees of challenging behaviour. However there is a continuing need for residential challenging behaviour units that use neurobehavioural models of rehabilitation.[8]

At the hub of the service network, there should be a Community Brain Injury Rehabilitation Centre, providing a number of services that meet the rehabilitation needs of the majority of people who suffer a brain injury and of their families. The centre should provide services such as day-patient rehabilitation programmes, outreach/community rehabilitation, a minor brain injuries clinic, a resource and information centre and a source of support for carers. Such a centre would also promote strong links with voluntary groups such as Headway. Furthermore, the centre should link with vocational rehabilitation services, as well as college education programmes. Very few regions have such a comprehensive community brain injury service, though there is evidence for the effectiveness of the key elements of this service.[9,10]

Critical Features of a Rehabilitation Service

Two other features are critical to a rehabilitation service – an interdisciplinary team and a goal-setting process.[11,12] The needs of brain-injured patients are complex and often cannot be met by one clinical discipline alone. The disciplines involved in rehabilitation include rehabilitation medicine, nursing, occupational therapy, speech and language therapy, clinical psychology/neuropsychology, physiotherapy, social work and psychiatry. The precise composition of the team will vary according to the nature of the service. In recent years the term 'interdisciplinary team' has been adopted to describe those teams who genuinely provide an integrated rehabilitation programme for patients. What defines an integrated programme most clearly is the operation of a patient-centred goal-setting system.[11,12] This means that goals for the rehabilitation programme are set collectively by the team, in conjunction with the patient and/or his or her advocate, rather than by individual disciplines in isolation. Whilst some goals may require input from only one discipline, for many goals the interventions of several team members will be necessary. Goals should be specific and measurable, with the time period for achievement clearly identified. The majority of goals at the post-acute stage should be written with reference to the activities/participation level of the ICF framework. Studies have demonstrated the value of patient-centred goal setting in improving patients' satisfaction with the rehabilitation process.[13]

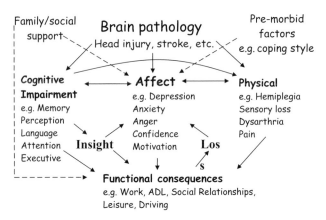

Figure 24.2 A summary of assessment template.

The Rehabilitation Process

The precise content of a rehabilitation programme varies according to individual need. However, the process always begins with an assessment, to determine the nature of any impairment in cognitive, emotional, behavioural or physical functioning and identify the functional consequences in terms of the ability to participate in activities of daily living, work, education, social and leisure activities. The task then is to formulate or map the relationship between the pathology, the impairments and the functional consequences. It is possible to do this in summary form (e.g. on a flipchart in a rehabilitation team meeting) where all elements of the assessment are listed, and a preliminary formulation of the causal relationships between impairment and functional elements can be drawn out. One example of a template used for this purpose at the Oliver Zangwill Centre for Neuropsychological Rehabilitation is provided in Figure 24.2.[11]

Linked to this assessment process is the setting of the rehabilitation goals. This should, wherever possible, directly involve the patient and his or her advocate. Long-term (i.e. end of programme) goals are identified along with a series of short-term goals that are the stepping stones to the achievement of the long-term goals. At regular goal-review meetings, plans of action relating to achieving short-term goals are set, with each plan of action describing clearly who will do what and by when. It is within these plans of actions that the various interventions to be applied by particular team members can be documented. Progress towards achievement of the short-term goals is recorded at each meeting. This can be done by noting whether a goal is achieved, partially achieved (some progress made, but goal not achieved as defined) or not achieved (no substantial progress made). Alternatively, a more detailed rating of progress can be made using the Goal Attainment Scaling system whereby a more detailed record of progress is made with reference to a scale using points relating to degrees of achievement (below or above the anticipated level).[12]

Cost-Effectiveness in Rehabilitation

Neurosurgical advances mean that increasing numbers of people are surviving brain injury. The costs of brain injury are wide ranging, beginning with the hospitalisation and medical care in the acute stages, and often extend into the community. On leaving hospital, a person may need supervision and care or, in some cases, placement in residential supported living. Medical costs may extend to treatment in the community and further hospitalisations may be required. The person may not be able to return to previous employment and therefore cease to contribute taxes and may need to claim disability benefits. Families may suffer financial loss initially during hospitalisation, which may include travel and parking costs, loss of earnings and child care. Family members may reduce their tax contributions through reducing working hours or giving up work to care for the person with a brain injury. Increased family stress as a result of brain injury is recognised and this can increase costs through absence from work or treatment for mental health problems. People with brain injury are significantly more at risk from mental health problems and alcoholism furthering the cost to health services.

Rehabilitation can address many of the above problems and reduce costs. However, in order to fund rehabilitation, authorities need to be convinced not only of its effectiveness *per se* but of the cost effectiveness.

Worthington, Ramos and Oddy[14] reviewed the evidence relating to the cost effectiveness of neuropsychological rehabilitation. They note that information on cost-effectiveness is often lacking from studies of intervention efficacy, including for neuropsychological rehabilitation interventions or services. However, there is some evidence suggesting that specialist rehabilitation services may be cost effective. For example, there is evidence that early admission to inpatient rehabilitation is associated with shorter hospital stays and improved clinical outcomes and is therefore cost-effective.[15] Wood in 1999 showed that for a group of 76 very severely brain-injured adults who underwent post-acute neurobehavioural rehabilitation within the first 2 years costs were reduced by over £20 000 per year (nearly £2 million in a lifetime) and for rehabilitation beginning more than 2 years after injury, by over £10 000 per year.[16] Furthermore, Worthington and colleagues completed a similar study with a larger sample of 133 patients, and found that rehabilitation costs were minimal compared to estimated lifetime savings, which were between £0.8 M and £1.1 M for adults admitted for neurobehavioural rehabilitation within a year of injury and between £400 K and £500 k for those admitted beyond 2 years.[17] Oddy and Ramos later reported similar figures for a further cohort of patients undergoing similar neurobehavioural rehabilitation programmes to those in Worthington and colleagues study, finding consistent levels of estimated savings (£0.57 to £1.13 M for those admitted within 12 months and £190 K to £860 K for those admitted after 12 months).[18]

Turner-Stokes et al. presented evidence that rehabilitation reduced dependency and care costs by up to £639 per week and that the highest reductions in care could be made in high-dependency groups.[19] Khan et al. introduced a traumatic brain injury programme during initial treatment in hospital, which included rehabilitation from the acute stages, education and involvement of the families and management by a TBI multi-disciplinary team in sub-acute rehabilitation. The programme resulted in a reduction in average length of hospital stay from 30.5 to 12 days and amounted to savings of over $21.8 million over a period of 6 years.[20]

The range of interventions and services for which there is compelling evidence of cost effectiveness remains limited, but the evidence that does exist does appear to indicate that rehabilitation services, particularly when they are provided relatively soon after injury, will produce better outcomes, and therefore reduce costs associated with ongoing disability.

In summary, rehabilitation is a collaborative process whereby the patient and his or her family work with an interdisciplinary team to maximise the patient's ability and opportunity to participate in those activities of everyday life that are valued by the patient. In the following chapters, the contributions of key members of the rehabilitation team are described, along with accounts of how specific cognitive impairments and behavioural problems should be treated.

References

1. Ward CD, McIntosh S. The rehabilitation process: a neurological perspective. In: Greenwood RJ, Barnes MP, McMillan TM, Ward, CD, eds. *Handbook of neurological rehabilitation*. Hove, UK: Psychology Press; 2003.

2. Wade D. Applying the WHO ICF framework to the rehabilitation of patients with cognitive deficits. In: Halligan P, Wade D, eds. *The effectiveness of rehabilitation for cognitive deficits*. Oxford: Oxford University Press; 2005.

3. McMillan TM. Neurorehabilitation services and their delivery. In: Wilson BA, ed. *Neuropsychological rehabilitation*. Lisse: Swets & Zeitlinger; 2003.

4. Herbert C. Planning, delivering and evaluating services. In: Goldstein LH, McNeil JE, eds. *Clinical neuropsychology: a practical guide to assessment and management for clinicians*. Chichester, UK: Wiley; 2004.

5. British Psychological Society. *Division of Neuropsychology report on clinical neuropsychology and rehabilitation services for adults with acquired brain injury*. Leicester, UK: BPS; 2005. www.bps.org.uk

6. Royal College of Surgeons. *Working party on the management of patients with head injury*. London: RCS; 1999.

7. Johnson R, Balleny H. Behaviour problems after brain injury: incidence and need for treatment. *Clin Rehabil* 1996;10:173–81.

8. Wood RL, Worthington AD. Neurobehavioural rehabilitation in practice. In: Wood RL, McMillan TM, eds. *Neurobehavioural disability and social handicap following traumatic brain injury*. Hove, UK: Psychology Press; 2001.

9. Powell J, Helsin J, Greenwood R. Community based rehabilitation after severe traumatic brain injury: a randomized controlled trial. *J Neurol Neurosurg Psychiatry* 2003;72:193–202.

10. Svendsen HA, Teasdale TW. The influence of neuropsychological rehabilitation on symptomatology and quality of life following brain injury: a controlled long-term follow-up. *Brain Injury* 2006;20:1295–306.

11. Wilson BA, Gracey F, Evans JJ, Bateman A. *Neuropsychological rehabilitation: theory, therapy and outcomes*. Cambridge: Cambridge University Press; 2009.

12. Evans JJ, Krasny-Pacini A. Goal setting in rehabilitation. In: Wilson BA, van Heugten C, Winegardner J, Ownsworth T, eds. *International handbook of neuropsychological rehabilitation*. Hove, UK: Psychology Press; 2017.

13. Holliday R, Cano S, Freeman JA, Playford ED. Should patients participate in clinical decision making? An optimised balance block design controlled study of goal setting in a rehabilitation setting. *J Neurol Neurosurg Psychiatr* 2007;78:576–80.

14. Worthington A, da Silva Ramos S, Oddy M. The cost-effectiveness of neuropsychological rehabilitation. In: Wilson BA, van Heugten C, Winegardner J, Ownsworth T, eds. *International handbook of neuropsychological rehabilitation*. Hove, UK: Psychology Press; 2017.

15. Kunik CL, Flowers L, Kazanjian T. Time to rehabilitation admission and associated outcomes for patients with traumatic brain injury. *Arch Phys Med Rehab* 2006;87:1590–6.

16. Wood RL, McCrea JD, Wood LM, Merriman RN. Clinical and cost effectiveness of post-acute

neurobehavioural rehabilitation. *Brain Injury* 1999;13:69–88.

17. Worthington A, Matthews S, Melia Y, Oddy M. Cost-benefits associated with social outcome from neurobehavioural rehabilitation. *Brain Injury* 2006;20 (9):947–57.

18. Oddy M, da Silva Ramos S. The clinical and cost-benefits of investing in neurobehavioural rehabilitation: a multi-centre study. *Brain Injury* 2013;27 (1):1500–7.

19. Turner-Stokes L, Paul S, Williams H. Efficiency of specialist rehabilitation in reducing dependency and costs of continuing care for adults with complex acquired brain injuries. *J Neurol Neurosurg Psychiatr* 2006; 77:634–9.

20. Khan S, Khan A, Feyz M. Decreased length of stay, cost savings and descriptive findings of enhanced patient care resulting from an integrated traumatic brain injury programme. *Brain Injury* 2002;16:537–54.

MDT and Rehabilitation of Head Injury

Judith Fewings, Ann-Marie Pringle, Thérèse Lebedis and Maggie Whyte

Introduction

The effectiveness of brain injury rehabilitation from early stages of recovery through acute, post-acute and community care is well documented.[1] Clinical guidelines recommend early assessment and rehabilitation from specialist multidisciplinary teams.[2-5] Key aspects of the multidisciplinary approach are highlighted as holistic and maximising the available resources (knowledge, experience, financial and physical) to work towards a common goal.[2] The British Society of Rehabilitation Medicine (BSRM) guidelines point to the benefits of an interdisciplinary team working towards an agreed set of goals and recommends systems for co-ordination of disciplines, communication with patients and families and education and training with teams.[3] Standards for major trauma centres and brain injury rehabilitation refer to the importance of acute multidisciplinary specialist trauma rehabilitation services.[3,6,7] The benefits of providing rehabilitation as an MDT are well recognised and do not only improve clinical outcomes and enhance patient safety but improve staff well-being and job satisfaction.[8,9]

The clinical roles of key members of the multidisciplinary team across the pathway of patient care are detailed in the following chapter.

Physiotherapy

Early physiotherapy intervention aims to maintain optimal respiratory function, thereby limiting secondary brain damage, avoid weaning delay, preserve the integrity of the musculoskeletal system and start the process of regaining motor control. For therapists to manage patients with TBI they must have an understanding of neural and muscle physiology, pathophysiology of brain injury and a working knowledge of all rehabilitation concepts and clinical experience. An accurate assessment needs to be made. A problem list and individual treatment plan is then constructed; no two head injured patients will have the same deficits/medical problems.[10,11]

The severity of the primary injury directly relates to the period of unconsciousness during which time they are more susceptible to secondary adaptations of the musculoskeletal system, compared with their conscious counterparts and thus poorer functional outcomes.[12]

Changes in management such as the introduction of Advanced Trauma Life Support (ATLS), National Institute for Health and Care Excellence (NICE) guidelines and specific protocol driven medical therapies have improved outcome and reduced mortality in patients with extensive neural injuries.[5,13] The development of regional trauma networks in the UK has also optimised time from injury to definitive treatment and comprehensive national audits and reporting systems are responsible for driving quality improvement and clinical governance.[14–16]

Respiratory Care

Physiotherapeutic interventions facilitate the maintenance of parameters to optimise cerebral oxygenation in the presence of raised intracranial pressure (ICP). The physiotherapist must monitor ICP throughout their treatment provision as the injured brain loses autoregulation and the Cerebral Perfusion Pressure (CPP) becomes directly related to the systemic Mean Arterial Blood Pressure (MAP) and the ICP.

$$CPP = \text{MAP} - \text{ICP}^{17}$$

Hypercarbia can result in cerebral vasodilation, increasing cerebral blood volume thereby raising ICP. Respiratory physiotherapy therefore must facilitate adequate oxygenation and avoidance of hypercarbia without precipitating any sustained rise in ICP or fall in MAP.

In the non-intubated TBI patient, supplemental oxygen must be administered to ensure adequate cerebral oxygenation. The decision whether or not to administer respiratory care to the intubated patient is multifactorial and multidisciplinary. Assessment should aim to establish whether the respiratory status will improve with physiotherapy intervention and also to ascertain the patient's stability in terms of their cardiovascular and intracranial parameters. Consideration must be given to the increased oxygen consumption and poor peripheral oxygen extraction present in the critically ill.[18,19] Rest periods have been shown to be essential in the care of the TBI patient to prevent sustained rises in ICP.[20]

Positioning

The optimum position, with respect to cerebral perfusion is head up 15°–30° with the neck in a neutral position; venous drainage is facilitated without compromise to systolic blood pressure thereby maximising CPP.[21] Critically ill patients frequently have decreased pulmonary functional reserve, this must be borne in mind when performing routine positional changes. There may be an increase in oxygen consumption of up to 50% following turning patients onto their side.[19] The traditional head down postural drainage positions are contraindicated in TBI patients as this increases ICP.[22] Caution is also required in positioning patients with bone flap defects, ensuring that no long-term pressure is applied to the affected area in a side-lying position. That said, judicious use of lateral side lying positioning has been shown to enhance recruitment and facilitate drainage from lung segments and may improve V/Q matching, optimising oxygenation.[23]

When ICP is uncontrolled by sedation alone, muscle relaxants may be used to reduce the metabolic demand, prevent the cough reflex and allow full control of the $PaCO_2$. However, the use of paralysis may contribute to other potential hazards; namely, early changes in skeletal muscle structure and potentially an increased risk of pneumonia.[24,25]

Where clinical assessment of the TBI patient indicates retained secretions, sputum clearance should be undertaken. Patients should be pre-oxygenated prior to positional changes, negating the increase in oxygen consumption, and the secretions removed. If the change in position is tolerated with no detrimental effects on CPP or ICP, it can be repeated on a 2–4 hourly basis if deemed necessary. If these simple manoeuvres do not result in improved oxygenation owing to tenacious/retained secretions, then active humidification and bronchoscopy by the medical staff should be considered.[26]

Manual Hyper-inflation

Manual chest techniques (MCT) and manual hyper-inflation (MHI) quickly and effectively remove sputum and reverse atelectasis.[27] **Caution** is required during MHI, MAP should be > 80 and the expiratory phase should be longer than the inspiratory phase.[18]

MHI consists of short periods of bagging, maintaining ventilatory tidal volumes, followed by five or six breaths of MHI with manual chest shaking and vibrations, repeated as necessary until secretions are loosened.[28]

The following parameters are necessary to avoid detrimental effects:

- Periods of Hyperinflation to be brief < 3.5 m
- Flow rate of 15 litres of 100% O_2 to a 2 litre bag
- Tidal volume 1.5 times the ventilator volume up to 1000 ml
- Peak Inflation Pressure less than or equal to 40 mmHg

In combination with other techniques, MHI can dramatically reduce treatment times. Patients have to be observed carefully during MHI as ICP can be raised secondary to increased intrathoracic pressure. However hyperventilation can assist in reducing ICP via decreasing $PaCO_2$. Manometers should therefore be included in the respiratory circuit. Concerns regarding detrimental effects of MHI (owing to raised ICP) have not been demonstrated.[27,28]

Suction

In ventilated TBI patients, suction is commonly regarded as a treatment that increases ICP; however, it is also viewed as a necessary procedure, which is required with a frequency sufficient to maintain a patent airway.[26] The transient increase in ICP caused can be mitigated with careful assessment and competent technique.

The following recommendations have been made to minimise potential hypoxaemia:

- Duration of catheter insertion 10–15 s
- Hyperoxygenate pre- and post-suctions using 100% O_2 or 20% above baseline.

The American Association of Respiratory Care Guidelines recommends 100% oxygen for 1 min post-suction.[26] The effectiveness of suction is dependent on adequate patient hydration, humidification and warming of inspired gases.[29]

Heat and Moisture Exchangers (HME) usually provide adequate humidification for ventilated patients in the short term (24–48 hours). However, the use of heated humidification should be instigated if the patient's secretions become thick, purulent or the patients past medical history and mechanism of injury suggests a potential risk (e.g. aspiration, asthma, smoker). The practice of instilling 5 ml of sodium chloride 0.9% aseptically and slowly prior to suctioning is widely used, but remains contentious. Adequate hydration, adequate humidification, use of mucolytic agents and effective mobilisation should be instituted prior to the consideration of saline instillation for patients with increased viscosity of their secretions.[30]

Manual Chest Techniques (MCT): Shaking, Vibrations and Percussion

Manual chest techniques (MCT) are frequently performed physiotherapeutic manoeuvres aiding sputum clearance along with other methods and positioning previously described. The evidence for its benefit however is controversial and sometimes conflicting.

Some studies show that simple interventions such as lateral positioning[31] and passive movements have significant impact on patients' oxygen consumption.[18] Others, however, have not shown any difference in oxygen consumption or cardiac index with MCT, indeed MCT have been credited with reducing Ventilator Acquired Pneumonia (VAP) and overall length of stay in ICU.[32]

Historically percussion in sedated, ventilated patients was attributed to a fall in ICP, its effect being greater if the patient was paralysed. The theory being that air flow transients in airways beneath a percussed segment. Vibrations performed manually by compressing the chest wall during expiration were found to increase peak expiratory flow rate by more than 50%.[33] The same technique during expiration on a ventilated breath has no effect on ICP but shaking during a MHI breath and MHI alone has been found to increase ICP.[25]

In the early stages following TBI, patients have a limited ability to tolerate even the most simple of interventions. Maintaining optimal conditions for brain recovery and avoiding secondary brain damage are the prime treatment maxims. Whilst airway and respiratory issues normally take precedence in the early stages following trauma, early attention to the musculoskeletal system is important in promoting recovery of head control and limb function.

NICE guidance[34] advocates commencing early rehabilitation in the ICU population at the point of physiological stability which enhances physical function and contributes to earlier discharge from critical care. Physiotherapy plays a pivotal role in both the acute and later phases of rehabilitative care for the TBI patient.

Musculoskeletal Integrity and Neuromuscular Status

Spasticity results from any lesion in the upper motor neuron pathway, causing absence (or disruption) of extrapyramidal inhibitory influence on alpha and gamma motor neurons. Reflex arcs are disinhibited giving rise to hyper reflexia and increased tone, typically in the antigravity muscles – upper limb flexors and lower limb extensors. A velocity-dependant increase in the tonic stretch is seen, that is greater resistance to faster stretch.[35]

Spasticity can occur early following TBI and may result in limb deformities compromising patient care and delaying early rehabilitation.[36]

Muscle stretch/lengthening is resisted by hypertonia. As a consequence muscles remain in a shortened position for prolonged periods of time which results in changes to the physical properties of muscle and associated soft tissues. Sarcomeres in series, responsible for determining distance and force of contraction, are reduced thereby decreasing its length and extensibility.[37] The muscle and soft tissue changes result in loss of joint range and movement.[11] Muscle function can also be compounded by pain associated with heterotopic ossification and the presence of skeletal fractures in the multiply injured. The risk in the TBI population has been found to be 20%.[38]

Stretch, either active or passive, is historically recommended to prevent contracture formation. The optimum degree and frequency is unknown and a meta-analysis found no significant effects when reviewing four recent trials[39]; however, prolonged stretch has been shown to reduce spasticity.[36] It is hypothesised that a sustained stretch on the shortened muscle tendon is responsible for modifying the physiological response of the muscle, that is damping its overactivity.[40] This is achieved through the process of splinting (applying a prolonged stretch through the application of a range of devices) which is now an established means of controlling contractures and spasticity in both adults and children.[41] Proactive splinting is frequently employed early in the course of TBI. This provides the prolonged stretch required to maintain joint range during the initial unconscious period and has been found to reduce spasticity in more chronic conditions.[42]

The optimum method of splinting (removable and non-removable) remains debatable. Removable casts/splints can be custom fashioned to allow passive range of movement exercises to maintain tissue and joint extensibility. Potential drawbacks of non-removable serial splints include primarily muscle atrophy, pain, increased DVT risk and pressure ulceration. It needs to be considered that the above methods hold the joint in a fixed position. Dynamic orthoses are being used more frequently in order to apply a sustained stretch whilst enabling the joint a degree of movement.[43] The most suitable method of splinting depends on the patient cohort, cognition and conscious level.[36] Comprehensive guidelines[41] reinforce the importance of multidisciplinary assessment and management by skilled postgraduate practitioners whilst providing a review of the current evidence base and calling for further research into this field.

From the management point of view, spasticity has two components amenable to treatment – biomechanical and neural.[44] The biomechanical aspect is managed by – passive movements, positioning, splinting and casting are all commonplace.[36,44] Alleviation of the neural component is achieved by antispasmodic drugs. Baclofen and Tizanidine are commonly used, others include Sodium Dantrolene and Clonidine. All these drugs have potential side effects, and some have been implicated in possibly delaying cognitive recovery following brain injury.[40,45]

In cases of focal spasticity or severe spasticity, Botulinum Toxin A (BTX-A) can be used. BTX-A is a powerful neurotoxin which inhibits presynaptic acetylcholine release at the neurotransmitter junction producing a localised temporary muscle weakness.[44] Its effects can be seen within 24–72 hours and lasts on average 3–4 months. International and European Consensus statements agree that its considered use in conjunction with passive movements and external sustained stretch devices; it has been shown to significantly reduce tone, allow toleration of the splints and improve functional recovery.[44,46,47]

Motor Control

The wide variety of treatment approaches in rehabilitation have their foundations in an array of motor control theories.[48] The challenge for the physiotherapist is to develop their own model of practice, where the treatment methods they select have a scientific, physiotherapeutic and practical knowledge base.

Forty-six per cent of ICU patients suffer from complications to their neuromuscular and cardiovascular systems due to prolonged immobilisation.[49] This leads to poor short-term outcomes and delays in both ventilator weaning and eventual ICU/hospital discharge.[50] Early mobilisation through structured programmes of rehabilitation has shown that they can be performed safely and are feasible in the literature and this is reinforced with National Guidelines.[3,34] The focus of research has primarily been the General ICU population;

however, results of recent studies appear to support early therapy interventions in Neuro ICU.[51]

Movement between different positions (postural sets) aims to stimulate proprioceptive input and thereby enhance efferent activity.[52] Excitation of the vestibulospinal tract involves recruitment of lower limb extensors, proximal musculature and head movement. This is closely linked with reticulospinal tract activity, influencing extensor tone and involving the cerebellum in maintaining equilibrium. Since the feet afford afferent input into the vestibulospinal tract, standing can be used as a therapeutic means of activation.

The tilt-table is a useful adjunct to facilitate early, safe standing. It is particularly useful and well tolerated for patients who are unconscious and require total support. Upright mobilisation benefits include improved bone density, cardiopulmonary function and gastrointestinal motility additionally the use of weight bearing helps maintain length in the plantarflexors.[53,54] Studies have demonstrated its potential to enhance arousal in the minimally concious.[55] Brain-injured recumbent patients have impaired autonomic orthostatic responses, initially only small angles of tilt should be used with continued monitoring of BP, SaO_2, HR, RR and skin colour. Malalignment should be avoided as this impairs normal proprioceptive input.[53]

Trunk control is equally as important as respiratory care and spasticity management in the rehabilitation of the head injured. The role of the trunk is fundamental to head control and limb function via the shoulder and pelvic girdles. Physiotherapy treatment of the trunk therefore needs to be incorporated; for this reason treatment plans frequently involve alternating sessions of standing (tilt-table initially, therapist facilitated later) and work in sitting.

A third of patients following TBI have visual deficits, effective positioning attained by the tilt-table and sitting enables normal head-neck alignment, stimulates visual and vestibular facilitated pathways[56] and promotes dynamic stability of anterior neck muscles. The anterior neck muscles are important for tongue movements and swallowing as they help stabilise the hyoid bone. Maintenance of neck and head range of movement (ROM) allows neuro visual rehabilitation to take place. Early active and passive orofacial movements are also encouraged as this helps with respiratory care, nutrition and communication recovery.

Movement modulation mediated by the cerebellum can be targeted to assist motor learning by means of task(s) repetition.[56] Movement and control of movement against gravity encourage balance control. As improvements in proximal trunk control, head control and selective lower limb movements occur, treatments gradually incorporate facilitation of gait. The therapist should continually strive to rehabilitate patients beyond their present functional ability in order to attain their maximal future functional status.

Posture and Seating

Posture and seating are important to normalise proprioceptive feedback, postural stability is necessary for functional activity.[57] Seating systems are frequently used for patients with severe neurologic impairment and are used as adjuncts to the previously mentioned treatments. Ankle range of movement and tone management are fundamental to wheelchair-dependant patients, the ability to achieve plantigrade contributes to ease and safety of transfer into the chair, and also reduces the risk of pressure areas associated with poor alignment and critical illness.[58]

By applying external supports to the patient in the most functional and least restrictive positions, a stable posture can be attained.[57] Appropriate orientation of the trunk in space is important to consider. Rearward tilting is used in many seating systems. The use of gravity to assist stability is considered vital in the severely posturally incompetent patient but used with caution to limit any further detrimental effects of social, visual and environmental isolation.[59] Additionally a wedge cushion, bilateral thoracic supports and head support along with the inclusion of a table can be used to build a stable posture.[57] Stability in the sitting position confers better orofacial control, swallowing and speech; social interaction and communication are enhanced reinforcing recovery of function and improving the patients' quality of life.[60]

Speech and Language Therapy

In the acute stages of recovery from brain injury, speech and language therapists are key in the assessment and intervention of difficulties with swallowing (dysphagia).

The consequences of dysphagia can be devastating and include malnutrition, aspiration and aspiration-associated pneumonia, choking and death. The incidence of swallowing disorders following traumatic brain injury is unknown, although one study identified dysphagia in 61% of patients admitted to an acute rehabilitation unit.[61] The main risk factors for dysphagia are: impaired level of consciousness, severe cognitive impairment, presence of a tracheostomy, and a period of ventilation in excess of 2 weeks.[62,63] Continuing cognitive and behavioural impairments influence the management of dysphagia and frequently delay the possibility of safe oral intake.[62,64]

The normal swallow has oral, pharyngeal and oesophageal stages.[64,65] These can be disrupted in a number of ways following TBI, including reduced lip closure, reduced range of tongue movement or reduced co-ordination of tongue movement (creating poor bolus control, slow oral transit times and inefficient oral clearance), delay in triggering the pharyngeal swallow (which may cause aspiration), reduced laryngeal elevation (resulting in residual food in the pyriform sinuses and at the laryngeal entrance) reduced laryngeal closure or absent swallow reflex (resulting in aspiration of food and liquid) and cricopharyngeal dysfunction (obstructing the passage of food into the oesophagus and resulting in solids or liquids collecting in the pharyngeal/laryngeal area).[62,63] Additional swallowing disorders can be caused by prolonged endotracheal intubation or emergency tracheostomy.[62]

The main clinical signs, which should prompt a swallowing assessment, are coughing during meals, gurgly voice quality, copious oral or pulmonary secretions, chest infection, obvious difficulty managing food orally and perceived delay in triggering the pharyngeal swallow.[62] Approximately 10% to 15% of dysphagic people with TBI are silent aspirators, however, and do not present with obvious signs.

Early evaluation of swallowing ability and aspiration risk is essential.[66,67] The speech and language therapist will usually undertake a bedside assessment of oral, pharyngeal and laryngeal function, and will evaluate the patient's communication status. Videofluoroscopy (VF), or modified barium swallow, is also often carried out in order to view what can only be assumed at the bedside assessment. Fibre-optic Endoscopic Evaluation of Swallowing (FEES) is available in many acute hospitals and will also provide an objective assessment of swallowing ability.[68] In both cases, patient compliance is essential.

The efficacy of dysphagia therapy after TBI is not well documented.[67,69] Thermal stimulation, where a cold stimulus is applied to the anterior faucial pillars, is commonly used to improve the swallow reflex.[65,70] Other dysphagia treatments in which the patient is an active participant are described elsewhere, but there is little evidence available as to how effective they are or how extensively they are used in patients with TBI.[65] The usual practice from early rehabilitation onwards is to encourage safe eating and drinking by modifying the patient's diet and the immediate environment. A supervised and regularly monitored regime involving practice amounts of thick puree is begun when considered safe to do so, with enteral feeding, usually via percutaneous endoscopic gastrostomy (PEG), meeting the main nutritional needs. With progress, the food gradually becomes more textured and amounts larger, with decreasing reliance on alternative methods of nutrition. Similarly, liquids can be thickened to varying degrees. The patient's seating position can be altered for maximal safety whilst eating, as can head position. Risk is minimised further by staff supervising and, if necessary, assisting dysphagic patients at mealtimes. It is important for family members and friends to understand the risks and the safe limits and to become involved in the rehabilitation process as early as possible.

The speech and language therapist working in brain injury rehabilitation is faced with the challenge of teasing out the communication deficits from any co-existing impairments and attempting to assist the patient towards regaining an acceptable level of interaction.

Disorders of Communication

Until the early 1970s, language dysfunction was not considered to be one of the main consequences of closed head injury, in contrast with impairments of memory and concentration.[71] Many authors agree that classical aphasic syndromes are relatively rare following TBI although the presence of word finding difficulties is recognised and Wernicke's aphasia has been reported in one or two papers.[71,72] Although many patients perform reasonably well on traditional tests of aphasia, deficits of basic language processing are by no means uncommon in brain injury. In addition to word finding difficulties, other characteristics of aphasia, such as paraphasias, impaired comprehension and reading and writing deficits are frequently encountered. Verbal fluency deficits are also common. Linguistic disorders tend to be more prevalent during the earlier stages of the patient's recovery and have frequently resolved by the time of discharge from hospital.

The ability to communicate verbally and non-verbally in a social context is often impaired following a TBI.[73,74] Difficulties with pragmatic communication skills, or how language is *used*, can persist long after any associated linguistic deficits. Deficiencies are frequently evident in turn-taking in conversation, initiating, maintaining and terminating conversation, using (and comprehending) facial expression, eye contact, tone of voice and gesture.[75] Patients are also reported as responding slowly or not at all, and appearing uninterested in the other speaker or their point of view.[76] Disorders of discourse are also very common. Discourse can be described as a series of related sentences used in communication interchanges, mainly in conversation but also in, for example narrative discourse such as story-telling, and procedural discourse during which a process is described, such as how to make spaghetti bolognaise. Impaired discourse skills can be characterised by an over-abundance of talk that is tangential and contains irrelevant and unrelated details, or a meagre amount of talk with little information content, difficulty staying on topic, difficulties generating questions or comments to sustain conversation, disordered sequencing of information, difficulties understanding or manipulating abstract language such as sarcasm, puns or metaphors.[72–77,85]

Verbal output can also be 'inaccurate and confabulatory', which is usually attributable to cognitive dysfunction rather than to a deficiency of linguistic processing or pragmatics.

'Cognitive communication disorder' is often used as a diagnostic label to cover any or all of the non-linguistic communication disorders following traumatic brain injury. The presence of additional cognitive deficits will have an adverse effect on communicative competence. Poor planning and impaired concentration can reduce the efficacy of sequencing and inclusion of relevant information in conversation or narrative. Reduced listening skills can impact upon the ability to absorb and integrate spoken language. Visual neglect and visuo-perceptual disorders affect reading and writing. Lowered arousal can diminish the available resources and energy to process complex communicative tasks and poor self-monitoring influences how well the person engages with others.[78]

Some authors attribute disorders of pragmatics and discourse following TBI to cognitive dysfunction, in particular to executive dysfunction.[71,78,79] Where communication disorders are non-linguistic in origin and are a direct consequence of other cognitive deficits, as above, the expectation is that the ability to communicate will improve when cognitive functioning does. Disorders of pragmatics and discourse are extensively described in the literature as a consequence of damage to the right cerebral hemisphere.[80] The characteristic features are more or less identical whether social communication is damaged by a TBI or a right hemisphere stroke. As disorders of basic language processing following TBI can reasonably be linked to trauma in the language centres of the dominant (usually left) hemisphere or their connections, it seems fitting that, in at least some cases, pragmatic disorders following TBI could result from damage to the functions of the right hemisphere.[81]

Disorders of speech, especially dysarthria, are common after a TBI, although there is disagreement in the literature regarding prevalence and recovery.[82] Depending on the neuropathology, any of the main subgroups of spastic, flaccid, ataxic, hypo- and hyperkinetic or a mixed dysarthria can be identified, with spastic dysarthria most common due to the regularity with which bilateral upper motor neurone damage occurs. There is considerable variability with regard both to the severity and the extent to which articulation, respiration, rate, resonance, volume and prosody are implicated. An additional complication is the possibility of dyspraxia affecting the articulation of speech sounds.

Assessment of Communication Skills

There is no universally recommended single method of assessing communication disorders following TBI. The population is a heterogeneous one and requires an individual approach. The patient's clinical presentation will change over time as a result of treatment, spontaneous recovery or a combination of both. A flexible approach to assessment of communication disorders is essential, as test selection and the timing of assessment will be influenced by a range of factors. Variables such as level of consciousness and arousal, agitation and restlessness, fatigue, concentration, emergence from PTA, levels of co-operation, insight, the extent of co-occurring cognitive deficits and the presence of identifiable specific communication deficits will determine whether the patient has reached the stage of being able to cope with the often lengthier and more demanding formal standardised tests or whether a more informal approach, which can be more easily adapted to cope with the patient's changing condition, is preferred.

Rehabilitation of Communication Disorders

Rehabilitation of communication disorders following TBI is a highly individualised, dynamic process. A multidisciplinary team approach is essential, as patients with a TBI frequently present with a range of disorders requiring input from several disciplines. Where possible, patients are encouraged to identify their own communication difficulties, highlighting those which they perceive to be the most disabling, although poor insight frequently inhibits this. The speech and language therapist will attempt to design a rehabilitation plan in accordance with the patient's needs, possibly focusing on or prioritising those deficits which would be most responsive to therapy. Techniques are often employed with the aim of remediating or restoring previous functions, as in word finding tasks and language therapy in general, or in articulation drills for dysarthria. Attempts are made to incorporate materials which are of personal interest or value to the patient in order to maximise motivation and participation. Compensatory techniques and assistive technology might be explored where further improvement is unlikely, for example in cases of severe dysarthria. For such patients a practical approach would be to train family members and friends as 'communication partners' in order to help them find optimal ways of conversing with and eliciting information from the person with a TBI. Detailed descriptions of approaches which have been used in the rehabilitation of impairments of pragmatic communication and discourse are provided elsewhere in the literature.[83,84]

The consequences of enduring communication impairments can be more devastating than those of physical deficits and are associated with failure to return to or maintain employment,[85] the gradual disintegration of family dynamics, often resulting in divorce,[86] and social isolation.[87] The importance of rehabilitation for communication disorders, and continued support for patients and their families, cannot be overstated.

Occupational Therapy

Occupational therapy enables people to achieve health, wellbeing and life satisfaction through participation in occupation (Royal College of Occupational Therapists).[88]

Kielhofner stated that humans have an occupational nature; humans can experience occupational dysfunction (difficulty engaging in daily activities and life roles); and that occupation can be used as a therapeutic agent.[89] Following brain injury, people may experience difficulties performing everyday activities. The varied and often complex nature of occupational dysfunction experienced following brain injury requires specialised assessment and treatment, provided by an occupational therapist with expertise in brain injury.[90]

Acute Care

In the acute phase and in early stages of recovery the occupational therapist will focus on the reduction of impairment and the prevention of secondary complications to maximise longer-term functional outcome. Continued evaluation of performance skills (motor, sensory, cognitive, psychological and social capacities) is used to establish a person's level of function, ability to engage in activity and to participate in meaningful occupations and life roles. Identifying meaningful and achievable goals guides intervention and supports person centred rehabilitation.

During periods of reduced arousal and alertness (e.g. coma, minimally conscious state) the occupational therapist will work with colleagues and the person's family and friends to establish a better understanding of the patient's cognitive ability and their level and pattern of arousal. Reactions to a variety of stimuli are observed in order to determine any consistent or meaningful responses and to establish an appropriate treatment programme. Multi-modal sensory stimulation programmes may be initiated to improve arousal and awareness, thus maximising a patient's potential for interacting with their environment in an appropriate way.[91] In the acute care setting this may be administered through structured observation of behaviours and responses to stimuli as identified via formal standardised assessments such as the Sensory Modality Assessment and Rehabilitation Technique (SMART).[92]

Occupational therapists use meaningful activities to increase alertness and awareness and to facilitate appropriate interaction with people and the environment. They may adapt the environment and provide external aids, such as call systems or TV controls which are adjusted to suit individual functional capacity and to aid independent means of controlling the environment. Other means of therapeutic support may be introduced, such as diaries to be used as memory aids. These measures can also serve to increase participation in the individual's recovery by family and friends who can guide what is relevant to be included in an individualised treatment programme.

Functional recovery is aided by the therapeutic application of activities. These include facilitated practice of daily living skills such as feeding and personal care tasks in order to enhance motor, sensory, psychological, cognitive and social functions. A daily routine may be established, balancing activity and rest according to individual needs and tolerances in order to maximise periods of alertness and to reduce fatigue. The environment will be managed to ensure appropriate levels of sensory input and regulate levels of stimulation.

Ascertaining the patient's level of cognitive ability is essential to anticipate long-term problems. For people with mild brain injury, the occupational therapist will be interested in cognitive impairment which may not be immediately obvious in the acute care setting but which may present the person with longer-term problems. Screening assessments may highlight these issues and the person is then referred to and/or provided with contacts and information about support services in the community if they are to be discharged home from the acute care setting. Referral for specialised community monitoring and rehabilitation may be appropriate and a more detailed cognitive assessment from a neuropsychologist may be recommended. The occupational therapist also plays an important role as part of the multidisciplinary team in assessing and monitoring levels of post-traumatic amnesia and providing appropriate interventions.

Motor and sensory function is assessed using a range of standardised assessments and structured observational methods in order to establish a baseline of abilities and to determine the impact on functional ability (occupational performance). It is essential that a coordinated multidisciplinary approach to the assessment and management of motor and sensory deficits is established to maximise outcome and minimise long-term complications such as contractures and pressure sores. These problems can be addressed through the implementation of a postural management programme in all aspects of the person's daily routines, and through the provision of equipment such as splints, specialised seating, wheelchairs, pressure relieving cushions and positioning aids. Splints or orthoses are made and or fitted to achieve and maintain normal alignment of the limb and muscle length, and to reduce the development of secondary complications. This, in turn, facilitates optimal physical function depending on the level of motor recovery.

For those with moderate or severe brain injury, recommendations for appropriate ongoing rehabilitation will be made by the occupational therapist and the multidisciplinary team. Options range from specialist in-patient brain injury rehabilitation services to community teams and case management services.

Preparation for transfer of care to home or further rehabilitation requires detailed planning. The occupational therapist may carry out home assessments to determine any ongoing support or equipment needs for a safe and effective discharge, and will ensure appropriate handover of the treatment plan to rehabilitation colleagues. A key worker system is used successfully in some acute care settings for information transfer in a seamless manner.

The occupational therapist also provides education and support for families, carers and friends throughout the acute phase to ensure appropriate and consistent input for the person with brain injury in all aspects of daily living and for their own support needs.

Post-Acute and Community Rehabilitation

Analysis of a person carrying out selected activities can determine where performance is limited, and can ascertain a person's potential for returning to previous or engaging in new occupations. This also enables the therapist to identify abilities and deficits, and forms the basis of a goal-orientated treatment plan.

People are generally goal directed in their actions and behaviour. Cognitive changes following brain injury can affect a person's interest, motivation and initiative to engage in new and previous activities. Goal directed therapy supports the achievement of personal goals via therapeutic interventions and rehabilitation is tailored to individuals needs. The person is more likely to be motivated to achieve a goal if it is something they are interested in and they are more likely to learn if therapy is goal orientated.

Intervention by the occupational therapist at this stage focuses on improving occupation and functional independence. Standardised assessments and behavioural observations are used to build a functional performance profile. Restorative and/or compensatory approaches may be used to improve function. Occupational therapy will use practice of daily activities incorporating strategy training to improve cognitive, motor, sensory psychological and social functions, for example schedules to structure and pace daily routines if fatigue is an issue, use of assistive technology (diary/electronic organisers/navigation aids) for memory and executive function deficits, coloured markers on the cooker controls or scanning training for visual difficulties, checklists to facilitate independence in personal care or graded activity programmes to improve motor functions. The occupational therapist will also facilitate practice of daily living activities to relearn essential skills, such as dressing, meal preparation, budgeting and shopping. This may include community mobility practice such as learning to use public transport, if driving is not possible. Occupational therapists can provide aids and adaptive equipment to support independent living, for example adapted feeding utensils, toilet rails, shower and bath seats, and give advice on positioning including the provision of splints, prescription of appropriate seating, wheelchairs and pressure relieving equipment. They may provide education and emotional support for patients, families and carers to assist in the development of awareness regarding the problems that affect daily living and participation in life roles.

For those people with profound brain injury, the occupational therapist will, alongside the multidisciplinary team, evaluate levels of awareness using a detailed multisensory evaluation. Once cognitive functions are identified, they will support the person in a minimally conscious or locked in state to engage with their environment in an appropriate manner. This may include the provision of electronic assistive technology and environmental control systems. Assessment can also help to determine whether a person remains in a vegetative state, in which case interventions will focus on disability management and maintaining basic care needs through, for example the provision of appropriate positioning and pressure care aids.

The occupational therapist plays a major role in facilitating the transition of care from hospital to community and will coordinate home and environmental assessments to identify any equipment, environmental modifications and support needs for discharge.

Community Rehabilitation

The primary focus of occupational therapy in the community setting is to maximise the person's ability to function in their own environment, and participate in their life roles. There is an emphasis on adjusting to limitations, improving quality of life and family and carer support. Resumption and participation in previous life roles (family, friends, social and work) can be affected by a number of consequences of brain injury including cognitive and physical impairment as well as psychosocial issues. People may experience difficulties with self-confidence, self-esteem, emotional issues, anxiety and social reintegration. Opportunity to practise tasks and incorporate techniques into daily routines is essential for learning.

Individually tailored treatment programmes may be extended to other activities of daily living (e.g. shopping and domestic tasks) through, for example facilitated practice; development of skills in the use of computers and information technology for learning education and communication; and to maintain participation in leisure activities – either old or new. The occupational therapist may provide education and support for behavioural, emotional and sexual issues and may assist social reintegration through introduction to support, social and interest groups. They may provide advice on the person's capacity to return to driving and any adaptations to vehicles that may be required. If driving is not possible, the occupational therapist will enable access to community facilities and the use of alternative transport options. For those people who have more severe physical difficulties, the occupational therapist will have a role in evaluating their abilities and making recommendations for assistive equipment and environmental adaptations, including wheelchairs, electrical assistive technology and environmental control systems.

Work is an essential and valued role in many people's lives. It may fulfil the occupational needs of those who wish to have paid employment, voluntary roles, social integration and personal satisfaction. Occupational therapists will integrate vocational rehabilitation into the person's rehabilitation programme and occupational therapists often provide specialised vocational rehabilitation services. Vocational rehabilitation focuses on raising awareness of the impact of brain injury on work-related skills, and facilitating a realistic exploration of vocational options. The occupational therapist may carry out functional capacity evaluations, and establish a retraining programme, which reduces the impact of impairments and increases independence, awareness and insight. The retraining programme will include strategies to compensate for difficulties and will develop functional performance, insight, attention, stamina, confidence and social skills to ensure effective integration to the workplace.

Brain injury can affect all areas of daily living and prevent participation in life roles. Occupational therapy, using occupation as an assessment tool and therapeutic medium, is essential at all stages of the person's journey in their recovery and adjustment to life following a brain injury.

Rehabilitation Prescription or Plan

A MDT care plan for patients detailing the rehabilitation needs and recommendations of patients with major trauma is a key performance indicator in UK major trauma centres (MTC)[6,7] with each MTC developing a rehabilitation prescription or plan to fit their service. NHS Grampian as part of the North of Scotland major trauma network piloted such a plan on patients through their MTC pathway and found that information enhanced communication and patient care; however, use of a paper version was over cumbersome. At the time of going to press, this is being developed in electronic form (further information at https://ww.nrhcc.scot/networks/trauma).

Good outcomes of traumatic brain injury require a number of professionals working in collaboration to maximise the effectiveness of rehabilitation. Key elements of this approach should include good communication, shared information and collaborative goals across the team.

References

1. Turner-Stokes L, Pick A, Nair A, Disler PB, Wade DT. Multi-disciplinary rehabilitation for acquired brain injury in adults of working age. *Cochrane Database Syst Rev* 2015; Issue 12.

2. Scottish Intercollegiate Guidelines Network (SIGN). *Brain injury rehabilitation in adults.* Publ. 130. Edinburgh: SIGN; 2013. www.sign.ac.uk

3. Royal College of Physicians and British Society of Rehabilitation Medicine. *Rehabilitation following acquired brain injury: national clinical guidelines.* Turner-Stokes L, ed. London: RCP, BSRM; 2003.

4. Scottish Intercollegiate Guidelines Network (SIGN). *Early management of patients with head injury.* Publ. 110. Edinburgh: SIGN; 2009. www.sign.ac.uk

5. National Institute for Health and Clinical Excellence. Head injury: assessment and early management. NICE Guideline (CG176); 2014.

6. Royal College of Physicians and British Society of Rehabilitation Medicine. *Specialist rehabilitation in the trauma pathway: BSRM core standards.* Turner-Stokes L, ed. London: RCP, BSRM; 2013.

7. National Institute for Health and Clinical Excellence. Major trauma service delivery. NICE Guideline (CG176); 2016.

8. Manser, T. Teamwork and patient safety in dynamic domains of healthcare: a review of the literature. *Acta Anaesthesiol Scand* 2009;53:143–51.

9. Epstein NE. Multidisciplinary in-hospital teams improve patient outcomes: a review. *Surgical Neurology International.* 2014;5 (Suppl 7):S295–S303.

10. Clini and Ambrosini. Early physiotherapy in the respiratory intensive care unit. *Respiratory Med* 2005;99(9):1096–104.

11. Campbell M. Rehabilitation for traumatic brain injury. In: *Physical therapy practice in context.* Edinburgh: Churchill Livingstone; 2000.

12. Stucki G, Steir-Jarmer M, Grill E, Melvin J. Rationale and principles of early rehabilitation after an acute injury or illness. *Dis Rehab* 2005;27(7/8):353–9.

13. ATLS Subcommittee, American College of Surgeons Committee on Trauma, International ATLS Working Group. Advanced trauma life support (ATLS): the ninth edition. *J Trauma Acute Care Surg* 2013;74:1363–6.

14. NHS Clinical Advisory Group for Major Trauma: Department of Health; 2010.

15. Neurosurgical National Audit Programme; 2014. www.hed.nhs.uk/SBNS/

16. Trauma Audit and Research Network (TARN). www.tarn.ac.uk/

17. Bullock R, Teasdale G. Head injuries – ABC of major trauma. *BMJ* 1990;300 (6738):1515–58.

18. Horiuchi K, Jordan D, Cohen D, Kemper MC. Insights into the increased oxygen demand during chest physiotherapy. *Crit Care Med* 1997;25 (8):1347–51.

19. Berney S, Denehy L. The effect of physiotherapy treatment on oxygen consumption and haemodynamics in patients who are critically ill. *Aust J Physiol* 2003;49:99–105.

20. Hough A. *Physiotherapy in respiratory care: a problem solving approach.* 2nd edn. Churchill Livingstone; 1996.

21. Feldman Z, Kanter MJ, Robertson CS, et al. Effects of head elevation on intracranial pressure, cerebral perfusion pressure and cerebral blood flow in head injured patients. *J Neurosurg* 1992;76(2):207–11.

22. Lee ST. Intracranial pressure changes during positioning of patients with severe head injury. *Heart Lung* 1989;18 (4):411–14.

23. Gossleink R, Bott J, Johnson M, et al. Physiotherapy for adult patients with critical illness: recommendations of European Respiratory Society and European Society of Intensive Care Medicine Task Force on Physiotherapy for critically ill patients. *Intensive Care Med* 2008;34:1188–99.

24. Batt J, Dos Santos CC, Cameron JI, Herridge MS. Intensive care unit-acquired weakness: clinical phenotypes and molecular mechanisms. *Am J Respir Crit Care Med* 2013;187:238–46.

25. Puthucheary ZA, Rawal J, McPhail M, Connolly B, Ratnayake G, Chan P, et al. Acute skeletal muscle wasting in critical illness. *J Am Med Assoc* 2013;310:1591–600.

26. Endotracheal suctioning of mechanically ventilated patients with artificial airways. American Association of Respiratory Care (AARC) Clinical practice Guideline; 2010.

27. Choi JSP, Jones AYM. Effects of manual hyperinflation and suctioning on respiratory mechanics in mechanically ventilated patients with ventilator-associated pneumonia. *Aust J Physiotherapy* 2005;51:25–30.

28. Frederique P, et al. Benefits and risks of manual hyperinflation in intubated and mechanically ventilated intensive care unit patients: a systematic review. *Criti Care Aug* 2012;16:R145.

29. Pathmanathan N, Beaumont N, Gratrix A. Respiratory physiotherapy in the critical care unit Continuing Education. *Anaesthes Crit Care Pain J* 2015;15(1):20-25.

30. Zahran EM, Abd El-Razik AA. Tracheal suctioning with versus without saline instillation. *J Am Sci* 2011;7(8):23–32.

31. Thomas PJ, Paratz JD, Lipman J, Stanton WR. Lateral positioning of ventilated intensive care patients: a study of oxygenation, respiratory mechanics, hemodynamics, and adverse events. *Heart Lung* 2007 36(4):277–86.

32. Malkoç M, Karadibak D, Yildirim Y. The effect of physiotherapy on ventilatory dependency and the length of stay in an intensive care unit. *Int J Rehabil Res* 2009;32(1):85–8.

33. McCarren B, Alison J, Herbert R. Manual vibration increases expiratory flow rate via increased intrapleural pressure in healthy adults: an experimental study. *Aust J Physiother* 2006;52:267–71.

34. National Institute for Health and Care Excellence. Rehabilitation after critical illness in adults. NICE Guideline (CG83); 2009.

35. Lance JW. Symposium synopsis. In Feldman RG, Young R, Koella WP, eds. *Spasticity: disordered motor control.* Chicago, IL: Year Book Medical Publishers; 1980.

36. Pathmanathan N, Beaumont N, Gratrix A. Respiratory physiotherapy in the critical

care unit Continuing Education. *Anaesthes Crit Care Pain J* 2015;15:20-25.

37. Williams PE. Use of intermittent stretch in the prevention of serial sarcomere loss in immobilised muscles. *Ann Rheum Dis* 1990;49:316.

38. Cipriano CA, Pill SG, Keenan MA. Heterotopic ossification following traumatic brain injury and spinal cord injury. *J Am Acad Orthop Surg* 2009;17:689–97.

39. Katalinic OM, Harvey LA, Herbert RD, Moseley AM, Lannin NA, Schurr K. Stretch for the treatment and prevention of contractures. *Cochrane Database Syst Rev* 2010;9:CD007455.

40. Gracies JM. Pathophysiology of spastic paresis. II: Emergence of muscle overactivity. *Muscle Nerve* 2005;31(5):552–71.

41. College of Occupational Therapists and the Association of Chartered Physiotherapists in Neurology (ACPIN). Splinting for the prevention and correction of contractures in adults with neurological dysfunction; 2015.

42. Jo HM, Song JC, Jang SH. Improvements in spasticity and motor function using a static stretching device for people with chronic hemiparesis following stroke. *Neurorehabilitation* 2013;32:369–75.

43. Doucet BM, Mettler JA. Effects of a dynamic progressive orthotic intervention for chronic hemiplegia: a case series. *J Hand Ther* 2013;26: 139–46.

44. Barnes MP, Johnson GR (eds). *Upper motor neurone syndrome and spasticity: clinical management and neurophysiology.* Cambridge: Cambridge University Press; 2008.

45. Lapeyre E, Kuks JB, Meijler WJ. Spasticity: revisiting the role and the individual value of several pharmacological treatments. *NeuroRehabil* 2010;27:193–200.

46. Esquenazi A, Novak I, Sheean G, Singer BJ, Ward AB. International consensus statement for the use of botulinum toxin treatment in adults and children with neurological impairments – introduction. *Eur J Neurol* 2010;17:1–8.

47. Simpson DM, Gracies JM, Graham HK, Miyasaki JM, Naumann M, Russman B, et al. Assessment: botulinum neurotoxin for the treatment of spasticity (an evidence-based review): Report of the Therapeutics and Technology Assessment Subcommittee of the American Academy of Neurology. *Neurology* 2008;70:1691–8.

48. Mathiowetz V, Haugen JB. Motor behaviour research: implications for therapeutic approaches to central nervous system dysfunction. *Am J Occ Ther* 1994;48 (8):733–45.

49. Topp R, Ditmyer M, King K, Doherty K, Hornyak J III. The effect of bed rest and potential of rehabilitation on patients in the intensive care unit. *AACN Clin Issues* 2002;13:263–76.

50. Stevens RD, Dowdy DW, Michaels RK, Mendez-Tellez PA, et al. Neuromuscular dysfunction acquired in critical illness: a systematic review. *Intensive Care Med* 2007;33:1876–91.

51. Gillick BT, Marshall WJ, Rheault W, Stoecker J. Mobility criteria for upright sitting with patients in the neuro/trauma intensive care unit: an analysis of length of stay and functional outcomes. *Neurohospitalist* 2011;1:172–7.

52. Allum JHJ, Bloem BR, Carpenter MG, et al. Proprioceptive control of posture: a review of new concepts. *Gait Posture* 1998;8:214–42.

53. Richardson DLA. The use of the tilt-table to effect passive tendo-Achilles stretch in a patient with head injury: *Physio Theory Pract* 1991;7:45–50.

54. Bourdin G, Barbier J, Burle J-F, et al. The feasibility of early physical activity in intensive care unit patients: a prospective observational one-center study. *Respir Care* 2010;55(4):400–7.

55. Krewer C, Luther M, Koenig E, Muller F. Tilt table for patients with severe disorders of consciousness: a randomized controlled trial. *PLoS One* 2015;10(12):e0143180.

56. Langhammer B, Stanghelle JK. Can physiotherapy after stroke based on the bobath concept result in improved quality of movement compared to the motor

relearning programme. *Physiother Res Int* 2011;16:69–80.

57. Pope PM, Bowes CE, Booth E. Advances in seating the severely disabled neurological patients. *Physio Ireland* 1994;15(1):9–14.

58. Williams AT, Leslie GD, Bingham R, Brearley L. Optimizing seating in the Intensive care unit for patients with impaired mobility. *Am J Crit Care* 2011;20 (1):19–27.

59. Rousseau K, Harrison A, Rochette A, Routhier F, et al. Impact of wheelchair acquisition on social participation. *Disability Rehab Assist Technol* 2009;4 (5):344–52.

60. Herman JH, Lange ML. Seating and positioning to manage spasticity after brain injury. *Neuro-rehabilitation* 1999;12:105–17.

61. Halper AS, Cherney LR, Cichowski K, Zhang M. Dysphagia after head trauma: the effect of cognitive-communicative impairments on functional outcomes. *J Head Trauma Rehabil* 1999;14(5):486–96.

62. Mackay LE, Morgan AS, Bernstein BA. Swallowing disorders in severe brain injury: risk factors affecting return to oral intake. *Arch Phys Medi Rehabil* 1999;80:365–71.

63. Logemann JA, Pepe J, Mackay LE. Disorders of nutrition and swallowing: intervention strategies in the trauma center. *J Head Trauma Rehabil* 1994;9(1):43–56.

64. Mayer V. The challenges of managing dysphagia in brain-injured patients. *Br J Commun Nurs* 2004;9(2):67–73.

65. Logemann J. *Evaluation and treatment of swallowing disorders.* Austin, TX: Pro-Ed; 1998.

66. Mackay LE, Morgan AS, Bernstein BA. Factors affecting oral feeding with severe traumatic brain injury. *J Head Trauma Rehabil* 1999;14(5):435–47.

67. Ward EC, Green K, Morton A-L. Patterns and predictors of swallowing resolution following adult traumatic brain injury. *J Head Trauma Rehabil* 2007;22(3):184–91.

68. Kelly AM, Hydes K, McLaughlin C, Wallace S. Fibreoptic endoscopic evaluation of swallowing (FEES): the role of speech and language therapy. Royal College of Speech and Language Therapists Policy Statement; 2007.

69. Schurr MJ, Ebner KA, Maser AL, Sperling KB, Helgerson RB, Harms B. Formal swallowing evaluation and therapy after traumatic brain injury improves dysphagia outcomes. *J Trauma* 1999;46 (5):817–23.

70. Hamdy S, Jilani S, Price V, Parker C, Hall N, Power M. Modulation of human swallowing behaviour by thermal and chemical stimulation in health and after brain injury. *Neurogastroenterol Motili* 2003;15:69–77.

71. McDonald S. Pragmatic language skills after closed head injury: ability to meet the informational needs of the listener. *Brain Lang* 1993;44:28–46.

72. King KA, Hough MS, Walker MM, Rastatter M, Holbert D. Mild traumatic brain injury: effects on naming in word retrieval and discourse. *Brain Inj* 2006;20:725–32.

73. Hough MS, Barrow I. Descriptive discourse abilities of traumatic brain-injured adults. *Aphasiology* 2003;17:183–91.

74. Dahlberg C, Hawley L, Morey C, Newman J, Cusick CP, Harrison-Felix C. Social communication skills in persons with post-acute traumatic brain injury: three perspectives. *Brain Injury* 2006;20:425–35.

75. Snow P, Ponsford J. Assessing and managing changes in communication and interpersonal skills following TBI. In: Ponsford J, Sloan S, Snow P, eds. *Traumatic brain injury: rehabilitation for everyday adaptive living.* Sussex, UK: Psychology Press; 1995.

76. Togher L, McDonald S, Code C. Communication problems following traumatic brain injury. In: McDonald S, Togher L, Code C, eds. *Communication disorders following traumatic brain injury.* Sussex, UK: Psychology Press; 1999.

77. Borgaro SR, Prigatano GP, Kwasnica C, Alcott S, Cutter N. Disturbances in affective communication following brain injury. *Brain Injury* 2004;18:33–9.

78. Body R, Perkins M, McDonald S. Pragmatics, cognition, and communication in traumatic brain injury. In: McDonald S, Togher L, Code C, eds. *Communication disorders following traumatic brain injury*. Sussex, UK: Psychology Press; 1999.

79. Martin I, McDonald S. Weak coherence, no theory of mind, or executive dysfunction? Solving the puzzle of pragmatic language disorders. *Brain Lang* 2003;85: 451–66.

80. Myers PS. Profiles of communication deficits in patients with right cerebral hemisphere damage: implications for diagnosis and treatment. *Aphasiology* 2005;19(12):1147–60.

81. Snow P, Douglas J, Ponsford J. Conversational discourse abilities following severe traumatic brain injury: a follow-up study. *Brain Injury* 1998;12:911–35.

82. Murdoch BE, Theodoros DG. Dysarthria following traumatic brain injury. In: McDonald S, Togher L, Code C, eds. *Communication disorders following traumatic brain injury*. Sussex, UK: Psychology Press; 1999.

83. Braverman SE, Spector J, Warden DL, et al. A multidisciplinary TBI inpatient rehabilitation programme for active duty service members as part of a randomized clinical trial. *Brain Injury* 1999;13:405–15.

84. Cicerone KD, Mott T, Azulay J, Friel JC. Community integration and satisfaction with functioning after intensive cognitive rehabilitation for traumatic brain injury. *Arch Phys Med Rehabil* 2004;85: 943–50.

85. Brooks N, McKinlay W, Symington C, Beattie A, Campsie L. Return to work within the first seven years of severe head injury. *Brain Injury* 1987;1:5–19.

86. Brooks N, Campsie L, Symington C, Beattie A, McKinlay W. The effects of severe head injury on patient and relative within seven years of injury. *J Head Trauma Rehabil* 1987;2:1–13.

87. Hammond FM, Hart T, Bushnik T, Corrigan J, Sasser H. Change and predictors of change in communication, cognition and social function between 1 and 5 years after traumatic brain injury. *J Head Trauma Rehabil* 2004;19:314–28.

88. Royal College of Occupational Therapists. Definitions of occupational therapy – essential briefing; 2015. www.rcot.co.uk/practice-resources

89. Kielhofner, G. *Conceptual foundations of occupational therapy*. 2nd edn. Philadelphia: F. A. Davis; 1997.

90. Malley D, Rowland D, Royal College of Occupational Therapists, Specialist Section Neurological Practice. Acquired brain injury: a guide for occupational therapists; 2013.

91. Wheeler S, Acord-Vira A. *Occupational therapy practice guidelines for adults with traumatic brain injury*. Bethesda, MD: American Occupational Therapy Association; 2016.

92. Gill-Thwaites H, Munday R. The sensory modality assessment and rehabilitation technique (SMART): a valid and reliable assessment for vegetative state and minimally conscious state patients. *Brain Injury* 2004;18(12):1255–69.

Chapter

26 Neuropsychological Rehabilitation

Jonathan J. Evans, Ceri Trevethan, Jackie Hamilton, Bruce Downey, Lindsey Beedie and Emma Hepburn

Introduction

Neuropsychological deficits following brain injury include cognitive impairment, difficulties with emotion, changes in self-identity, impairment in insight, behavioural challenges and personality change. The following chapter reviews rehabilitation for neuropsychological problems and includes specific reference to mild traumatic brain injury and traumatic brain injury in children.

Neuropsychological Rehabilitation for Cognitive Impairments

Cognitive impairments in memory, attention, executive functioning, language or perception cause many of the day-to-day problems after head injury. Rehabilitation interventions for cognitive impairments will usually be just one component of a broader programme aimed at enabling the head-injured person to achieve agreed functional goals. Nevertheless, there is an emerging evidence base relating to how best to manage specific cognitive impairments. Following a brief discussion of the importance of assessment, this section will describe the approaches that are recommended in relation to each of the major cognitive domains.

Cognitive Assessment and Rehabilitation Planning

The aim of assessment is to determine the nature of any impairment in cognitive, emotional, behavioural or physical functioning and identify the functional consequences in terms of the patient's ability to participate in activities of daily living, work, education, social and leisure activities. Several members of the rehabilitation team contribute to the assessment of cognitive functioning, including clinical psychologists, speech and language therapists and occupational therapists. All of the team members should contribute to the identification of problems with functional everyday activities, but occupational therapists have a particularly important role to play through direct observation/assessment of patients carrying out activities of daily living and, if appropriate, vocational tasks.

The patient's awareness of his or her impairment and the consequences for everyday life should also be examined. The factors that may contribute to impaired insight/ awareness after brain injury are many and varied. Clare presents a biopsychosocial model of awareness in Alzheimer's disease, though the principles apply to most neurological conditions.[1,2] Another useful model is the hierarchical model of Crosson et al. which suggests that awareness may be intellectual, emergent or anticipatory.[3] Intellectual awareness refers to knowing that you have an impairment, but not necessarily recognising the occurrence of problems as they occur. Emergent awareness refers to 'online' awareness of problems as they occur, whilst anticipatory awareness refers to using knowledge of deficits to anticipate problems and taking steps to prevent problems occurring. There are a variety of tools that can be used to examine insight, including the Insight Interview.[4]

Assessment of mood, emotion and behaviour is critical to rehabilitation planning for several reasons. Firstly, mood disorders are common after brain injury and so represent an important therapeutic target in their own right. Secondly, mood disorders may have an impact on cognition and so assessment of mood is important for the interpretation of performance on cognitive tests. Finally, mood disorder rather than cognitive impairment may be the major limiting factor in terms of the patient's ability to participate in activities of daily living and it is therefore important to establish this, so that therapeutic efforts can be appropriately directed.

The task then is to formulate or map the relationship between the pathology, the impairments and their functional consequences. One way of doing this is for team members, in a summary of assessment meeting, to use a standard template where all elements of the assessment are listed, and a preliminary formulation of the causal relationships between impairment and functional elements can begin to be drawn out (see a summary of assessment template, Figure 24.2).

Perhaps the most critical aspect of planning for rehabilitation is setting the rehabilitation goals. In most circumstances it is best if goals are written in terms of functional outcomes, but under each of the goals for which it is relevant, there should be documentation of plans of action relating to the management of cognitive impairments that are obstacles to the achievement of the long-term goal. Evans and Krasny-Pacini[5] describe the process of goal setting in detail.

Approaches to Rehabilitation for Cognitive Impairments

Rehabilitation for cognitive impairments can be approached in several ways. The World Health Organization International Classification of Functions (ICF) considers health in terms of body structures, body functions, activities and participation. We use this framework as the context for the diagrammatic formulation approach presented in Figure 24.2. This is also relevant to thinking about rehabilitation interventions. So, we could aim to target rehabilitation efforts at body structures with pharmacological therapies, or interventions aimed at brain repair such as stem cell implantation, but these remain primarily in the realms of research rather than routine clinical treatments. We could target specific cognitive functions with the aim of restoring normal functioning, or teaching strategies that may compensate for deficits across a wide range of situations. Alternatively we may need to address specific everyday tasks and activities, introducing task-specific strategies (including external aids) for managing cognitive impairments in each specific task or activity in turn. Let us imagine that we have a patient who has memory problems that cause difficulties in his daily life including work activities. If we can improve his memory functioning in a general way, then improvement in all aspects of his functioning which have been affected by impaired memory should follow. However, if we cannot improve memory per se, we may need to look at the specific tasks (one by one if necessary) that are affected and enable the patient to compensate for impaired memory in relation to each task. The former approach, if effective, would be more efficient, but if we cannot improve memory in a very general way, then the latter approach will be more likely to bring about real improvements in everyday functioning, albeit potentially limited to those specific situations that are targeted in the rehabilitation context.

To determine which approach to rehabilitation is most appropriate, it is important to refer to the evidence base in relation to the treatment of specific cognitive impairments. This evidence base remains limited, but is large enough that several systematic reviews have been conducted and clinical guideline documents produced.[6–12] In the sections below, the evidence as it relates to the cognitive domains of memory, attention, executive functioning, language and perception will be considered. However, before turning to the specific cognitive domains it is important to return to the issue of insight and awareness.

As noted, awareness is a critical issue in rehabilitation, much of which is dependent upon the patient independently implementing strategies to compensate for deficits in everyday life. If a patient lacks insight, then careful attention should be paid to the factors that are likely to be responsible. For some, insight difficulties arise from poor attention that prevents self-monitoring and hence the patient fails to notice problems as they occur (something that is particularly relevant in relation to poor social communication). Similarly, impaired memory may mean that the patient cannot remember the nature or frequency of errors. Deficits in executive functioning may mean that the patient cannot anticipate the consequences of actions. For some there may be a lack of demand on cognitive skills – think how little responsibility patients in an inpatient rehabilitation ward have for independent organising, planning, remembering and initiation of activities. The patient who has not yet returned to work may find it hard to appreciate the cognitive demands that are made in the course of everyday work until actually placed in that situation (or a closely analogous one). For others, denial of disability may represent a means of coping with the overwhelming consequences of injury. The intervention will vary depending on the cause of the insight problem. However, for most patients with insight difficulties, some combination of education about brain injury, supported exposure to functional difficulties and psychological support emphasising positive coping will be appropriate.[13] Work aimed at improving insight must be clearly set in the context of positive, functional goals, though it is often the case that the patient's ultimate goal may not be achievable. For some patients it may not be possible to improve insight and it will be necessary to focus on modifications to the environment that have the effect of reducing cognitive demands on the patient.

Let us turn then to the specific cognitive domains and discuss, with reference to the evidence base, the approaches that are recommended.

Memory

There is very little evidence that memory can be improved through simple mental exercise or practice at remembering (e.g. practising remembering lists or objects, playing computer games) – people can get better at memory exercises, but this may not translate into improvements in everyday functioning. There is much stronger evidence to support the use of strategies/aids that act as cognitive prostheses, compensating for memory impairment. Cicerone et al.[7] and Velikonja[10] concluded that, for those with mild impairment, training in the use of 'internal' memory strategies as well as the use of external memory aids such as notebooks or diaries should be standard practice. Internal strategies include the use of visual imagery and other mental association strategies aimed at improving the encoding of information.[14] For those with more severe impairment, external memory aids including the use of electronic reminding devices are recommended. The most extensively evaluated electronic reminding system is NeuroPage,[15] but a number of different forms of reminding technology have been shown to improve remembering of everyday activities.[16] In memory rehabilitation, one size does not fit all. It is important to work with the patient/family to construct a system of memory aids/strategies designed to meet the range of specific everyday remembering demands the patient has placed upon them (or wants to take on).

Attention

Despite some early promising evidence that training specific attentional functions using computerised cognitive training programmes might be beneficial, there is very little evidence that such training programmes generalise to performance on functional activities.[17] Recent review and guideline documents note that use of de-contextualised computer training is not recommended because of the lack for generalisation to everyday functions.[17] However a number of other specific recommendations have been made,[17] including: use of meta-cognitive strategies (discussed further in the next section on executive functions) which involve the learning of mental strategies or routines to help stay on track in tasks; training dual-tasking by practice on combining functional tasks to promote task automation; treat mood and sleep disorders that may interfere with concentration using cognitive behaviour therapy; modify or manage the environment to reduce attentional demands. Ponsford and colleagues[17] also concluded that methylphenidate could improve speed of processing in people after TBI (as measured on standardised tests), though noted that the impact on everyday functioning is not yet established. By working directly on functional activities, patients may develop strategies to compensate for attentional difficulties or, in some cases, become skilled at a particular task such that the task requires less conscious attention and is less subject to errors caused by poor attention. Often strategies learned in relation to one functional situation can be applied in other situations. For example, using a 'speak aloud' strategy to manage attention when performing a task sequence could be applied to several situations.[18]

Executive Functioning

The term 'executive functions' relates to the cognitive skills required to plan, problem solve and achieve intended goals effectively. Several studies suggest that problem-solving training can be useful, at least for some patients.[19] It is likely that this would only be beneficial for those who are more mildly impaired, though the question of who can benefit has not been systematically examined. The training involves patients being taught to follow a sequence of stages involved in problem solving (recognising problem, defining goal, identifying possible solutions, choosing solution, making plan, implementing plan, monitoring progress). Goal Management Training (GMT) uses a self-instructional approach and is based on teaching the patient the concept of using a 'mental blackboard' to write intended goals/tasks on, and then to develop a mental checking routine to more effectively maintain attention to tasks and intended goals. This is a good example of a meta-cognitive strategy that now has sufficient evidence for its efficacy to be recommended in several guideline documents.[20] The use of external alerting (via SMS text messaging) in combination with GMT has been shown to be beneficial.[21,22] The NeuroPage system referred to above has also been shown to be useful at prompting action in a patient with an initiation deficit.[23] Careful consideration of the nature of the deficit that is contributing to poor problem solving or task management can be helpful in selecting the appropriate intervention approach.

Visuo-spatial Functions

Very few disorders of visual or spatial perception have been subject to rehabilitation studies with the exception of unilateral neglect, which is much less common after head injury than after stroke. Neglect does, however, provide a good example of how theories of attention, perception and action are coming together to influence the development of rehabilitation interventions. Visual scanning training is now recommended as a practice standard.[7] Recent studies have also suggested that limb-activation training should also be considered. This involves training the patient to make at least minimal movements of the left limb in left hemispace, an intervention that is hypothesised to reduce neglect as a result of activating right hemisphere representations of left personal and peri-personal space and reducing the inhibitory activation of the intact left hemisphere.[7]

Language and Communication

Rehabilitation for language deficits has the longest tradition and the most extensive database upon which to draw conclusions regarding the effectiveness of rehabilitation, though there has been considerable variation in the conclusions that have been drawn by those who have reviewed the evidence. As with unilateral neglect, much of the aphasia therapy research relates to people after stroke; however, most recent reviews conclude that aphasia therapy can be effective.[7,24] Aphasia therapy refers to interventions for specific language deficits identified from careful assessment of precise areas of impairment sometimes based on cognitive-neuropsychological models of language. One of the criticisms of such approaches has been that they do not necessarily bring about changes in people's ability to participate in everyday activities requiring language (e.g. social conversation). It has been argued therefore, that rehabilitation should focus on the broader concept of functional, or social, communication (i.e. the activities and participation level of the ICF framework). This is particularly relevant for people who have suffered a head injury, as after head injury a range of impairments other than specific language deficits may impact on communication. Difficulties such as impulsivity, impaired perception of emotion in others, poor attention and monitoring leading to poor turn-taking or tangential speech can all impact on communication even when basic language skills are intact and therefore need to be addressed as part of the rehabilitation programme.[25]

Conclusions

We live in exciting times when it comes to neuropsychological rehabilitation. The evidence base concerning the effectiveness of treatment approaches is beginning to be substantial enough to provide recommendations on what standard clinical practice should be for each of the major domains of cognitive impairment. Treatments based on sound theoretical models of normal cognition are emerging. But equally important, awareness is growing that any treatment for a specific cognitive impairment must also have a clear relationship with improvements in the ability to participate in activities of everyday life.

Rehabilitation of Emotional Disorders

Emotional changes are common after TBI. Some of these changes will be a normal reaction and adjustment to the injury and its consequences and it is important for professionals to understand and allow for the natural progress of grief and adjustment. However a large proportion of individuals post–brain injury develop a diagnosable mood disorder. Within the UK population prevalence surveys indicate a 5.9% prevalence rate for Generalised Anxiety Disorder (GAD) and 3.3% for depression[26]; however, studies on the TBI population indicated significantly higher rates. In a systematic review by Zaninotto et al.[27] estimates for rates of depression were reported as high as 77%, whilst Kreutzer et al.,[28] Jorge et al.[29] and Seel et al.[30] found rates of 42%, 33% and 27% respectively in TBI patients. Neuropsychological testing also demonstrated that depressed patients had a greater degree of cognitive impairment. Whelan-Goodinson et al.[31] found rates of 65% for depression and 38% for anxiety up to 5.5 years post-injury. Osborn et al.[32] found 11% of people were diagnosed with GAD and 37% reported clinically significant levels of anxiety following TBI and were most prevalent 2 to 5 years post-injury.

Studies have shown that individuals with a history of TBI are 1.55 to 4.05 times more likely to die by suicide than the general population.[33] They have also been found to have a higher level of suicidal ideation of 25%[33] compared to general population estimates of 2.1%–10%.[34] There is a heightened risk of post-traumatic stress disorder (PTSD) although symptoms overlap including impaired concentration, sleep, temper and fatigue. Calson et al. found, in their systematic review, an incidence rate of between 14% and 56% for non-military trauma related TBI.[35]

The development of mood disorder post-TBI is likely due to a combination of factors including the cognitive and physical effects of injury leading to consequences such as changes in employment, relationships, activities and social support. Pre-morbid risk factors such as pre-existing mood disorders, life stressors and maladaptive coping behaviours can also contribute. In addition neuroanatomical changes as a result of the injury are also likely to impact, though involvement is not fully understood. It is thought that disruption to the structures or circuits involving the prefrontal cortex, amygdala, hippocampus, basal ganglia and thalamus may have an impact as well as disruption to the neurotransmitter system.[36]

The identification and treatment of mood disorders are an integral part of brain injury rehabilitation and can impact on the individual's ability to engage in other areas of their rehabilitation. Assessment of mood disorders should occur at every stage of the rehabilitation journey, including the earlier stages where factors such as PTSD may have an increased impact on an individuals' ability to engage in their rehabilitation. A multi-faceted approach to assessment should be used. Relying solely on one measure is likely to be unhelpful due to the overlap of cognitive symptoms post-injury and the symptoms of anxiety/depression which could lead to an overestimation of mental disorder.[37] Rather, a formulation approach should be used considering pre-morbid factors, areas of damage, cognitive profile, the individuals account of their experience and if possible information from significant others and observations from other professionals involved in the individuals care. Normal adjustment processes should be considered to avoid over pathologising normal and understandable emotional reactions to the injury and its consequences. Education and support should be provided to the individual and others involved in their care alongside monitoring to ensure a mood disorder does not develop over time.

Treatment of mood disorders in brain injury is complex, and it is unlikely that one treatment in isolation will be effective.[37] Interventions have typically involved cognitive behavioural therapy (CBT), systemic and behavioural approaches. Often a combination of therapeutic approaches are required, alongside pharmacological interventions. The psychological intervention may require a comprehensive overall rehabilitation programme alongside individual therapy in order to be effective.

Cognitive consequences of brain injury such as reduced processing speed, memory, executive functioning and attention deficits may mean that the delivery of therapy requires adjustment. This may take the form of shorter sessions, written information, increased structure to the session and involvement of others as a memory aid for the session content or to provide support with home tasks. Often it is the principles of CBT that are applied in treatment rather than a full manualised approach. Due to the use of a non-standard approach and the challenges of identifying a homogeneous sample in TBI, studies examining the efficacy of therapeutic approaches can be challenging.

Evidence for effective use of CBT in anxiety is positive with some randomised controlled trials (RCTs) showing good results.[38] In a systematic review of psychological interventions for treating neuropsychiatric consequences of acquired brain injury, Verberne et al. cited four high-quality studies which showed decreased anxiety in people with acquired brain injury after CBT.[39] There is also evidence for the use of CBT in treating depression with people with TBI.[40] Ponsford reports a RCT to evaluate a programme of adapted CBT which found reduced symptoms of anxiety and depression and gains in psychosocial functioning present at 18 weeks post-intervention.[41]

Over recent years Acceptance and Commitment Therapy (ACT) has become more widely used for the treatment of psychological difficulties, particularly those associated with chronic health conditions. ACT does not aim to change the content of difficult experiences, as often health status itself cannot be changed, rather therapy focuses on being able to manage difficult thoughts and experiences whilst continuing to engage in behaviours consistent with the individual's value system. For people with brain injury, this approach may facilitate adaption to the changes that have arisen as a result of the brain injury enabling continuing engagement in the aspects of life that they most value. Reviews have highlighted the likely appropriateness of ACT for use within a brain injury population.[42,43] Other approaches have shown some utility in psychological intervention for people with TBI including mindfulness[44] and compassion focused therapy.[45]

Self-Identity and Brain Injury

Self-identity can be described as a cluster of attitudes and beliefs we have about ourselves at any given moment.[46] Self-identity is therefore the view or construction we have of ourselves. Sense of self is based on both our past and present, as well as our anticipated future and is a multifaceted and fluid construct that can change over time. Self-identity is also closely associated with our social identity. Factors contributing to the construction and models of self-identity are described by Ownsworth, proposing that self-identity is social in nature, as individuals derive their self-identity from group membership.[47]

Brain injury presents a challenge to self-identity as it is frequently associated with loss or change in social, emotional, cognitive and physical functioning as well as loss or change of roles, social relationships and, sometimes, physical appearance. These changes are thought to pose a threat as they can alter or challenge our identity. Ben-Yishay describes a catastrophic reaction that is a response to the threat of post-injury discrepancies between pre-injury self representation and post-injury reality.[48] The reconstruction of identity into an organised, compelling and reasonably realistic identity is proposed to be central to the process of rehabilitation.[49]

Self-identity is therefore an important factor to consider in working with people with brain injury and should be central to holistic neuropsychological rehabilitation programmes. For example, the Oliver Zangwill centre's Y shaped model of rehabilitation is based on the self-identity discrepancies that occur after a brain injury.[50] Whilst traditionally outcomes after brain injury have been measured in psychological wellbeing, cognitive or functional outcomes, changes in self-identity have been suggested to be an important factor in adaptation and adjustment to brain injury and therefore should be considered by the multi-disciplinary team providing rehabilitation for people with traumatic brain injury.

Group Rehabilitation

The use of groups has been a well-established feature of brain injury rehabilitation since the 1940s and 1950s. Groups are often used within holistic rehabilitation, alongside individualised elements of the programme. For example the Oliver Zangwill centre use group learning as part of their intensive outpatient programme, including intervention for cognition, mood management and communication.[50]

One of the core components of holistic neuropsychological rehabilitation is the establishment of a therapeutic milieu, a supportive and therapeutic social context. Ben-Yishay argues that this social context helps clients develop their sense of identity that they can apply to other social contexts.[48]

There are several ways that group approaches may impact beneficially on an individual. As self-identity is linked to group membership it is proposed that group approaches have a role to play in reconstructing identity after brain injury.[47] Research suggests that group intervention following brain injury is twice as likely to lead to positive self concept than individually delivered rehabilitation.[51] Brain injury can be associated with stigma and shame, and meeting others who do not fit with our perception of brain injury may help widen perceptions of what a brain injury means and normalise experiences, thereby destigmatising brain injury and reducing associated shame. Von Mesenkampf et al. report a number of benefits to the participants in their group therapeutic intervention for TBI including normalising effects, helping with acceptance, finding a new identity and positive mental health changes.[52] In their review, Patterson et al. conclude that patients perceive group interventions to be beneficial for sharing experiences and reducing isolation, receiving help and feedback and, assisting with adjustment and adaptation to life after TBI.[53]

Group approaches may also have beneficial effects on other aspects of rehabilitation. Group membership is thought to allow experiential social learning in a safe environment, that can then be transferred to other areas of a person's life. Increasing social connectivity has been identified as a primary goal of ABI survivors.[54] Group approaches can provide social opportunities and group membership that extend beyond the confines of the rehabilitation setting, allowing opportunities to establish friendship and meaningful daily activities that can impact positively on quality of life beyond time limited health care provision.

Behavioural Management Following Traumatic Brain Injury

If you, a loved one, be it a family member or friend, was ill or had some type of disability: How would they want to be supported and spoken to when ill, distressed and frightened?[55]

Neurobehavioural and personality changes after traumatic brain injury (TBI) are the product of complex interactions which involve neurological disabilities, social demands, previously established behaviour patterns and personal reactions to a combination of these factors.[56] Compared to impairments of specific abilities, for example reading or memory, disturbances of emotion or behaviour, often accompanied by executive dysfunction, are more likely to result in extensive changes in a person's life.[56] The complexity of this area is highlighted by the need to consider neurological, psychological and social aspects of the impact of TBI including interpersonal relationships, social participation and vocational activity[57] which undermine the capacity for independent living, affect family dynamics and roles and limit rehabilitation and community reintegration.[58,59]

Behavioural disturbance following TBI can present as inappropriate vocalisation (e.g. frequent screaming, shouting), intolerance to medical management or equipment, directed or diffuse aggressive, disinhibited or sexualised behaviour.[60] Agitated TBI patients may pose a risk to themselves, their family, staff members,[60] and occasionally to other patients. Behavioural change following TBI can also present as apathy or lack of initiation, resulting in withdrawal from activities, which are less visible, but equally important to recognise as forms of challenging behaviour.[56]

Reported prevalence of neurobehavioural change (NBC) varies from 10% to 96% of patients, with estimates varying according to the exact definition used and the setting studied.[59] NBC is a major burden on families and carers with immediate and long-term impact.[58,60] NBC can also be a significant source of stress for staff teams.

Behaviour Management

Whenever NBC is identified, the first essential step is always to assess for and rule out medically treatable sources of agitation or distress, for example pain/discomfort, alcohol/substance withdrawal, mood disorder, urinary retention, constipation.[60,62]

The next question is whether behaviour is challenging to the point that assessment and intervention is required?[63] A framework can be applied to structure how information is collected, to manage clinical decision-making and evaluate therapeutic interventions at any stage in the brain injury pathway[63] (see Figure 26.1).

Specialist neuropsychological assessment, advice regarding behavioural management and cognitive rehabilitation, is recommended.[61] The Clinical Neuropsychologist may be involved in co-ordinating a behavioural management plan, to be consistently delivered by all those interacting with the patient.[61] They also have a pivotal role in ensuring systematic information-sharing and provision of psychoeducation about TBI generally and in relation to each unique case. De-escalation techniques are recommended,[64] but there is no universally accepted model and the core skill set is not clearly defined.[65] A format for a de-escalation plan and an example of use is illustrated in Figure 26.2.

For serious aggressive behaviour, pharmacological intervention may be considered, but must be individually tailored, commenced at low doses with surveillance for adverse effects.[60] Drugs with sedative effects should be avoided where possible although can occasionally be considered with psychiatric advice.[61] Specialist behavioural assessment and management should be provided alongside pharmacological intervention.[62,63]

The primary goal of behavioural assessment is to identify factors which drive and maintain the specific behaviour of concern and to understand the function of the behaviour. Assessment involves collecting a variety of information from multiple sources (see Figure 26.1). Neuropsychological assessment provides a profile of strengths and weaknesses specific to the individual. In relation to executive dysfunction, formal assessment may not highlight the true functional impact of TBI, so observation and interviews with the person, their network and staff

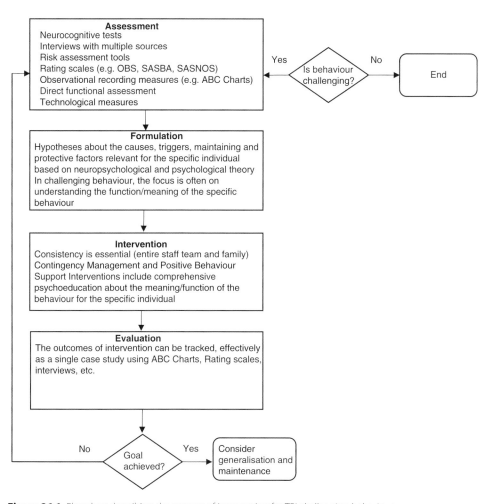

Figure 26.1 Flowchart describing the process of intervention for TBI challenging behaviour.

team are also vital.[66] Rating scales such as the Overt Behaviour Scale (OBS)[67] (available for free download from http://tbims.org/), St Andrews Swansea Neurobehavioural Scale (SASNOS)[68] and St Andrews Sexual Behaviour Assessment (SASBA)[69] make valuable contributions.[66] Risk assessment should also be considered. Observational recording measures, such as training staff and family to complete Antecedent Behaviour Consequence (ABC) Charts (Figure 26.3) whenever an episode of the specified behaviour occurs, or a detailed process of Functional Analysis are also required.[66] Increasingly, technology, such as biofeedback, is also being employed to track and modify NBC[70] as discussed in Chapter 27 of this book.

TBI results in a range of cognitive, emotional, behavioural, physical and functional impairments which interact to produce complex and unique profiles and therefore people with TBI can present with similar types of NBC, yet the underlying causes can vary widely. A formulation-based approach provides a clear understanding of the function(s) of the behaviour and how it is being maintained. This process involves generating hypotheses

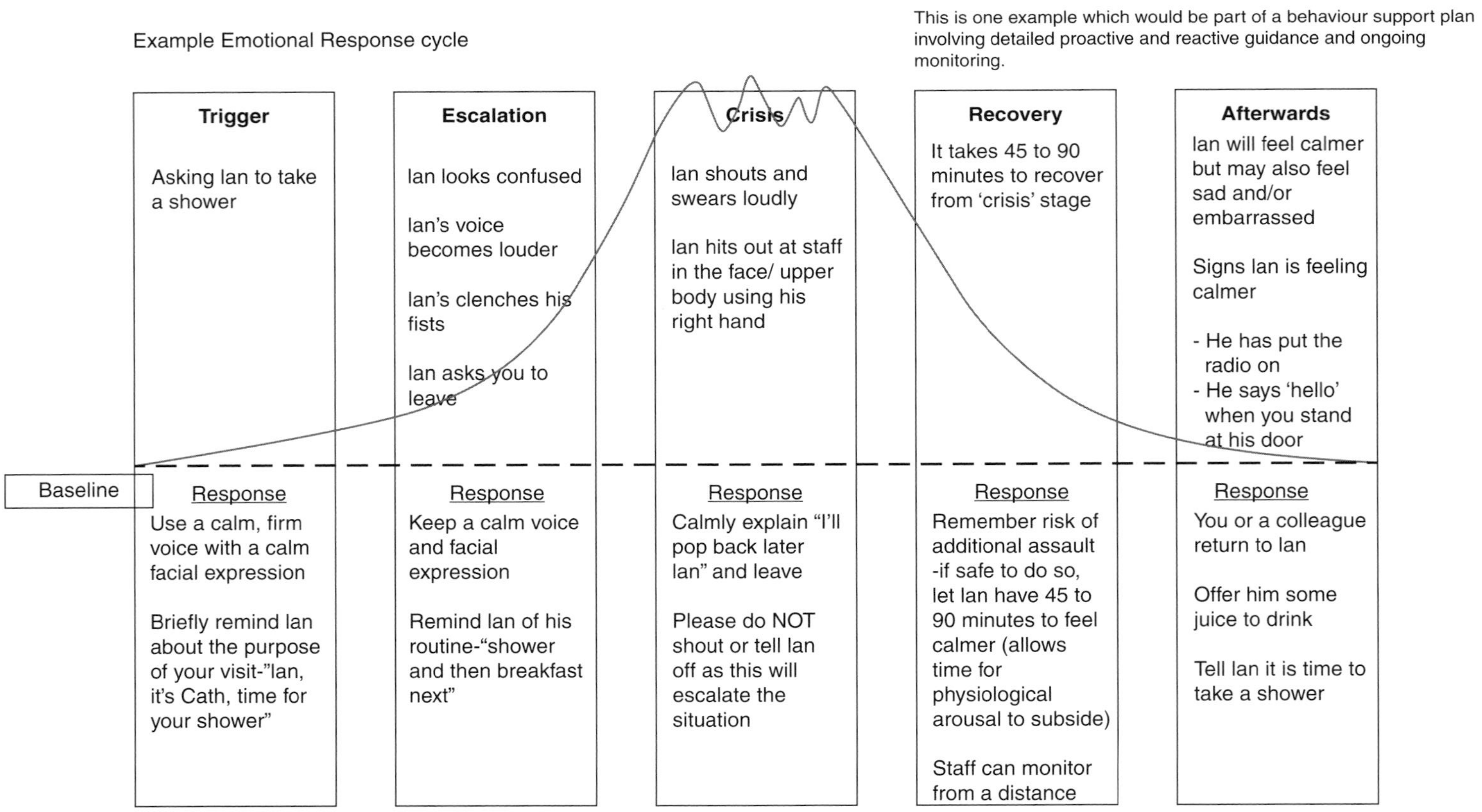

Example Emotional Response cycle

This is one example which would be part of a behaviour support plan involving detailed proactive and reactive guidance and ongoing monitoring.

Trigger	Escalation	Crisis	Recovery	Afterwards
Asking Ian to take a shower	Ian looks confused Ian's voice becomes louder Ian's clenches his fists Ian asks you to leave	Ian shouts and swears loudly Ian hits out at staff in the face/ upper body using his right hand	It takes 45 to 90 minutes to recover from 'crisis' stage	Ian will feel calmer but may also feel sad and/or embarrassed Signs Ian is feeling calmer - He has put the radio on - He says 'hello' when you stand at his door
Response Use a calm, firm voice with a calm facial expression Briefly remind Ian about the purpose of your visit-"Ian, it's Cath, time for your shower"	**Response** Keep a calm voice and facial expression Remind Ian of his routine-"shower and then breakfast next"	**Response** Calmly explain "I'll pop back later Ian" and leave Please do NOT shout or tell Ian off as this will escalate the situation	**Response** Remember risk of additional assault -if safe to do so, let Ian have 45 to 90 minutes to feel calmer (allows time for physiological arousal to subside) Staff can monitor from a distance	**Response** You or a colleague return to Ian Offer him some juice to drink Tell Ian it is time to take a shower

Baseline

Figure 26.2 Example emotional response cycle.

NAME: (D.O.B:)   BEHAVIOUR RECORDING SHEET

Date/Time of incident	Setting and Triggers. Where was the patient, what was she/he doing? Who else was present? What were they doing/saying?	Target Behaviour:	Consequence. How did others react? Hoe did the patient respond?
Example: 13/03/18 9 am	John was sitting in the lounge waiting for his breakfast. Three other residents were also in the lounge, but not seated near him. Staff member approached John, facing him, and placed toast and tea on the table in front of him.	John reached with left hand towards the staff member and nipped on the right arm as she was placing these items on the table.	Staff member said "ouch," removed John's hand, and moved out of his reach. John was still reaching out towards the staff, and was laughing. Staff member then went to attend to another resident in the lounge.

Figure 26.3 Antecedent Behaviour Consequence (ABC) chart.

about the causes, triggers and maintaining factors of the person's psychological, interpersonal and behavioural problems. The formulation is then used to inform and drive intervention(s).[66]

Recent reviews indicate that behavioural approaches such as positive behaviour supports (PBS) and contingency management are effective across a range of settings.[68] Individualised PBS techniques can include maximising choice in planning activities, using a timetable, daily feedback to emphasise strengths and achievements, education about TBI and anxiety management training. Contingency management includes interventions such as not responding to aggression, if safe to do so, and providing social interaction and reinforcement when the person shows desired, non-aggressive behaviours in order to reinforce these.[66] Such interventions are most effective when delivered in a neurobehavioural setting with a therapeutic milieu; a social climate and culture which increases awareness, improves motivation, encourages success, minimises cognitive impairment and routinely reinforces appropriate behaviour and skills consistently by the entire multidisciplinary team.[66] Neurobehavioural rehabilitation delivered in this way can save care costs in the long term.[71]

Evaluation, such as comparing data before and after intervention, is important so the success of the intervention can be measured and adjustments made to improve effectiveness of the approach.

Behavioural Challenges of Post-traumatic Amnesia

Post-traumatic amnesia (PTA) describes a post-injury period of confusion and memory loss – after regaining consciousness, during which the patient is disorientated and unable to learn new day-to-day information.[72] Key features can include disorientation, loss of memory, poor attention, distractibility and slowed reaction time. Patients in PTA may also sleep for long periods, be emotionally labile, restless, anxious, have difficulty following instructions, be agitated or aggressive. They may be independently mobile and able to speak and respond appropriately to some questions, therefore it would be easy to conclude that their level of consciousness is not impaired. However, if observed closely, although their level of arousal may be within normal limits, their awareness is not. There may be brief periods or 'islands' when the patient appears orientated and to be retaining information, which may be a sign of emerging from PTA; however, fluctuations can occur over a long time period. During this time, if aggressive or other challenging behaviour is observed, it can often be interpreted as purposeful when it is a result of impaired awareness, confusion, fear or disorientation.[72]

Prospective assessment of PTA involves regular assessment of functions relating to PTA status and can involve careful questioning and interview and/or standardised tests which focus on orientation and memory. This can be complex particularly as the patient has a very short attention span.[72] The Galveston Orientation and Amnesia Test (GOAT)[73] and Westmead Scale[74] (available for free download from http://psy.mq.edu.au/pta) are suitable and involve brief, daily, repeated assessment of orientation and memory/new learning. PTA is also often assessed retrospectively, by interview, as prospective assessment is not always possible. Patients are asked to recall when they remember waking up. It is important to acknowledge that this memory may reflect an 'island' of memory or patients may report information that their family have discussed with them, rather than their true memory of events.[72] However, both retrospective and prospective methods have value.[75]

When patients who are in, or are emerging from, PTA present with agitated, aggressive or challenging behaviour one to one supervision and observation is recommended,[61] alongside referral for specialist neuropsychological advice. Managing the patient in a quiet environment, for example small or single room, avoiding over-stimulation, for example ensure music/TV is not on constantly or at a loud volume, limiting visitor numbers, limiting visit lengths and promoting frequent rest periods are all recommended.[61,72]

Providing the staff team, family and patient (when timely) with information about PTA and TBI is essential. Information should ideally include a combination of information about PTA (e.g. the Headway leaflet on PTA available at www.headway.org.uk) and about the specific triggers for the individual patient, as part of a behavioural management plan.

Reduced Insight and Self-Awareness

Clinically, self-awareness can be defined as an understanding of one's abilities and limitations and how this impacts on task performance in everyday living.[76] Self-awareness deficits have been reported in up to 97% of people with brain injury[76] and can occur due to PTA or associated with dysexecutive syndrome. Impaired self-awareness is crucial to consider because of its potential role as a risk factor for neurobehavioural disturbance and because self-awareness deficits can negatively impact on engagement with rehabilitation resulting in poorer interpersonal, social and vocational outcomes.[76]

Psychoeducation for the patient, family and staff team is essential. Appropriate timing of this for patient and family needs consideration. Models of self-awareness[77,78] can be useful resources to highlight the impact of impaired awareness and to demonstrate that there are different types and levels of self-awareness which can develop during rehabilitation. For example, demonstrating that although a patient may be able to acknowledge that their planning abilities have been affected, they are not yet able to monitor their performance 'online' during a task and predict possible problems in advance. Neuropsychological assessment of self-awareness can also be relevant to assessment of capacity, particularly regarding questions about patients declining rehabilitation or requesting discharge against professional advice[61] (see Chapter 22).

Feedback interventions, which aim to enhance performance through feedback on assessment results, progress in therapy, and attainment of goals have been demonstrated to produce modest improvements in self-awareness.[76]

Personality Change

Changes in personality following brain injury can reflect an exaggeration of pre-existing characteristics, such as an assertive person becoming aggressive or a sociable person becoming overly talkative, or can represent a distinct change in personality following TBI. Changes associated with reduced impulse control, reduced empathy, emotional lability, irritability, aggression, socially inappropriate and sexually disinhibited behaviours are all potential examples. Changes in mood and mental state can also overlap with personality change in TBI. For example, irritable or agitated behaviour could be linked to a combination of mood disorder, executive dysfunction and personality change.[78] Personality change after TBI can be further complicated by self-awareness deficits and deficits in emotion regulation.

The complexity of the interplay between the neurological, psychological and social/participation factors as well as the impact of family functioning, highlights the importance of seeking specialist neuropsychological assessment. As well as identifying the person's profile of strengths and weaknesses, this process can enable the rehabilitation team to support person-centred goal-setting and to openly acknowledge potential barriers to rehabilitation progress. The process of neuropsychological assessment and formulation, using relevant resources,[79,80] can help the patient, family and staff make sense of the factors contributing to the change in personality. This process can support the family and patient at a time when relationships are strained as all involved are attempting to adjust to their new roles and identities.

Small and growing evidence is emerging that over time, usually at least 3 years post-injury, some people with TBI may experience some positive personality change and growth following their struggle to understand and accept their experiences.[81] In future, there is hope this research may yield new avenues for intervention, for at least some of those experiencing TBI.

Mild Traumatic Brain Injury and Post-concussion Syndrome

This section describes the post-acute assessment and treatment of patients who present to services with ongoing symptoms following mild traumatic brain injury. Throughout literature, the terms minor head injury, concussion, mild head injury and mild traumatic brain injury (MTBI) are often used interchangeably; however, these terms are not synonymous.[82] Within this section the term MTBI will be used referring to the effects of closed brain injury in adults.

Epidemiology and Definitions

MTBI is the most common type of traumatic brain injury, typically caused by falls, road traffic collisions, assaults and sports accidents. Worldwide, the incidence rates for MTBI are between 100 and 300 per 100 000 population with mild injuries accounting for between 70% and 90% of all traumatic brain injuries (TBIs).[83]

The definition of what constitutes a MTBI varies, dependant on criteria used; however, following comprehensive review of the scientific literature the World Health Organization (WHO) recommended the following definition:

> 'Mild traumatic brain injury is an acute brain injury resulting from mechanical energy to the head from external force. Operational criteria for clinical identification include:
>
> (i) One or more of the following: confusion or disorientation, loss of consciousness for 30 min or less, post-traumatic amnesia for less than 24 hours and/or other transient neurological abnormalities such as focal signs, seizure and intracranial lesion not requiring surgery;
>
> AND
>
> (ii) GCS score of 13–15 after 30 min post–head injury or later upon presentation for health care. These manifestations of MTBI must not be due to drugs, alcohol, medications, caused by other injuries or treatment for other injuries (e.g. systemic injuries, facial injuries or intubation), caused by other problems (e.g. psychological trauma, language barrier or coexisting medical conditions) or caused by penetrating craniocerebral injury'.[83]

It should be noted that this definition acknowledges that MTBI can occur in the absence of loss of consciousness (LOC), significant amnesia or other focal abnormalities, in line with current research findings, and that concussion, by definition, constitutes a MTBI.

Difficulties with Classification and Assessment in Post-acute Phase

Indices used to gauge severity of brain injury including LOC, PTA and GCS have been demonstrated to be less reliable in predicting outcome after MTBI than following more severe brain injury.[82,84] Indeed, unconsciousness and measurable PTA have been found to be relatively uncommon in cases where an alteration in mental status or other defining features of MTBI are clearly evident.[82] The GCS is not sensitive to the common symptoms (headache, nausea, dizziness and sensitivity to light and noise) or alterations in mental status associated with MTBI (e.g. confusion, amnesia, poor concentration).

Often the patient with MTBI presents to medical services seeking help for ongoing difficulties days (or even weeks or months) following injury. Thus measures indicating severity such as LOC and PTA may be difficult to establish as account of the injury is retrospective, the patient may not have memory of the incident and there may not have been witnesses present. The presence of structural abnormalities on CT and MRI gives a subcategory of injury, referred to as complicated MTBI, with an associated slower recovery.[82] Usually injuries where there is skull fracture or substantive haematoma are not generally considered mild.[85]

Imaging

Scan sensitivity needs to be considered in diagnosis of MTBI. CT has been found to have poor sensitivity in the overwhelming majority of MTBI cases with MRI being more sensitive for detection of all stages of subarachnoid haemorrhage, contusions and axonal injury.[86] However, MRI still may not document tissue damage even when the history and neuropsychological findings indicate impairment supporting a diagnosis of MTBI.[87] Advanced neuroimaging techniques such as fMRI, PET or SPECT have shown promising results in detection of abnormalities in MTBI where conventional CT and MRI findings are negative.[86] Whilst it is important to be aware of these issues, in reality, many individuals who sustain MTBI do not undergo imaging at any point in their journey and therefore self-reported symptoms are the main source of information available to the clinician.

Non-specific Symptoms and Diagnosis

The diagnosis of MTBI is based in large part on subjective symptoms reported by the patient. Symptoms are diverse and frequently include headache, sleep disturbance, fatigue, feeling slowed down, mental fog, irritability, depression and anxiety, subjective cognitive impairments (e.g. difficulties with information processing, concentration, word finding and memory), dizziness, and sensitivity to light and noise.[88,89] Although there are commonalities, individuals may experience any number of symptoms at different times and to varying degrees. Such symptoms are often collectively referred to as post-concussion syndrome (PCS), although the diagnosis of PCS should essentially be reserved for those patients whose symptoms fall outside the normal pattern of expected recovery after MTBI in severity and persistence.

Recovery and Outcome

Symptoms following MTBI typically present at the time of initial injury or appear within the first few days. In the overwhelming majority of uncomplicated cases, symptoms remit fairly quickly, with estimates of symptom and cognitive recovery ranging from several hours to several weeks.[90] The majority of studies report recovery for most within 3–12 months.[82,85,91] Those with structural abnormalities on imaging and those who experience PTA are more likely to show more severe symptoms and slower recovery in the acute phase; however, neither is predictive of subacute or long-term outcome in the majority of MTBI patients.[92] Repeated MTBI has been shown to increase the risk of symptoms lasting longer[93] and there have been rare cases of death or severe disability where a second injury has occurred before full recovery.[82] Studies examining concussion in sport have suggested long-term effects on attention[94] and memory.[95]

Persistent Post-concussion Syndrome

There are a small but significant number of individuals whose symptoms fall outside the normal pattern of expected recovery after MTBI.

It is estimated that around 10%–20% of patients with MTBI continue to complain of long-term post-concussive symptoms.[96] Iverson warns of overestimate due to the non-specificity of symptoms which may be associated with pre-existing or comorbid conditions,[97] although others propose this is an underestimate, suggesting up to 50% individuals with MTBI have long-term cognitive impairment.[98]

This diagnosis is controversial as there is continuing debate as to whether the presence, intensity and duration of these symptoms are due to an organic (neurologic) process, psychological reaction to the brain injury or other non-injury-related factors. These issues are complex and can be clinically challenging.

Several studies have demonstrated that sociodemographic and other non-injury-related variables have at least equal, and perhaps greater, significance in predicting long-term outcome after MTBI.[83,98] Ponsford and colleagues[98] investigated factors contributing to persisting problems following MTBI and concluded that ongoing problems were more likely in individuals who had a history of previous head injury, neurological or psychiatric problems, were female, and who's injury had occurred in a motor vehicle accident. Other factors found to be associated with risk of poor functional outcome are pre-existing medical or psychological problems, alcohol and drug problems, high levels of psychosocial stress at time of injury and poor social support systems after injury.[83] In addition, ongoing litigation has been cited as negatively influencing outcome.[99]

The symptoms that make up the core criteria for the formal diagnosis of PCS are highly nonspecific and have been found to occur at similar rates after other forms of physical trauma.[99] Indeed, several studies have demonstrated relatively high rates of PCS symptoms in various samples – from patients with chronic pain, depression or fibromyalgia to personal injury claimants and even normal, healthy individuals.[100] Thus diagnosis can be challenging and given the non-specificity of symptoms, consideration of alternative diagnostic explanations for ongoing symptoms should be considered by the assessing clinician.[85]

The impact of PCS on daily functioning and working life can be significant. Studies on return to work of patients with PCS have estimated those failing to return to work 1–2 years after injury as between 17% and 53%.[97]

In summary, currently available evidence does not support neuronal damage as the main underlying mechanism in PCS but a range of other factors, including psychological, socio-demographic and motivational factors. In line with this, and gathering increasing support, is the recommendation that a wider formulation of all relevant factors to the patient's symptoms is more appropriate than the diagnostic label of PCS and therefore direction of treatment should be considered within a biopsychosocial model.

Treatment of MTBI

The symptoms following MTBI can be distressing and worrying, especially if the patient does not know what to expect. A systematic review[101] identified a small number of studies on early intervention which provided some evidence that early, limited educational intervention and providing reassurance about the lack of significant brain injury and the high probability of a good recovery, coupled with advice and encouragement on gradual return to regular activities, reduce long-term complaints. Clinical guidelines recommend all patients should be offered reassurance about the nature of their current symptoms and advice on gradual return to normal activities after uncomplicated MTBI.[85] Headway have produced a helpful booklet on minor head injury and concussion, and a Factsheet specifically for GPs, both of which outline common symptoms and practical suggestions (www.headway.org.uk). They detail that alcohol should be avoided in first few days after injury because brain injury can reduce tolerance to alcohol and that individuals should avoid returning to work too quickly. If symptoms are prolonged and disabling, it may be appropriate for the patient to be referred to a neurologist or neuropsychologist for further assessment and treatment. Neuropsychological intervention will include a number of different approaches tailored to the individual, based on the formulation of the patients problems and may include therapy for psychological factors, cognitive rehabilitation and a wider team approach (e.g. engagement of occupational therapy for fatigue management).

Rehabilitation Following Traumatic Brain Injury in Children

The majority of children will experience a knock to their head at some point throughout their childhood. Fortunately, for most, these injuries are not of sufficient severity to warrant hospitalisation and they simply return to everyday activities. However, a sizeable minority of those children that present to paediatric accident and emergency departments as a result of head-injury are often subsequently recognised as having suffered a traumatic brain injury (TBI). In situations where this is the case, it is not uncommon for children to be left with a range of physical, cognitive and behavioural difficulties that can negatively impact upon everyday functioning and their social, emotional, intellectual, and academic development. In this sense, it is widely appreciated that paediatric TBI produces vulnerability to unwelcome and dramatic change in developmental trajectories that can seriously undermine a child's later life outcomes.

Across the spectrum of difficulties that can manifest in everyday life, impairments in cognitive functioning play an important mediating role. In this context, children that have suffered a TBI are noted to be especially vulnerable to experiencing problems with attention, speed of information processing, various aspects of memory (including working memory, verbal memory, visual memory, and prospective memory), and executive functioning.[102,103] Should a child acquire even one of these deficits in isolation, then there is significant potential for that child's behaviour and learning or capacity to function effectively in their day-to-day environment to be compromised. Any combination of impairments, as is often the case in TBI, increases the likelihood of experiencing problems in multiple areas of life.

The scale of the problem should not be underestimated either; paediatric TBI incidence estimates vary, with highest at 486 children per 100 000.[104] Even if the most conservative incidence estimate of 50 children per 100 000 was accepted, this would equate to around 3 million children worldwide suffering a TBI each year.[105] TBI is widely recognised as a leading cause of acquired disability in childhood that comes with significant economic costs for individuals, families and society as a whole.[106]

Appreciating the increased risk of personal loss, not to mention the significant global public health challenge that paediatric TBI represents, a fundamental aim of neuropsychological review is directed towards ensuring that required interventions designed to remediate TBI sequelae are implemented in as timely a manner as possible. Unfortunately however, at this point in time there is a shortage of empirical intervention studies designed to tackle the constellation of everyday life problems that TBI children and their families may face.[107,108] In this sense, the evidence-base for paediatric neuropsychological intervention might reasonably be considered as lagging, behind its adult counterpart. Encouragingly however, intervention-based studies describing positive results continue to emerge; with individual studies and literature reviews highlighting promise when it comes to treating problems with behaviour,[109] attention,[110,111] memory,[112] executive functioning[113] and academic functioning.[114] Recognising that family functioning can influence outcome following paediatric TBI, it is encouraging that family-focused interventions have described improvements in problem-solving skills, family relationships, the behaviour of the child and cognitive outcome post-treatment.[115,116] Given the finding that access to rehabilitation is a key variable exerting influence over eventual outcome,[117] it is heartening that the knowledge-base, from upon which to build practice, is constantly growing.

Of course it is important to recognise that, fortunately, not all children that experience TBI will suffer impairments. Indeed, the consequences of TBI in childhood is a complicated individualised process that is influenced by a number of factors including the type of injury, age at injury, the child's premorbid functioning, various psychosocial variables (such as family functioning, adjustment and socio-economic status) and injury severity, with those sustaining moderate and severe injuries identified as being most vulnerable to experiencing enduring neuropsychological impairments.[118] Bearing the above findings in mind, it is imperative that those involved in the child's rehabilitation take account of those factors that influence residual sequelae when prognosticating about the expected long-term outcome and developing individually tailored intervention programmes.

In terms of those factors that mediate outcome, the observation that younger children, especially those with more serious brain injuries, are particularly vulnerable to experiencing poorer outcomes would appear worthy of special mention here. The impact of early TBI may not become fully apparent until the child fails to achieve developmental expectations in late childhood or early adulthood. This further highlights the need for a long-term developmental perspective to rehabilitation to be taken in the case of paediatric TBI. Moreover, the fact that a meaningful minority of children that sustain mild TBIs can experience long-term problems with cognition and psychosocial functioning[119] underlines need for vigilance and longer-term monitoring of outcomes even in the case of mild TBI. Increased risk of psychiatric disorder,[120] of suffering underemployment and poorer quality of life,[121] and heightened risk of becoming involved in criminal activities during adulthood[122] all strengthen need for long-term follow-up in paediatric TBI populations. Considering such findings, together with the fact that when it comes to children you are naturally dealing with an ongoing process of physical, social, emotional, cognitive and intellectual development, it is not uncommon for the practicing paediatric neuropsychologist to continue to review the status of children affected by TBI for many years after the initial injury has occurred. Crucially, the process of review enables appropriate developmentally sensitive interventions to be prescribed at the right time and coordinated support plans to be updated accordingly.

It is perhaps unsurprising given extensive variability in outcome following paediatric TBI, and identified need for monitoring of functioning, that models of service delivery recommending clinical follow-up across developmental trajectories have been proposed.[123] In this context, it is crucial that affected children and families have access to a range of professional support across social, educational and health care sectors; with points of significant life transition (e.g. moving from primary school into secondary school education) being particularly important occasions where review of child and family needs should be undertaken and interventions provided accordingly.

In summary, TBI is a common cause of mortality and long-term disability in children that can have a devastating effect upon a child's subsequent development and functioning for the rest of their lives. If we are to adequately support children to achieve their post-injury potential and live as enriched a life as possible, comprehensive family-orientated and community-focused rehabilitation interventions designed to counteract the array of cognitive, behavioural and psychosocial deficits that often surface post-TBI are required.

Summary

Neuropsychological intervention for patients with traumatic brain injury involves holistic, formulation-based assessment and intervention and may include cognitive rehabilitation, behavioural programmes or psychological therapy. Patients with mild brain injury and post-concussive symptoms benefit from neuropsychological formulation and intervention and there is a wide range of evidence for neuropsychological intervention for children with TBI.

References

1. Clare L. The construction of awareness in early stage Alzheimer's disease: a review of concepts and models. *Br J Clin Psychol* 2004;43:155–75.

2. Ownsworth T, Clare L, Morris R. An integrated biopsychosocial approach to understanding awareness deficits in Alzheimer's disease and brain injury. *Neuropsychol Rehabil* 2006;16:415–38.

3. Crosson B, Barco PP, Velozo CA, Bolesta MM, Werts D, Brobeck T. Awareness and compensation in post-acute head injury rehabilitation. *J Head Trauma Rehabil* 1989;4:46–54.

4. Malouf T, Langdon R, Taylor A. The insight interview: a new tool for measuring deficits in awareness after traumatic brain injury. *Brain Injury* 2014;28:1523–41.

5. Evans J, Krasny-Pacini A. Goal setting in rehabilitation. In: Wilson BA, Winegardner J, Van Heugten CM, Ownsworth T., eds. *Neuropsychological rehabilitation: the international handbook.* Abingdon, UK: Routledge;2017.

6. Wilson BA. Towards a comprehensive model of cognitive rehabilitation. *Neuropsychol Rehabil* 2002;12:97–110.

7. Cicerone KD, Langenbahn DM, Braden C, et al. Evidence-based cognitive rehabilitation: updated review of the literature from 2003 through 2008. *Arch Phys Med Rehabil* 2011;92:519–30.

8. Ponsford J, Bayley M, Wiseman-Hakes C, et al. INCOG recommendations for management of cognition following traumatic brain injury, Part II: Attention and information processing speed. *J Head Trauma Rehabil* 2014;29:321–37.

9. Tate R, Kennedy M, Ponsford J, et al. INCOG recommendations for management of cognition following traumatic brain injury, Part III: Executive

function and self awareness. *J Head Trauma Rehabil* 2014;29:338–52.

10. Velikonja D, Tate R, Ponsford J, et al. INCOG recommendations for management of cognition following traumatic brain injury, Part V: Memory. *J Head Trauma Rehabil* 2014;29: 369–86.

11. Scottish Intercollegiate Guideline Network. *Brain injury rehabilitation in adults: a national clinical guideline.* Edinburgh: SIGN;2013.

12. American Congress of Rehabilitation Medicine. *Cognitive rehabilitation manual: translating evidence based recommendations into practice.* Virginia: ACRM;2014.

13. Wilson BA, Gracey F, Evans JJ, Bateman A. *Neuropsychological rehabilitation: theory, therapy and outcomes.* Cambridge: Cambridge University Press;2009.

14. Craik FIM, Winocur G, Palmer H, et al. Cognitive rehabilitation in the elderly: effects on memory. *J Int Neuropsych Soc* 2007;13:132–42.

15. Wilson BA, Emslie H, Quirk K, Evans JJ. Is Neuropage effective in reducing everyday memory and planning problems? A randomised control crossover study. *J Neurol Neurosurg Psychiatry* 2001;70:477–82.

16. Jamieson M, Cullen B, McGee-Lennon M, Brewster S, Evans JJ. The efficacy of cognitive prosthetic technology for people with memory impairments: a systematic review and meta-analysis. *Neuropsychol Rehabil* 2014;24:419–44.

17. Ponsford J, Bayley M, Wiseman-Hakes C, Togher L, Velikonja D, McIntyre A, Janzen S. Tate R INCOG recommendations for management of cognition following traumatic brain injury, Part II: Attention and information processing speed. *J Head Trauma Rehabil* 2014;29(4):321–37.

18. Park N, Barbuto E. Treating attention impairments. In: Halligan P, Wade, D, eds. *The effectiveness of rehabilitation for cognitive deficits.* Oxford: Oxford University Press;2005.

19. Evans JJ. Can executive impairments be effectively treated? In: Halligan P, Wade D, eds. *The effectiveness of rehabilitation for cognitive deficits.* Oxford: Oxford University Press;2005.

20. Tate R, Kennedy M, Ponsford J, Douglas J, Velikonja D, Bayley M, Stergiou-Kita M. INCOG w traumatic brain injury, Part III: Executive function and self awareness. *J Head Trauma Rehabil* 2014;29(4):338–52.

21. Tornås S, Løvstad M, Solbakk A-K, Evans J, Endestad T, Hol PK, Schanke A-K, Stubberud J. Rehabilitation of executive functions in patients with chronic acquired brain injury with goal management training, external cuing, and emotional regulation: a randomized controlled trial. *J Int Neuropsychol Soc* 2016;22,436–52.

22. Gracey F, Fish JE, Greenfield, E, Bateman, A, Malley D, Hardy G, Ingham J, Evans JJ, Manly T. A randomized controlled trial of assisted intention monitoring for the rehabilitation of executive impairments following acquired brain injury. *Neurorehabil Neural Repair* 2017;31(4):323–33.

23. Evans JJ, Emslie H, Wilson BA. External cueing systems in the rehabilitation of executive impairments of action. *J Int Neuropsychol Soci* 1998;4: 399–408.

24. Brady MC, Kelly H, Godwin J, Enderby P, Campbell P. Speech and language therapy for aphasia following stroke. *Cochrane Database Syst Rev* 2016;Issue 6: CD000425.

25. Douglas, J, Togher L. Managing acquired social communication disorders. In: Wilson BA, Winegardner J, Van Heugten CM, Ownsworth T, eds. *Neuropsychological rehabilitation: the international handbook.* Abingdon, UK: Routledge;2017.

26. Stansfield S, Clark C, Bebbington P, King M, Jenkins R, Hinchcliffe S. Common mental disorders. In: McManus S, Bebbington P, Jenkins R, Brugha T, eds. *Mental health and wellbeing in England: Adult Psychiatric Morbidity Survey.* Leeds, UK: NHS Digital; 2014.

27. Zaninotto AL, Vicentini JE, Fregni F, Rodrigues PA, Botelho C, Souza de Lucia MC, Paiva WS. Updates and current perspectives of psychiatric assessments after traumatic brain injury: a systematic review. *Front Psychiatr* 2016;7:95–108.

28. Kreutzer JS, Seel RT, Gourley E. The prevalence and symptom rates of depression after traumatic brain injury: a comprehensive examination. *Brain Injury* 2001;15(7):563–76.

29. Jorge RE, Robinson RG, Moser D, Tateno A, Crespo-Facorro B, Arndt S. Major de-pression following traumatic brain injury. *Arch Gen Psychiatr* 2004;61 (1):42–50.

30. Seel RT, Kreutzer JS, Rosenthal M, Hammond FM, Corrigan JD, Black K. Depression after traumatic brain injury: a National Institute on Disability and Rehabilitation Research Model Systems multicenter investigation. *Arch Phys Med Rehabil* 2003;84(2):177–84.

31. Whelan-Goodinson R, Ponsford J, Johnston L, Grant F. Psychiatric disorders following traumatic brain injury: their nature and frequency. *JHead Trauma Rehabil* 2009;24:324–32.

32. Osborn AJ, Mathias JL, Fairweather-Schmidt AK. Prevalence of anxiety following adult traumatic brain injury: a meta-analysis comparing measures, samples and postinjury intervals. *Neuropsychology* 2016;30(2):247–61.

33. Mackelprang JL, Bombardier CH, Fann JR, Temkin NR, Barber JK, Dikmen SS. Rates and predictors of suicidal ideation during the first year after traumatic brain injury. *Am J Public Health* 2014;104(7):100–7.

34. Nock MK, Borges G, Bromet EG, Cha CB, Kessler RC, Lee S. Suicide and suicidalbehavior. *Epidemiol Rev* 2008;30 (1):133–54.

35. Carlson KF, Kehle SM, Meis LA, Greer N, MacDonald R, Rutks I, Sayer NA, Dobscha SK, Wilt TJ. Prevalence, assessment, and treatment of mild traumatic brain injury and posttramatic stress disorder: a systematic review of the evidence. *J Head Trauma Rehabil* 2011;26:103–15.

36. Schwarzbold M, Diaz A, Martins ET, Rufino A, Amanle LN, Thais ME, Quevedo J, Hohl A, Linhares MN, Walz, R. Psychiatric disorders and traumatic brain injury. *Neuropsychiatr Dis Treatment* 2008;4:797–816.

37. Fleminger S, Oliverl DL, Williams WH, Evans J. The neuropsychiatry of depression after brain injury. *Neuropsychol Rehabil* 2003;13:65–87.

38. Bryant RA, Moulds M, Guthrie R, Nixon RD. Treating acute stress disorder following mild traumatic brain injury. *Am J Psychiatr* 2003;160(3): 585–7.

39. Verberne DPJ, Spauwen PJJ, van Heugten CM. Psychological interventions for treating neuropsychiatric consequences of acquired brain injury: asystematic review. *Neuropsychol Rehabil* 2018;13:1–34.

40. Fann JR, Bombardier CH, Vannoy S, Dyer J, Ludman E, Dikmen S,Temkin N. Telephone and in-person cognitive behavioral therapy for major depression after traumatic brain injury: arandomized controlled trial. *J Neurotrauma* 2014;32 (1):45–57.

41. Ponsford J. Interventions for anxiety and depression. In: McMillan T, Wood R, eds. *Neurobehavioural disability and social handicap following traumatic brain injury.* Hove, UK: Psychology Press;2017.

42. Whiting DL, Deane FP, Simpson GF, McLeod HJ, Ciarrochi J. Cognitive and psychological flexibility after a traumatic brain injury and the implications for treatment in acceptance-based therapies: a conceptual review. *Neuropsychol Rehabil* 2015;27:2.

43. Soo C, Tate RL, Lane-Brown A. A systematic review of acceptance and commitment therapy (ACT) for managing anxiety: applicability for people with

acquired brain injury. *Brain Impairment* 2011;12:54–70.

44. Bédard M, Felteau M, Marshall S, Cullen N, Gibbons C, Dubois S, Maxwell H, Mazmanian D, Weaver B, Rees L, Gainer R, Klein R, Moustgaard A. Mindfulness-based cognitive therapy reduces symptoms of depression in people with a traumatic brain injury: results from a randomized controlled trial. *J Head Trauma Rehabil* 2014;29 (4):13–22.

45. Ashworth F, Gracey F, Gilbert P. Compassion focused therapy after traumatic brain injury: theoretical foundations and a case illustration. *Brain Impairment* 2011;12(2):128–39.

46. Hamacheck D. *Encounters with the self.* New York: Holt, Reinhart and Winston;1992.

47. Ownsworth T. *Self-identity after brain injury (neuropsychological rehabilitation: a modular handbook).* Hove, UK: Psychology Press;2014.

48. Ben-Yishay Y. Post-acute neuropsychological rehabilitation: aholistic approach. In: Christensen AL, Uzzell BP, eds. *International handbook of neuropsychological rehabilitation.* New York: Kluwer Academic/ Plenum;2000.

49. Biderman D, Daniel Side E, Reyes A, Marks B. Ego-identity: can it be reconstituted after a brain injury? *Int J Psychol* 2006;41:355–61.

50. Wilson B, Gracey F, Malley D, Bateman A, Evans J. The Oliver Zangwill Centre approach to neuropsychological rehabilitation. In: Wilson FGB, Evans J, Bateman A, eds. *Neuropsychological rehabilitation: theory, models, therapy and outcome.* Cambridge: Cambridge University Press;2009.

51. Ownsworth T, Haslam C. Impact of rehabilitation on self-concept following traumatic brain injury: an exploratory systematic review of intervention methodology and efficacy. *Neuropsychol Rehabil* 2016;26(1):1–35.

52. Von Mensenkampff B, Ward M, Kelly G, Cadogan S, Fawsit F, Lowe N. The value of normalization: group therapy for individuals with brain injury. *Brain Injury* 2015;29(11):1292–9.

53. Patterson F, Fleming J, Doig E. Group-based delivery of interventions in traumatic brain injury rehabilitation: a scoping review. *Disabil Rehabil* 2016;38 (20):1961–86.

54. Martin R, Levack WM, Sinnott KA. Life goals and social identity in people with severe acquired brain injury: an interpretative phenomenological analysis. *Disabil Rehabil* 2015;37(14):1234–41.

55. O'Brien S. Expert by experience – a personal reflection of the experience of mental health services: overcoming unsafe and aversive practices. *Clin Psychol Forum* 2017;290:5–8.

56. Worthington A, Wood RLl. Behaviour problems. In: Tyerman A, King NS, eds. *Psychological approaches to rehabilitation after traumatic brain injury.* Oxford: BPS Blackwell;2008.

57. Gainotti G. Emotional and psychosocial problems after brain injury. *Neuropsychol Rehabil* 1993;3:259–77.

58. Alderman N, Wood RL, Neurobehavioural approaches to the rehabilitation of challenging behaviour. *Neurorehabilitation* 2013;32:761–70.

59. Tam S, McKay A, Sloan S, Ponsford J. The experience of challenging behaviours following severe TBI: a family perspective. *Brain Injury* 2015;29:813–21.

60. Scottish Intercollegiate Guidelines Network (SIGN). Brain injury rehabilitation in adults;2013. www .sign.ac.uk/sign-130-brain-injury-rehabilitation-in-adults.html

61. British Society for Rehabilitation Medicine (BRSM). National Clinical Guidelines: rehabilitation following acquired brain injury (under review);2003. www .headway.org.uk/media/3320/bsrm-rehabilitation-following-acquired-brain-injury.pdf

62. Department of Health. Positive and proactive care: reducing the need for restrictive interventions;2014. www.gov.uk/government/uploads/system/uploads/attachment_data/file/300293/JRA_DoH_Guidance_on_RP_web_accessible.pdf

63. NHS Protect. Meeting needs and reducing distress;2015. www.maybo.co.uk/file/2135/meeting_needs_and_reducing_distress.pdf

64. National Institute for Health and Care Excellence (NICE). Head injury: assessment and early management;2014 (updated 2017).www.nice.org.uk/guidance/cg176

65. National Institute for Health and Care Excellence (NICE). Violent and aggressive behaviours in people with mental health problems;2017. www.nice.org.uk/guidance/qs154

66. Alderman N. Challenging behaviour. In: McMillan TM, Alderman N, eds. *Neurobehavioural disability and social handicap following traumatic brain injury.* Abingdon, UK: Routledge;2017.

67. Kelly G, Todd J, Simpson G, Kremer P, Martin C. The Overt Behaviour Scale (OBS): a tool for measuring challenging behaviours following ABI in community settings. *Brain Injury* 2006;20:307–19.

68. Alderman N, Wood RLl, Williams C. The development of the St Andrew's Swansea Neurobehavioural Outcome Scale: validity and reliability of a new measure of neurobehavioural disability and social handicap. *Brain Injury* 2011;25:83–100.

69. Knight C, Alderman N, Johnson C, Green S, Birkett-Swan L, Yorstan G. The St Andrew's Sexual Behaviour Assessment (SASBA): development of a standardised recording instrument for the measurement and assessment of challenging sexual behaviour in people with progressive and acquired neurological impairment. *Neuropsychol Rehabil* 2008;18:129–59.

70. O'Neill B, Findlay G. Single case methodology in neurobehavioural rehabilitation: preliminary findings on biofeedback in the treatment of challenging behaviour. *Neuropsychol Rehabil* 2014;24:365–81.

71. Alderman N, Wood RLl. Neurobehavioural approaches to the rehabilitation of challenging behaviour. *NeuroRehabilitation* 2013;32:761–70.

72. Wilson BA, Herbert CM, Sheil A. *Behavioural approaches in neuropsychological rehabilitation: optimising rehabilitation procedures.* East Sussex, UK: Psychology Press;2003.

73. Levin HS, O'Donnell VM,Grossman RG. The Galveston Orientation and Amnesia Test. *J Nervous Mental Dis* 1979;167:657–84.

74. Marosszeky NEV, Ryan L, Shores EA, Batchelor J, Marosszeky JE. *The PTA Protocol: guidelines for using the Westmead Post-Traumatic Amnesia (PTA) Scale.* Sydney: Wild and Wooley;1997.

75. McMillan TM, Jongen ELMM, Greenwood RJ. Assessment of post-traumatic amnesia after severe closed head injury: retrospective or prospective? *J Neurol NeurosurgPsychiatr* 1996;60:422–7.

76. Schmidt J, Lannin N, Fleming J, Ownsworth T. Feedback interventions for impaired self-awareness following brain injury: asystematic review. *J Rehabil Med* 2015;43:673–68.

77. Crosson C, Barco PP, Velozo C, Bolesta MM, Cooper PV, Werts D, Brobeck TC. Awareness and compensation in post acute head injury rehabilitation. *J Head Trauma Rehabil* 1989;4:46–54.

78. Toglia J, Kirk U. Understanding awareness deficits following brain injury. *NeuroRehabilitation* 2000;15:57–70.

79. Evans JJ. Theoretical influences on brain injury rehabilitation. Presented at the Oliver Zangwill Centre 10thAnniversary Conference; 2006.www.ozc.nhs.uk

80. Winson R, Wilson B, Bateman A. *The brain injury rehabilitation workbook.* New York: Guilford Press;2017.

81. Grace JJ, Kinsella EL, Muldoon OT, Fortune DG. Post-traumatic growth following acquired brain injury: a systematic review and meta-analysis. *Front Psychol* 2015;6:1162.

82. Mcrea MA. *Mild traumatic injury and postconcussion syndrome: the new evidence base for diagnosis and treatment.* New York: Oxford University Press;2008.

83. Cassidy JD, Caroll LJ, Peloso PM, Borg J, von Holst HL, et al. Incidence, risk factors and prevention of mild traumatic brain injury: results of the WHO Collaborating Centre Task Force on Mild Traumatic Brain Injury. *J Rehabil Med* 2004;43 (Suppl):28–60.

84. Lucas, JA. Traumatic brain injury and postconcussive syndrome. In: Snyder JP, Nussbaum PD, eds. *Clinical neuropsychology: a pocket handbook for assessment.* Washington, DC: American Psychological Association;1998.

85. Scottish Intercollegiate Guidelines Network (SIGN 130). Brain injury rehabilitation in adults: a national clinical guideline;2003. www.sign.ac.uk/assets/sign130.pdf

86. Wintermark M, Sanelli PC, Anzai Y, Tsiouris AJ, Whitlow CT. Imaging evidence and recommendations for traumatic brain injury: conventional neuroimaging techniques. *J Am Coll Radiol* 2015;36(2):1–11.

87. Wilkinson I, Lennox G. *Essential neurology.* Malden, MA: Blackwell;2005.

88. Lovell MR, Iverson GL, Collins MW, Podell K, Johnstone KM, Pardini D, et al. Measurement of symptoms following sports-related concussion: reliability and normative data for the post-concussion scale. *Appl Neuropsychol* 2006;13 (3):166–74.

89. Georgiades C, Clarke D. *Minor brain injury: a guide to causes, symptoms and strategies.* Nottingham, UK: Headway Brain Injury Association;2004.

90. McCrea M, Guskiewicz KM, Marchall SW, et al. Acute effects and recovery time following concussion in collegiate football players: the NCAA concussion study. *JAMA* 2003;290:2556–63.

91. King NS, Tyerman A. Neuropsychological presentation and treatment of head injury and traumatic brain damage. In: Halligan PW, Kischka U, Marshall JC, eds.

Handbook of clinical neuropsychology. Oxford: Oxford University Press;2003.

92. Iverson GL, Lange RT, Gaetz M, Zasler ND. Mild traumatic brain injury. In: Zasler ND, Katz DI, Zafonte RD, eds. *Brain injury medicine: principles and practice.* New York: Demos Medical Publishing;2006.

93. Iverson GL, Gaetz M, Lovell MR, Collins MW. Cumulative effects of concussion in amateur athletes. *Brain Injury* 2004;18:433–43.

94. Wall SE, Williams WH, Cartwright-Hatton S, Kelly TP, Murray J, Murray M, Owen A, Turner M. Neuropsychological dysfunction following repeat concussions in jockeys. *JNeurolNeurosurgPsychiatr* 2006;77:518–20.

95. McMillan TM, McSkimming P, Wainman-Lefley J, Maclean LM, et al. Long-term health outcomes after exposure to repeated concussion in elite level: rugby union players. *JNeurolNeurosurgPsychiatr* 2016;88:512–19.

96. Rutherford WH. Postconcussion symptoms: relationship to acute neurological indices, individual differences and circumstances of injury. In: Levin HS, Eisenberg HM, Benton AL, eds. *Mild head injury.* New York: Oxford University Press; 1989.

97. Iverson GL, Lange RT. Post-concussion syndrome. In: Schoenberg MR, Scott JG, eds. *The little black book of neuropsychology: a syndrome-based approach.* New York: Springer;2011.

98. McInnes K, Friesen CL, MacKenzie DE, Westwood DA, Boe SG. Mild traumatic brain injury (mTBI) and chronic cognitive impairment: a scoping review. *PLoS One* 2017;12(4):e0174847.

99. Ponsford J, Willmott C, Rothwell A, Cameron P, Kelly AM, Curran C, Ng K. Factors influencing outcome following mild traumatic brain injury in adults. *J Int Neuropsychol Soc* 2000;6 (5):568–79.

100. Iverson GL, Lange RT. Examination of post-concussion-like' symptoms in

healthy population. *Appl Neuropsychol* 2003;10(3):137–44.

101. Borg J, Holm L, Peloso PM, Cassidy JD, Carroll LJ, von Holst H, et al. Non-surgical intervention and cost for mild traumatic brain injury: results of the WHO Collaborating Centre Task Force on Mild Traumatic Brain Injury. *J Rehabil* 2004;43(suppl):76–83.

102. Middleton, JA. Practitioner review: psychological sequelae of head injury in children and adolescents. *J Child Psychol Psychiatr* 2001;42(2):165–80.

103. Yeates KO. Traumatic brain injury. In: Yeates KO, Ris MD, Taylor HG, Pennington BF, eds. *Paediatric neuropsychology: research, theory and practice.* 2nd edn. London: The Guilford Press;2010.

104. Mitra B, Cameron PA, Butt W, Rosenfeld JV. Children or young adults? A population-based study on adolescent head injury. *ANZ J Surg* 2006;76:343–50.

105. Dewan MC, Mummareddy N, Wellons JC3rd, Bonfield CM. The epidemiology of global pediatric traumatic brain injury: qualitative review. *World Neurosurg* 2016;91:497–509.

106. World Health Organization. *Neurological disorders: public health challenges.* Geneva, Switzerland: WHO Press;2006.

107. Catroppa C, Soo C, Crowe L, Woods D, Anderson V. Evidence-based approaches to the management of cognitive and behavioural impairments following pediatric brain injury. *Future Neurol* 2012;7:719–31.

108. Ross KA, Dorris L, McMillan T. A systematic review of psychological interventions to alleviate cognitive and psychosocial problems in children with acquired brain injury. *Develop Med Child Neurol* 2011;53(8):692–701.

109. Ylvisaker M, Turkstra L, Coehlo C, Yorkston K, Kennedy M, Sohlberg MM, Avery J. Behavioural interventions for children and adults with behaviour disorders after TBI: a systematic review of the evidence. *Brain Injury* 2007;21 (8):769–805.

110. Adlam A-LR, Limond J, Lah S. Rehabilitation of attention disorders: children. In: Wilson BA, Winegardner J, van Heugten CM, Ownsworth T, eds. *Neuropsychological rehabilitation: the international handbook.* London: Routledge;2017.

111. Backeljauw B, Kurowski BG. Interventions for attention problems after pediatric traumatic brain injury: what is the evidence? *Phys Med Rehabil* 2014;6 (9):814–24.

112. Parker G, Haslam C, Fleming J, Shum D. Rehabilitation of memory disorders in adults and children. In: Wilson, BA, Winegardner J, van Heugten CM, Ownsworth T, eds. *Neuropsychological rehabilitation: the international handbook.* London: Routledge;2017.

113. Catroppa C, Anderson V. Planning, problem-solving and organizational abilities in children following traumatic brain injury: intervention techniques. *Pediatr Rehabil* 2006;9(2):89–97.

114. Butler RW. Cognitive rehabilitation. In: Hunter SJ, Donders J, eds. *Pediatric neuropsychological intervention.* New York: Cambridge University Press;2007.

115. Braga LW, Da Paz Junior AC, Ylvisaker M. Direct clinician-delivered versus indirect family-supported rehabilitation of children with traumatic brain injury: A randomized controlled trial. *Brain Injury* 2005;19(10):819–31.

116. Wade SL, Michaud L, Brown TM. Putting the pieces together – preliminary efficacy of a family problem-solving intervention for children with traumatic brain injury. *J Head Trauma Rehabil* 2006;21(1):57–67.

117. Anderson V, Catroppa C, Morse S, Haritou F, Rosenfeld J. Identifying factors contributing to child and family outcome at 30 months following traumatic brain injury in children. *J Neurol Neurosurg Psychiatr* 2005;76:401–8.

118. Trenchard SO, Rust S, Bunton P. A systematic review of psychosocial outcomes within 2 years of paediatric traumatic brain injury in a school-aged

population. *Brain Injury* 2013;27 (11):1217–37.

119. Lloyd J, Wilson ML, Tenovuo O, Saarijärvi S. Outcomes from mild and moderate traumatic brain injuries among children and adolescents: A systematic review of studies from 2008–2013. *Brain Injury* 2015;29(5):539–49.

120. Max JE, Friedman K, Wilde EA, Bigler ED, Hanten G, Schachar RJ, Saunders AE, Dennis M, Ewing-Cobbs L, Chapman SB, Yang TT, Levin HS. Psychiatric disorders in children and adolescents 24 months after mild traumatic brain injury. *J Neuropsychiatr Clin Neurosci* 2015;27(2):112–20.

121. Anderson V, Brown S, Newitt H, Hoile H. Educational, vocational, psychosocial, and quality-of-life outcomes for adult survivors of childhood traumatic brain injury. *J Head Trauma Rehabil* 2009;24(5):303–12.

122. Williams H, Cordan G, Mewse AJ, Tonks J, Burgess CN. Self-reported traumatic brain injury in male young offenders: a risk factor for re-offending, poor mental health and violence? *Neuropsychol Rehabil* 2010;20(6):801–12.

123. Scottish Acquired Brain Injury Network: SABIN. Paediatric acquired brain injury best practice statements. NHS Scotland; in press.

Chapter 27

Assistive Technology and Rehabilitation

Brian O'Neill, Catherine Best and Matt Jamieson

Introduction

Technologies are human creations that augment human ability. Information processors are our most advanced technologies, providing both a useful metaphor in understanding cognitive function,[1] and digital devices which can augment impaired cognition.[2]

The view of the brain as comprising distinct modules of function has held sway in behavioural neurology and neuropsychology since the inception of these disciplines.[3] Backed by lesion and imaging studies, this conceptualisation has allowed the development of reliable cognitive tests, and therefore an understanding of how impairment of functional modules predicts everyday functional behaviour. This chapter reviews evidence that specific technologies can be used to support impairments of the specific mental functions impaired by brain injury. Suggestions are offered on how digital technologies might be used in clinical practice to overcome the cognitive impairments, improve independent activity, and encourage greater participation. We will include published studies of assistive technology for cognition (ATC) that have been tested in clinical populations, thus excluding concept systems and prototypes. We also exclude devices developed to remediate functions, and devices to support communication (AACs), and devices that are solely for monitoring of health or safety status. We will focus on devices that support cognitive function when used.

Technologies to support cognitive function are booming. With rapid development and obsolescence, the longevity of this chapter rests on our focus on the interface between human mental functions and technological functions. Desktops, laptops, personal digital assistants (PDAs) and smartphones have served as the technical underpinnings of reminders to support executive function. In this case, reminding is the technological function, which has been evidenced to be effective in supporting executive function. Evidence for specific technological functions will continue to indicate their usefulness for a given cognitive deficit, even when the underpinning technology changes.[2]

The World Heath Organisation International Classification of Functioning, Disability and Health (ICF) places less emphasis on aetiology or diagnosis, and posits that if impairment remains constant, modifying the environment with technology can improve activity or participation.[4] The ICF's 11 specific mental functions (see Table 27.1) offer an assessment framework that is familiar to most clinicians. Disablement in daily life, such as missing medications, failure to attend appointments, social isolation secondary to poor planning and difficulty organising for the day, inattention-related risks such as taps being left on or doors unlocked, poor co-ordination of shopping/meals, food in the fridge going out of date or memory-related neglect of laundry and cleaning, indicates the need for neuropsychological assessment. By measuring the functions we can gain a profile of strengths and weaknesses that indicates technologies to trial.[2,5–7]

Table 27.1 The ICF 11 specific mental functions

	Specific mental function	Typically presenting problems
1	**Attention**	Poor safety awareness; kitchen accidents; cannot concentrate
2	**Memory**	Vague history; conversational poverty; loss of items; self-neglect
3	Psychomotor	
4	**Emotion**	Lability; avoidance; easily frustrated; aggression; social difficulties
5	Perception	
6	Thought	
7	**Higher-level cognition**	Apathy; disorganisation; difficulty sequencing; poor judgement; missing appointments; poor medication compliance
8	Language	
9	Calculation	
10	Sequencing movements	
11	**Experience of self & time**	Disorientation; poor insight; getting lost

Note: Those currently addressed in bold.[4]

Effectiveness of ATC

The typical constellation of mental function impairments after traumatic brain injury indicates a focus on studies examining supports for *Attention, Memory, Emotion, Higher-level cognition,* and the *Experience of self and time.*

Attention Functions

Attention is the mental function of focusing on an external stimulus or internal experience for the required period of time. ATC has been used to shift visuospatial attention, support sustained attention and direct attention to internal representations, such as their goals.[6] Brain injury is associated with difficulty sustaining attention and being highly distractible.

Robertson and colleagues theorised that attention is maintained by endogenous process and exogenous stimulation.[8] An exciting film easily supports sustained attention. Reading the phonebook at bedtime requires significant endogenous resources. Phasic alerting, by tones, or vibration via mobile phones or other electronic devices, is an exogenous support for attention.[9-11] Other ATCs redirect attention by sending participants messages with content that calls attention to their goals by text[12] or by voice messaging.[13] The messages include cues to pre-agreed goals and thus redirect attention to the participants' internal goal representations. They have been shown to improve on-task behaviour. There is good evidence for the effectiveness of content-free cueing in improving task performance, but weaker evidence for its impact on goal-directed behaviour. Use, once established, tends to be maintained.[14]

Memory Functions

Memory functions are employed when registering, storing and retrieving information. In this section we will address supports for episodic memory systems which underpin our autobiography, as distinct from prospective, memory discussed above.

There are two main types of ATC supporting episodic memory: cameras and multimedia reminiscence devices. SenseCam was developed by Microsoft Research, Cambridge as an outward-facing stills camera, taking photos at set intervals or when changing light levels triggered a photo-sensor. The regular review of the automatically captured images has been found to improve autobiographical memory in conditions where amnesia is prominent, such as limbic encephalitis,[15] Korsakoff's syndrome[16] and Alzheimer's disease.[17] These systems are commercially available as Narrative Clip (http://getnarrative.com/) or SnapCam (https://uk.ioncamera.com/snapcam/).

Alm et al. reported on the development and use of a touch screen interactive multimedia reminiscence tool. Users interact with the system, to activate familiar images or sound samples, to trigger personal memories, which the user can then discuss.[18] Studies with people with dementia suggested that the system was useable and enjoyed. Effect on memory recall rate or facilitation of conversation has yet to be reported. Overall, the empirical support for ATC for memory functions is limited and studies have been qualitative or single subject designs with risk of bias.

Emotional Functions

Emotional functions are related to the feeling and affective components of the processes of the mind, such as the cognitive regulation of emotion. Emotion dysregulation has been related to highly problematic social functioning after brain injury[19,20] and to the poor life choices of persons with brain injury.[21]

Technological functions that support emotion include distraction, and biofeedback. Personal stereos have been used to distract users with schizophrenia from the distressing effects of auditory hallucinations.[22] While neuropsychiatric consequences of severe head injury are common, the applications of such technologies in this population is unreported.

Biofeedback devices have been used to treat anxiety disorders.[23] O'Neill and Findlay reported two cases of chronic emotional dysregulation, and challenging behaviours after brain injury. Following daily 20 min sessions of emWave2 biofeedback on heart rate variability the frequency of externalised aggression, and self-injury respectively, decreased significantly.[24] This finding and acceptability to users justified a randomised control cross-over study and positive preliminary results have been reported.[25]

Distressed behaviour secondary to disorientation in dementia has been treated using a device with the functions affect-awareness and distraction. The system, in the form of a robot seal called *Paro* (a big-eyed furry harp seal pup) affords caregiving, and distracts from other concerns, and senses aspects of the user's physiology, and behaviour and reinforces anxiety-alleviating behaviours such as stroking. Initial clinical trials indicate that significant improvements in emotional state and quality of life resulted from integrating Paro into care facilities for persons with dementia.[26] The approach offers promise for treating distress secondary to hypoxic and severe traumatic brain injury, but no trials have yet been reported.

Awareness of state is a prerequisite for regulation. Similarly, prediction of problematic emotional states allows us to possibly prevent them. O'Neill et al. recruited two individuals with unpredictable impulsive aggression to wear smart watches that sensed galvanic skin response, heart rate, temperature and movement, and related this data to routine recordings of overt aggression. In both cases, incidents were predicted with an accuracy of about 80%, and several hours lead. Future work aims to assess the effect of feedback on physiological indicators of escalation and prompts to aid emotion regulation. Such systems might augment inpatient neurobehavioural rehabilitation (e.g. www.thedtgroup.org/brain-injury /for-professionals) for problematic social behaviour.[28]

Higher-Level Cognitive Functions

The greatest quantity and quality of evidence for assistive technology for cognition is for its effectiveness in supporting the higher-level cognitive functions of time management and planning.

Time management functions are prospective memory functions that ensure a behaviour stops, and another begins at a specific time, for example stopping ongoing activity and leaving for a doctor's appointment. Examples include aural or visual reminders to perform a given task at a particular time using voice recorders with a timer, text messaging to mobile phones, voice messages to phones, smartphone alerts or scheduling software on a PC and PDAs.[5-7] Thus if patients with neurological illness are having difficulty remembering medication regimes, or appointments, despite being motivated to do so, then prospective memory failure is likely. The simplest, evidenced intervention is to ask the person to use their phone to set a distinctive reminder, with text instruction, for example *'take morning medications'* repeating daily. Help to set up the reminder is often required.

The prompts can be either explicit statements of what action to perform,[29] or implicit, content-free cues.[11]

While there are significant difficulties in randomised controlled trials in this area, reviews of evidence for prospective memory aids have indicated strong support. A recent review performed a meta-analysis including seven group studies, and concluded there was strong evidence for the efficacy of prospective memory prompting devices for people with acquired brain injury or degenerative diseases.[7]

Technology that assists planning by acquiring context awareness and providing step-by-step support during task performance is increasingly well evidenced. Mihailidis et al. developed and tested the COACH system to support users with dementia with hand washing. A situated camera, over the sink, captures visual data on the position of the users' hands and gives auditory prompts of corrective steps if significant deviations are noted.[30] Lancioni et al. developed and trialled the VICAID palm top system to micro-prompt people with intellectual disability through vocational tasks. Key features included the simplified user interface (single button), visual and auditory prompts, and rewards for successful task completion through feedback to the user.[31] Lancioni et al. have used a smartphone to provide reminders and instructions to people with intellectual and sensory disabilities to perform daily activities.[32] O'Neill et al. examined the use of a computer system called Guide, that emulates carer prompts and questions, and responded to the users' verbal responses in a naturalistic supportive dialogue.[33] Guide has been shown to support reha-bilitation relevant sequences, to support a person with brain injury to follow a morning routine,[34] and to support two people with severe cognitive impairment to use blood glucose checking technology.[35] O'Neill et al. reported data from 24 individuals with severe cognitive impairment after brain injury, randomly assigned to Guide, or rehabilitation as usual. They found that there were significantly reduced carer interventions in morning routines for the Guide condition after daily use for 3 weeks (https://guide-research.com/).[36]

In summary, there have been over[30] published studies on reminding technologies, encompassing both macro-prompting (event reminders), and micro-prompting approaches (sequence support reminders) that, taken together, indicate moderate support for the effectiveness of assistive technology to support organisation and planning.

Experience of Self and Time Functions

Experience of self and time functions is related to the awareness of a person's identity, body, and position in the reality of their environment, and of time. People with brain injury are often acutely disoriented to facts from their own autobiographies, current time and place, and treatment rationale. Technologies in this area chiefly support awareness of self in relation to recent events, and location (i.e. navigation).

Disorientation to brain injury status, and rationale for treatment is a common distressing presentation. Brown et al. used tablet computers to present five patients with persisting disorientation at 4 months, videos of family members describing where they were and why, the aims of the rehab stay to address deficits, and goals set. On an orientation questionnaire, participants showed significant improvement in ability to recall information pertaining to awareness of deficit in 4 of 5 users.[37] Scripted orientation videos holds promise for addressing awareness difficulties, but larger trials are needed.

Text prompts to mobile phones have been successfully used to help remind participants of their rehabilitation goals.[38] Similarly, the summary of psychological formulation, arrived at in therapy has helped an individual increase awareness of their behavioural tendencies, and in so doing reduced interpersonal disputes.[39]

Robinson et al. developed two devices that use Global Positioning Systems (GPS) to locate and direct a pedestrian to a desired destination.[40] Other navigation aids use information in the environment to cue context-dependent directions. For example, Chang et al. used a series of tags to provide the basis for context-dependent navigation using a handheld device.[41] Morris et al. developed an intelligent mobility platform that generates a representation of location using sensors and guides the user on this basis.[42] Finally, Liu et al. also developed an ATC that guides the user based on an internal (pre-programmed) map of the environment.[43] Overall, evidence for the effectiveness of these navigation devices is limited to technical trials and usability studies without case control; the majority of studies of technologies to help with navigation are thus qualitative.[44]

Awareness of deficit is a significant barrier to engagement in rehabilitation. A randomised control trial invited 54 participants with TBI to carry out a meal preparation task four times and to then receive one of three types of feedback: watching a video of performance plus verbal feedback, verbal feedback or experiential feedback. The study found that video plus verbal feedback was most effective in improving awareness, without impacting emotional status.[45] Tablet computers offer portability, a short lag between filming and review, and thereby a practical means of supporting insight.

In summary, the strongest available evidence of the effectiveness of ATCs is for supporting prospective memory and planning. There is some support for the use of ATC to support emotion regulation and to facilitate attention to personal goals. And the use of portable tablets to present orientation information or feedback on performance promises support for orientation and insight.

Facilitating Use

People with cognitive impairment are making increasing use of smartphones and tablet ATC.[46] Barriers to their use may be overcome and engagement facilitated through personalisation to user motivations, level of insight and preferences.

Users vary in their motivation to use ATC, even in studies where they have been shown to be effective.[47] Previous experience of technology, the perceived stigma of using a support, and insight into their unaided task performance each affect motivation to engage. Users will also vary in their motivation to perform the target behaviours. Technologies have the potential to not only help users complete tasks they would otherwise be unable to, they can help to initiate and to maintain new behaviours. Text message prompts can lead to lasting change in health behaviours in healthy populations[48] and are most effective if received near the moment of decision-making[49] or if messages are personalised to the individual or the current situation.[50] In people with substance misuse, a frequent TBI co-morbidity, just-in-time prompting uses input from the user and environment to assess risk, providing simple encouragement when risk is low, or prompting an intervention when risk increases.[49] Just-in-time adaptive interventions include prompting use of tangible resources for problem solving;[51,52] enhancing specific self-efficacy;[53] facilitating seeking support from others,[54] even reducing the need for the user to actively seek help.[55] The feasibility of these interventions is allowed by advances in sensing technologies, situational modelling, and personal technologies that collect data about users' behaviour.[50] There is increasing interest in the use of sensing technologies to deliver adaptive interventions in brain injury rehabilitation,[24,56] where a key aim is to support people to organise their time to be functional and rewarding. As well as supporting prospective memory by prompting at the right time, devices can also support the independent initiation and engagement in the scheduling of activities. Stawarz and colleagues developed a medication reminding system that fostered habit formation by using event based prompts, instead of more common time based prompts, for example to set your daily schedule each morning after breakfast.[57] Such design for habit formation utilises behavioural antecedents or triggers, motivation to engage in a behaviour, and technology support for performance of the behaviour (in line with persuasive design frameworks such as that by Fogg et al.[58]

Anosognosia challenges rehabilitation delivery. Commencing interventions before the client has accepted the need for support often potentiates rehabilitation failure.[59] Additionally, therapists prompts are common antecedents of aggressive behaviour,[60] presumably as interpersonal directives can be noxious. On the other hand receiving cues from a device can increase feelings of autonomy. An example of this is the GUIDE system that delivers personalised prompts to aid in the performance of complex sequences such as personal care routines. This system has been shown to be as effective as a human caregiver support for morning routines, yet removes the need for carers to be in patients' rooms, which can be perceived as intrusive.[27] Similarly, people can perceive reminders from family or carers as nagging, but accept the same prompts as texts to a phone, apparently seeing themselves as active agents, using a phone.

Increasing the accessibility of scheduling software increases scheduling behaviour.[61] Web interface design guidelines have been developed to ensure that people with cognitive impairment have enough time to understand content; can navigate easily (via clear titles and headings); easily comprehend text; and help to avoid or easily correct mistakes.[62] Cognitive impairments after brain injury give rise to different accessibility requirements for assistive technologies. The top four recommendations collated from the literature were use of pictures, icons, or symbols along with text; clear and simple text; use of consistent navigation and design on every page; and use of headings, titles, and prompts.[63]

These guidelines ought to influence choices when selecting or creating an ATC. For example, where information presented is restricted by the screen size of portable devices, the evidence suggests that a narrow/deep user interface (several layered screens each with less information) is preferable,[64] and scheduling applications to broad/shallow approach (few screens each with a lot of information).[65,66] Another design choice is the degree of pro-activity of apps in attempting to engage the user's attention. Unsolicited push-notifications risk being annoying, but were found to result in participants with brain injury setting many more reminders, without being negatively appraised.[61] Verbally mediated interfaces (e.g. voice assistants) promise cognitive support with reduced distraction from the ongoing task. Theory-based design to improve the accessibility of assistive technologies.

For both high- and low-impairment groups, it is insufficient to prescribe and pro-gramme a device, and send users away with it. An iterative process of selection, systematic instruction, support and individual tailoring is required. Intensive systematic instruction facilitates the use of ATCs.[67]

Conclusion

We hope to have demonstrated that early research shows effectiveness of devices for supporting aspects of attention, prospective memory, the organisation of behaviour and insight. The lag between technological development, and clinical trials may hopefully be met by increasing interest amongst health care professionals, academics and industry, to support trials. We realise that the skill set for this work, is niche. As such, we invite interested professionals to get in touch for advice on available technologies, the use of small sample and single case experimental designs to demonstrate effectiveness in those they serve.

We conclude with cautious optimism regarding this new set of potentially powerful rehabilitation tools. Humans produce technologies to extend their abilities. The technical environment and social practices are continuously refined to support cognition and behaviour. Our environment now includes portable electronic devices that closely emu-late brain function, and are widely used by healthy people to augment their cognitive abilities. These same devices, now normal and valued, hold great potential to meet the needs of those with cognitive and functional impairment. This potential will only be fully realised by clinicians who are aware of ATC, and implement its use to help their patients meet their needs.

References

1. Finger S. *Minds behind the brain: a history of the pioneers and their discoveries.* New York: Oxford; 2000.

2. O'Neill B, Gillespie A. *Assistive technology for cognition: a handbook for clinicians and developers.* Hove, UK: Psychology Press; 2014.

3. Fodor JA. *The modularity of mind.* Cambridge, MA: MIT Press; 1983.

4. World Health Organization. International classification of functioning, disability and

health (ICF); 2002. www.who.int/classifica
tions/icf/en/

5. De Joode E, van Heugten C, Verhey F, van Boxtel M. Efficacy and usability of assistive technology for patients with cognitive deficits: a systematic review. *Clin Rehabil* 2010;24:701–14.

6. Gillespie A, Best C, O'Neill B. Cognitive function and assistive technology for cognition: a systematic review. *J Int Neuropsychol Soc* 2012;18:1–19.

7. Jamieson M, Cullen B, McGee-Lennon M, Brewster B, Evans JJ. The efficacy of cognitive prosthetic technology for people with memory impairments: a systematic review and meta-analysis. *Neuropsychol Rehabil* 2014;24(3–4):419–44.

8. Robertson IH, Mattingley JB, Rorden C, Driver J. Phasic alerting of neglect patients overcomes their spatial deficit in visual awareness. *Nature* 1998;395: 169–72.

9. Manly T, Hawkins K, Evans J, Woldt K, Robertson IH. Rehabilitation of executive function: facilitation of effective goal management on complex tasks using periodic auditory alerts. *Neuropsychologia* 2002;40(3):271–81.

10. Rich LP. *Prompting self-monitoring with assistive technology to increase academic engagement in students with attention-deficit/hyperactivity disorder symptoms.* Unpublished PsyD thesis, Hofstra University, New York; 2009.

11. Fish J, Evans JJ, Nimmo M, Martin E, Kersel D, Bateman A, Manly, T. Rehabilitation of executive dysfunction following brain injury: 'content-free' cueing improves everyday prospective memory performance. *Neuropsychologia* 2007;45(6):1318–30.

12. Yeates G, Hamill M, Sutton L, Psaila K, Gracey F, Mohamed S, O'Dell J. Dysexecutive problems and interpersonal relating following frontal brain injury: Reformulation and compensation in cognitive analytic therapy (CAT). *Neuropsychoanalysis* 2008;10(1): 43–58.

13. Hart T, Hawkey K, Whyte J. Use of a portable voice organizer to remember therapy goals in traumatic brain injury rehabilitation: a within-subjects trial. *J Head Trauma Rehabil* 2002;17(6):556–70.

14. Svoboda E, Richards B, Yao C, Leach L. Long-term maintenance of smartphone and PDA use in individuals with moderate to severe memory impairment. *Neuropsychol Rehabil* 2015;25(3): 353–73.

15. Berry E, Kapur N, Williams L, Hodges S, Watson P, Smyth G., Wood K. The use of a wearable camera, SenseCam, as a pictorial diary to improve autobiographical memory in a patient with limbic encephalitis: a preliminary report. *Neuropsychol Rehabil* 2007;17(4–5):582–601.

16. Svanberg J, Evans JJ. Impact of SenseCam on memory, identity and mood in Korsakoff's syndrome: a single case experimental design study. *Neuropsychol Rehabil* 2014;24(3–4): 400–18.

17. Woodberry E, Browne G, Hodges S, Watson P, Kapur N, Woodberry K. The use of a wearable camera improves autobiographical memory in patients with Alzheimer's disease. *Memory* 2015;23 (3):340–349.

18. Alm N, Astell A, Ellis M, Dye R, Gowans G, Campbell J. A cognitive prosthesis and communication support for people with dementia. *Neuropsychol Rehabil* 2004;14 (1–2):117–34.

19. Bond MR, Brooks DN, McKinlay W. Burdens imposed on the relatives of those with severe brain damage due to injury. *Acta Neurochir* 1979;28(suppl):124–5.

20. Gosling J, Oddy M. Rearranged marriages: marital relationships after head injury. *Brain Injury* 1999;13(10):785–96.

21. Wood RL. Understanding neurobehavioural disability. In Wood RL, McMillan TM, eds. *Neurobehavioural disability and social handicap following traumatic brain injury.* Hove, UK: Psychology Press; 2001.

22. McInnis M, Marks I. Audiotape therapy for persistent auditory hallucinations. *Br J Psychiatr* 1990;157(6):913–14.

23. Reiner R. Integrating a portable biofeedback device into clinical practice for patients with anxiety disorders: results of a pilot study. *Appl Psychophysiol Biofeedback* 2008;33(1):55–61.

24. O'Neill B, Findlay G. Single case methodology in neurobehavioural rehabilitation: preliminary findings on biofeedback in the treatment of challenging behaviour. *Neuropsychol Rehabil* 2014;24 (3–4):365–81.

25. Habib F, O'Neill B, Evans JJ. Biofeedback in treatment of challenging behaviour after brain injury. Poster at the 11th Conference of the Neuropsychological Rehabilitation Special Interest Group of the World Federation for NeuroRehabilitation (WFNR), Limasol, Cyprus; 2014.

26. Bemelmans R, Gelderblom GJ, Jonker P, de Witte L. Effectiveness of robot Paro in intramural psychogeriatric care: a multicentre quasi-experimental study. *J Am Med Directors Assoc* 2015;16 (11):946–50.

27. O'Neill B, Best C, O'Neill L, Ramos, SDS, Gillespie A. Efficacy of a micro-prompting technology in reducing support needed by people with severe acquired brain injury in activities of daily living: a randomized control trial. *J Head Trauma Rehabil* 2017;29.

28. Worthington AD, Matthews S, Melia Y, Oddy M. Cost-benefits associated with social outcome from neurobehavioural rehabilitation. *Brain Injury* 2006;20 (9):947–57.

29. Wilson BA, Emslie HC, Quirk K, Evans JJ. Reducing everyday memory and planning problems by means of a paging system: a randomised control crossover study. *J Neurol Neurosurg Psychiatr* 2001;70 (4):477–82.

30. Mihailidis A. The efficacy of an intelligent cognitive orthosis to facilitate handwashing by persons with moderate to severe dementia. *Neuropsychol Rehabil* 2008;14(1–2):135–71.

31. Lancioni GE, O'Reilly MF, Seedhouse P, Furniss F, Cunha B. Promoting independent task performance by persons with severe developmental disabilities through a new computer-aided system. *Behavior Modification* 2000;24(5):700–18.

32. Lancioni GE, Singh NN, O'Reilly MF, Sigafoos J, Alberti G, Zimbaro C, Chiariello V. Using smartphones to help people with intellectual and sensory disabilities perform daily activities. *Front Public Health* 2017;5:282.

33. O'Neill B, Moran K, Gillespie A. Scaffolding rehabilitation behaviour using a voice mediated assistive technology for cognition. *Neuropsychol Rehabil* 2010;18:1–19.

34. O'Neill B, Best C, O'Neill L, Gillespie A. Automated prompting technologies in rehabilitation and at home. *Social Care Neurodisability* 2013;4(1):17–28.

35. Moir J, Evans JJ, O'Neill B. Assistive technology for supporting diabetes self-management in persons with cognitive impairment following acquired brain injury. Unpublished.

36. O'Neill B, Gillespie A. Assistive technology, disability and rehabilitation. In: McMillan TM, Wood RLL, eds. *Neurobehavioural Disability and Social Handicap Following Traumatic Brain Injury*. 2nd ed. Hove, UK: Psychology Press, 2017.

37. Brown P, Clark A, Seddon E, O'Neill B. Scripted orientation videos and awareness of deficit. Poster at the 10th Conference of the Neuropsychological Rehabilitation Special Interest Group of the World Federation for NeuroRehabilitation (WFNR), Maastricht, Netherlands; 2013.

38. Culley C, Evans JJ. SMS text messaging as a means of increasing recall of therapy goals in brain injury rehabilitation: a single-blind within-subjects trial. *Neuropsychol Rehabil* 2010;20(1):103–19.

39. Yeates G, Hamill M, Sutton L, Psaila K, Gracey F, Mohamed S, O'Dell J. Dysexecutive problems and interpersonal relating following frontal brain injury: reformulation and compensation in

cognitive analytic therapy (CAT). *Neuropsychoanalysis* 2008;10(1):43–58.

40. Robinson L, Brittain K, Lindsay S, Jackson D, Olivier P. Keeping In Touch Everyday (KITE) project: developing assistive technologies with people with dementia and their carers to promote independence. *Int Psychogeriatr* 2009;21 (3):494–502.

41. Chang YJ, Tsai SK, Wang TY. A context aware handheld wayfinding system for individuals with cognitive impairments. In: *Proceedings of the 10th international ACM SIGACCESS conference on computers and accessibility.* New York: Association for Computing Machinery; 2008.

42. Morris A, Donamukkala R, Kapuria A, Steinfeld A, Matthews JT, Dunbar-Jacob J, Thrun S. A robotic walker that provides guidance. In *Robotics and automation: Proceedings ICRA'03.* Vol. 1. New York: IEEE; 2003.

43. Liu X, Makino H, Maeda Y. Basic study on indoor location estimation using visible light communication platform. In *Engineering in medicine and biology society.* New York: IEEE; 2008.

44. Harniss M, Brown P, Johnson K. Cognitive technologies for wayfinding. In: O'Neill B, Gillespie A, eds. *Assistive technology for cognition.* Hove, UK: Psychology Press; 2014.

45. Schmidt J, Fleming J, Ownsworth T. Lannin NA Video feedback on functional task performance improves self-awareness after traumatic brain injury a randomized controlled trial. *Neurorehabil Neural Repair* 2013;27(4):316–24.

46. Jamieson M, McGee-Lennon M, Cullen B, Brewster S, Evans J. Issues influencing the uptake of smartphone reminder apps for people with acquired brain injury. In: *Proceedings of the 17th international ACM SIGACCESS conference on computers and accessibility.* New York: ACM; 2015.

47. Kerssens C, Kumar R, Adams AE, Knott CC, Matalenas L, Sanford JA, Rogers WA. Personalized technology to support older adults with and without

cognitive impairment living at home. *Am J Alzheimer's Dis Other Dementias* 2015;30 (1):85–97.

48. Abroms LC, Whittaker R, Free C, Van Alstyne JM, Schindler-Ruwisch JM. Developing and pretesting a text messaging program for health behavior change: recommended steps. *JMIR mHealth and uHealth* 2015;3(4):e107.

49. Kumar S, Nilsen WJ, Abernethy A, Atienza A, Patrick K, Pavel, M., Spruijt-Metz, D. Mobile health technology evaluation: the mhealth evidence workshop. *Am J Preventive Med* 2013;45 (2):228–36.

50. Nahum-Shani I, Smith SN, Tewari A, Witkiewitz K, Collins LM, Spring B, Murphy S. Just in time adaptive interventions (jitais): an organizing framework for ongoing health behavior support. Technical report 14-126. Methodology Center, Penn State; 2014.

51. King AC, Hekler EB, Grieco LA, Winter SJ, Sheats JL, Buman MP, Cirimele, J. Harnessing different motivational frames via mobile phones to promote daily physical activity and reduce sedentary behavior in aging adults. *PLoS One*;2013;8 (4):e62613.

52. Lin JJ, Mamykina L, Lindtner S, Delajoux G, Strub HB. Fish'n'Steps: encouraging physical activity with an interactive computer game. In Dourish P, Friday A, eds. *Ubiquitous computing.* Berlin: Springer; 2006.

53. Dennison L, Morrison L, Conway G, Yardley L. Opportunities and challenges for smartphone applications in supporting health behavior change: qualitative study. *J Med Internet Res* 2013;15(4):e86.

54. Rotheram-Borus MJ, Tomlinson M, Gwegwe M, Comulada WS, Kaufman N, Keim M. Diabetes buddies peer support through a mobile phone buddy system. *Diabetes Educator* 2012;38(3):357–65.

55. Nundy S, Dick JJ, Goddu AP, Hogan P, Lu C-YE, Solomon MC, Peek ME. Using mobile health to support the chronic care model: developing an institutional

initiate. *Int J Telemed Appl* 2012. doi:10.1155/2012/871925

56. Lee SI, Adans-Dester C, O'Brien A, Diaz GV, Black-Schaffer R, Patel S, Bonato P. Using wearable motion sensors to estimate longitudinal changes in movement quality in stroke and traumatic brain injury survivors undergoing rehabilitation. *Arch Phys Med Rehabil* 2016;97(10):e117.

57. Stawarz K, Cox AL, Blandford A. Don't forget your pill! Designing effective medication reminder apps that support users' daily routines. In *Proceedings of the 32nd annual ACM conference on human factors in computing systems*. New York: ACM; 2014.

58. Fogg BJ. A behavior model for persuasive design. In *Proceedings of the 4th international conference on persuasive technology*. New York: ACM; 2009.

59. Van den Broek MD. Why does neurorehabilitation fail? *J Head Trauma Rehabil* 2005;20(5):464–73.

60. Alderman N, Knight C, Morgan C. Use of a modified version of the Overt Aggression Scale in the measurement and assessment of aggressive behaviours following brain injury. *Brain Injury* 1997;11(7):503–23.

61. Jamieson M, O'Neill B, Cullen B, Lennon M, Brewster S, Evans J. ForgetMeNot: active reminder entry support for adults with acquired brain injury. In: *Proceedings of the 2017 CHI conference on human factors in computing systems*. New York: ACM; 2017.

62. Web Content Accessibility Guidelines 1.0. www.w3.org/TR/WCAG10/

63. Friedman MG, Bryen DN. Web accessibility design recommendations for people with cognitive disabilities. *Technol Disabil* 2007;19(4):205–12.

64. Hu R, Feng JH. Investigating information search by people with cognitive disabilities. *ACM Trans Accessible Comput* 2015;7 (1):1-30.

65. De Joode E, Proot I, Slegers K, van Heugten C, Verhey F, van Boxtel M. The use of standard calendar software by individuals with acquired brain injury and cognitive complaints: a mixed methods study. *Disabil Rehabil Assist Technol* 2012;7 (5):389–98.

66. Jamieson M. Investigating assistive technology to support memory for people with cognitive impairments. PhD dissertation, University of Glasgow; 2016.

67. Powell LE, Glang A, Pinkelman S, Albin R, Harwick R, Ettel D, Wild MR. Systematic instruction of assistive technology for cognition (ATC) in an employment setting following acquired brain injury: a single case, experimental study. *NeuroRehabilitation* 2015;37(3):437–47.

Chapter 28

Outcomes and Prognosis

Helen M. K. Gooday

Introduction

Brain injury remains a major cause of disability and death, especially in young people. In survivors, the extent of recovery depends largely on the severity of the injury. Residual disabilities include both cognitive and physical impairments with the most rapid recovery often occurring within the first 6 months after injury, but improvement may continue for years.

Outcome after TBI also depends on many other factors including patient and injury characteristics such as premorbid state (e.g. older age, comorbidities, personality, cognitive functioning), mechanism of trauma, presence and severity of extracranial injuries, patient response, quality of care and the social environment.

Linking patient and injury characteristics at presentation to outcome is the science of prognosis. Clinicians treating patients often make therapeutic decisions based on their assessment of prognosis, and assessment of prognosis is also important in relation to counselling patients and relatives. Despite this, clinicians are often reluctant to make predictions in relation to the outcome of individual patients.

Severity Measures

A wide variety of measures have been used to assess the severity of the brain injury. Some of the most commonly described ones are detailed below.

Coma/Level of Awareness

The longer the duration of coma (as measured by the time to follow commands) the more likely a worse outcome.[1] In particular, a duration of coma greater than 4 weeks makes a good recovery unlikely. Loss of consciousness for 30 min or less is often associated with mild brain injury. Although a low initial Glasgow Coma Scale (GCS) score is correlated with worse outcomes, specificity is lacking indicating that some patients with a low GCS can achieve a good recovery and vice versa.

Post-traumatic Amnesia (PTA)

PTA is defined as a period of time from the initial brain injury until the individual's memory for ongoing events becomes reliable, consistent and accurate. In general, a longer duration of PTA correlates with a worse outcome. A PTA of less than an hour is regarded as a mild brain injury and a PTA exceeding 4 weeks reflects an extremely severe injury.

MRI Scan

MRI scanning sequences have been utilised to try and offer prognostic information at an early stage (see Chapter 5). A number of studies have been undertaken which have looked at MRI scan results from 2–4 weeks after injury and outcome.[2–8] A recent systematic review and meta-analysis of studies evaluated the predictive value of acute MRI lesion patterns for discriminating clinical outcome in moderate and severe TBI. It found a strong association between brain stem lesions on MRI and unfavourable long-term prognosis. Injury to any region of the brain stem was significantly predictive of both all-cause mortality and unfavourable neurological outcome. Classification of the depth of brain injury visualised on MRI by radiological scores was also predictive of unfavourable outcome. However, it was noted that there was a high risk of bias in the current body of literature, and that large, well-controlled studies were necessary to better quantify the prognostic role of early MRI in moderate and severe TBI.[9] One study of patients with diffuse axonal injury found all those with diffuse axonal injury on MRI scan had severe disability at 1 year post-injury.[7] At present, there is limited evidence that MRI scanning can improve outcome prediction in mild TBI.[10] It is hoped that MRI and newer neuroimaging tools such as diffusion tensor imaging will be increasingly useful in relation to providing prognostic information.[11]

CT Scan

The presence of subarachnoid haemorrhage, cisternal effacement, significant midline shift, extradural haematoma or subdural haematoma on an acute care CT scan is associated with worse outcomes. Owing to individual patient factors, including the burden of secondary insults, more specific conclusions about the implications of the lesions cannot be drawn.[12] However, data from CT scan results now provides an important contribution to computer-based prognostic modelling, as described in the CRASH trial.[13]

Outcome Measures

A range of different tools are also used to assess outcome after brain injury. These are discussed below.

The Glasgow Outcome Scale (GOS)

The GOS[14–16] was commonly used before other scales were developed, and is the most widely used outcome measure in brain injury research. The five categories of the original scale are dead, vegetative, severely disabled, moderately disabled and good recovery. An extended version of the scale (GOSE) divides each of the latter three categories into two providing a scale from 1 to 8 (Table 28.1).[15]

The Disability Rating Scale (DRS)

The DRS[17] measures disability levels following severe brain injury from coma to the community (Table 28.2). The measure is commonly employed in the brain injury outcome literature. The total score ranges from 30 (death) to 0 (no disability) with a range of intermediary levels including mild, partial, moderate and severely extreme limitation and two grades of vegetative state. These all have numerical values derived from summation of individual components of the scale.

Table 28.1 The Glasgow Outcome Scale[4]

GOS	GOSE	
1	1	*Death*
2	2	*Vegetative State* (see text)
3		*Severe disability; conscious but dependent*
	3	Communication is possible, minimally by emotional response; total or almost total dependency with regard to activities of daily life.
	4	Partial independence in activities of daily life, may require assistance for only one activity, such as dressing; many evident post-traumatic complaints and/or signs; resumption of former life and work not possible
4		*Moderate disability; independent but disabled*
	5	Independent in activities of daily life, for instance can travel by public transport; not able to resume previous activities either at work or socially; despite evident post-traumatic signs, resumption of activities at a lower level is often possible
	6	Post-traumatic signs are present; however, resumption of most former activities either full-time or part-time
5		*Good recovery*
	7	Capable of resuming normal occupation and social activities; there are minor physical or mental deficits or complaints
	8	Full recovery without symptoms or signs

Source: Reproduced with permission from the BMJ Publishing Group.

Other more functionally based measures include the Barthel Index,[18] the Functional Independence Measure (FIM) and the Functional Assessment Measure (FAM).[19,20] For specific rehabilitation programmes, use of goal achievement often provides a more reliable and sensitive outcome measure, for example goal attainment scaling (GAS).[21,22]

Threshold Values

Although there is now an enormous body of literature which demonstrates factors that are likely to lead to a good or poor prognosis after brain injury, this generally only provides information about populations of patients, and cannot necessarily be applied to individual patients. This is therefore of limited value to clinicians.

The concept of 'threshold values' is of much greater practical usefulness in relation to providing prognostic information to individual families or patients. A 'threshold value' is a value of a predictor variable above or below which a particular outcome is especially unlikely. For example, several studies have reported that no patients with PTA exceeding 3 months achieved a good recovery as defined by the GOS. Thus, 3 months would be considered a threshold value for the duration of PTA, at least in terms of excluding the possibility of a good recovery on the GOS. As the length of a patient's PTA extends beyond 3

Table 28.2 The Disability Rating Scale

Arousability, awareness and responsibility		
Eye opening	**Communication ability (verbal, written, letter board or sign)**	**Best motor response**
0 Spontaneous	0 Orientated	0 Obeying
1 To speech	1 Confused	1 Localising
2 To pain	2 Inappropriate	2 Withdrawing
3 None	3 Incomprehensible	3 Flexing
	4 None	4 Extending
		5 None
Cognitive ability for self-care activities (Does patient know how and when? Ignore motor disability?)		
Feeding	Toileting	Grooming
0 Complete	0 Complete	0 Complete
1 Partial	1 Partial	1 Partial
2 Minimal	2 Minimal	2 Minimal
3 None	3 None	3 None
Level of functioning (consider both physical and cognitive disability)		*'Employability' (as a full-time worker, homeworker or student)*
0 Completely independent		0 Not restricted
1 Independent in special environment		1 Selected job, competitive
2 Mildly dependent		2 Sheltered workshop, non-competitive
3 Moderately dependent		3 Not employable
4 Markedly dependent		
5 Totally dependent		
Categorisation of outcome scores (limitations, severity)		
0 None	4–6 Moderate	17–21 Extremely severe
1 Mild	7–11 Moderately severe	22–24 Vegetative state
2–3 Partial	12–16 Severe	25–29 Extreme vegetative state
		30 Dead

Source: Reproduced with permission from Elsevier © 1982.

months, clinicians can counsel family members about realistic expectations for the future. On the other hand, if 2 months have not yet elapsed since the injury, clinicians can give hope to families even if the patient is still in PTA. Threshold values can be seen as 'milestones' in a patient's recovery.[12]

Prognostic Models

Prognostic models are statistical models that combine data from patients to predict outcome, and they are more likely to be accurate than simple clinical predictions. Data collected in the Medical Research Council (MRC) CRASH trial was used to develop prognostic models to obtain valid predictions of relevant outcomes in patients with traumatic brain injury.[13] Extensive work by the IMPACT study group, which analysed individual patient data from more than 10 000 patients with severe or moderate TBI merged from 11 studies, confirmed age, GCS motor score, pupillary response and CT characteristics as the most powerful independent prognostic variables.[23] With advances in statistical modelling and the availability of large datasets, it has been possible to develop prognostic models that are increasingly useful in clinical practice, research and the assessment of quality in health care.[24]

Disability and Outcome after Brain Injury

More than 150 000 patients with a brain injury are known to be admitted to hospital each year in the UK. Estimates of the frequency of subsequent disability in such patients previously ranged from two or three to 45 per 100 000 population per year.[25–28] This variation reflected limitations in previous studies, particularly the lack of data on patients with an apparently mild injury, who account for 80% of admissions.[25] Using extrapolated data from the population a prospective study conducted in Glasgow identified the incidence of disability admitted with a brain injury was 100–150 per 100 000 population, much greater than previously anticipated.[29] The study also showed that increased severity of injury on admission was associated with increased rate of death or vegetative state, and a decreased rate of good recovery: however the initial severity of injury was not related to late disability, which occurred in almost half of each group. Survival with moderate or severe disability was common after mild head injury (47%) and similar to that after moderate (45%) or severe injury (48%).

Prolonged Disorders of Consciousness: Vegetative and Minimally Conscious States

After severe injury many patients regain an independent existence and may return to premorbid social and occupational activities.[30] Inevitably, some remain severely disabled requiring long-term care, including a very small proportion (<2%) who go on to experience prolonged disorders of consciousness (PDOC).

The vegetative state (more recently termed the unresponsive wakefulness syndrome[31]) is a clinical condition of complete unawareness of the self and the environment accompanied by sleep–wake cycles with either complete or partial preservation of hypothalamic and brain stem autonomic functions.[32,33] The persistent vegetative state (PVS) can be judged to be permanent 12 months after traumatic injury in adults and children. The Minimally Conscious State (MCS) is a condition of severely altered consciousness in which there is minimal but definite behavioural evidence of self- or environmental awareness.[34]

Accurate diagnosis is important in relation clinical management, as decisions typically include the possibility of treatment being withdrawn. However, current clinical methods of diagnosis lack accuracy and it has been suggested that guidelines should be modified to include functional imaging as an independent source of diagnostically relevant information.[32]

Data on prognosis for patients in a vegetative state remains limited. There is evidence that time spent in the vegetative state, age and type of brain injury affect prognosis with younger patients showing better recovery rates. Functional neuroimaging can be used to rule out a diagnosis of vegetative state with quantitative measurements of brain activity positively correlated with recovery.[35–37] In adults who are in a vegetative state at 1 month post-injury, 33% will die by 12 months, 15% will remain in PVS and 52% will recover consciousness, although only 7% will make a good recovery as defined by the GOS.[38] The limited information available suggests that improvement is more likely in patients in a MCS compared with patients in a PVS, with greater likelihood of emerging from MCS.[39] Positron emission tomography (PET) imaging may be more accurate than functional MRI, and therefore of greater utility in relation to diagnosis and prognosis.[40]

Outcome after Severe and Moderate Brain Injury

A systematic review of published, peer-reviewed literature showed that, in adults, moderate and severe TBIs were associated with cognitive deficits 6 months or longer post-injury.[41] A prospective, multicentre Dutch study of patients with moderate and severe TBI showed a relatively high 6 month mortality rate for both severe (46%) and moderate (21%) brain injuries.[42] At 1 year post-injury, 45% of moderate and 52% of severe TBI survivors still experienced disability (as defined by a score of six or less on the GOSE). It was noted that the patients were more elderly than in previous comparable studies, which was thought to explain the relatively disappointing results.

Outcomes after moderate TBI have previously been described as being less uncertain than after severe TBI, with more than 90% of individuals with moderate TBI achieving either moderate disability or good recovery.[43,44] There are certain risk factors associated with the poorer outcomes: lower GCS scores, older age and abnormalities on the CT scan.[43,44] When these are present, patients are more likely to have moderate or severe degrees of disability. However, the above studies have shown that even individuals who make a good recovery often have residual neuro-behavioural problems.

Outcome after Mild Brain Injury

There is no universally agreed definition of mild brain injury. In 1993 the American Congress of Rehabilitation Medicine Head Injury Special Interest Group on Mild Traumatic Brain Injury defined mild traumatic brain injury as an injury to the head or mechanical forces applied to the head involving loss of consciousness for less than 30 min (possibly no loss of consciousness) with post-traumatic amnesia for less than 24 hours.[45] Some researchers have differentiated complicated and uncomplicated mild TBI.[46] A complicated mild TBI is diagnosed if the person has a GCS score of 13–15 but shows some brain abnormality (e.g. oedema, haematoma or contusion) on a CT scan.

Patients who sustained a mild brain injury were previously believed to have no organic sequelae, and symptoms of post-concussion syndrome were considered to be psychiatric or psychological in nature, or due to malingering.[47,48] It is now known that a small proportion of patients who have had a mild TBI do have long-lasting neurological and cognitive impairment. It has been shown that the outcome from mild TBI depends on a combination of pre-injury, injury and post-injury factors.[49] A systematic review of meta-analyses on the cognitive sequelae of mild TBI showed that overall recovery occurred by 90 days post-injury for most individuals and by 7 days post-injury for athletes.[50] Post-concussional syndrome is discussed in more detail in Chapter 26.

Compounding Effects of Secondary Insults

Primary traumatic damage to the brain may be made worse by the superimposition of 'secondary insults'. These can occur soon after the injury, during transfer to the hospital and during the subsequent treatment of the brain-injured patient. Such insults may be of either intracranial or systemic origin (i.e. hypotension, hypoxaemia, pyrexia) and may arise during initial management or later in intensive care. Secondary insults were characterised in the 1970s and 1980s, when a number of researchers reported that in severely brain-injured patients hypoxia was found in 30% and arterial hypotension in 15% on arrival in the emergency department. Secondary insults also occur within the intensive care environment. Gopinath et al. used a jugular venous catheter to identify episodes of jugular venous desaturation and reported that episodes of desaturation were strongly associated with a poor neurological outcome. Just a single desaturation increased the incidence of poor outcome from 55% to 75%.[51] More recently, the occurrence of secondary insults prior to or on admission to hospital in TBI patients was shown to be strongly related to poorer outcome.[52] Much of the focus of modern brain injury management is therefore directed at minimising the incidence and severity of such insults. These are discussed in detail in other chapters of this book.

Long-Term Outcome

Risk for Dementia and Other Neurological Disorders

For the past 20 years there has been considerable interest in the relation between traumatic brain injury and the future development of cognitive impairmen.[53,54] It has been suggested that traumatic brain injuries reduce 'cognitive reserve', resulting in increased vulnerability to developing dementia.[55] An epidemiological association between TBI and the development of Alzheimer's disease later in life has been demonstrated.[56] There have been few large scale studies with long-term follow-up. A recent large population-based observational cohort study in Denmark showed that TBI was associated with an increased risk of dementia, even for those who had sustained a mild TBI.[57] This contrasts with a previous systematic review, which found no evidence that patients who had a mild TBI were at risk of dementia.[58] In addition to the direct pathophysiological consequences of TBI on the brain, it was noted that TBI is associated with higher rates of depression, alcohol abuse, and sedentary lifestyle, which are all risk factors for dementia.[59] It has been suggested that traumatic encephalopathy is a spectrum disorder that shares clinical and neuro-pathological hallmarks with other neurodegenerative disorders, such as Alzheimer's disease, Parkinson's disease, frontotemporal dementia, and Lewy body dementia.[60] TBI is known to be a cause of epilepsy.[61] TBI might also confer a long-term risk for stroke[62,63] and Parkinson's disease,[64–66] and is associated with an increased long-term mortality rate[67] in including an increased risk of suicide.[68] It is well recognised that repeated concussive or subconcussive blows as experienced by various athletes, and particularly boxers, sometimes induce the development of neurological signs and progressive dementia.[69] This condition, initially known as 'dementia pugilistica', and more recently termed chronic traumatic encephalopathy (CTE), may develop some years after the last injury and is most likely to develop in boxers with long careers who have been dazed, if not knocked out, on many occasions. In a detailed study of the brains of 15 ex-boxers, one of the characteristic patterns of damage was the presence of many neurofibrillary tangles diffusely throughout the cerebral cortex and the brain stem.[70] These tangles broadly conformed to the topographic pattern found in Alzheimer's disease.

More recently, other athletes involved in contact sports who have sustained repeated minor concussion have been studied using neuroimaging and neuropsychological assessment. There is evidence that three or more concussions are associated with small but measurable cumulative effects, and increased risk for future concussions.[71]

Researchers have described distinct pathological features of CTE as well as a wide range of clinical symptom presentations. These clinical symptoms are highly variable, non-specific to individuals described as having CTE pathology in case reports, and are often associated with many other factors.[72] This is currently an area of intense interest, and research is currently under way in Scotland to look at the health records of amateur footballers in a large prospective study.[73]

Genetic Factors and Outcome from Head Injury

Apolipoprotein E4 (APOE 4) is a lipid transporter in the brain and cerebrospinal fluid.[74] It is the product of a single gene. The presence of APOE 4 alleles, especially in the homozygous condition, appear to be associated with worse outcome after TBI,[75] although other studies have had contradictory results. APOE 4 is believed to play a role in the inflammatory response and neuronal repair following trauma. It has been associated with age-related cognitive impairment, decreased synapse–neurone ratio, increased susceptibility to neuro-toxins and hippocampal atrophy.[76] A meta-analysis published in 2008 indicated that the presence of the APOE4 allele was not associated with the initial severity of brain injury following TBI but was associated with increased risk of poor long-term outcome at 6 months after injury.[77] There is also some limited data to suggest that APOE e4 allele is associated with poor global outcomes after TBI in children.[78]

Special Populations: Older Age

With increasing longevity, and an increase in the elderly population, management of, and outcome from TBI in elderly people is increasingly important. The main cause of TBI in this population is falls, followed by motor vehicle accidents.[79] Older patients have a worse outcome after a TBI, and the lower the admission GCS, the more likely an unfavourable outcome. In particular, in patients over 65, the chances of a good recovery after severe TBI are unlikely. There are many potential reasons for this, ranging from the nature of the injuries in the elderly (e.g. subdural haematomas) to age-related changes in the brain (e.g. decreased functional reserve, less elasticity of blood vessels). Several authors have noted that, in terms of outcome, a moderate TBI in the elderly resembles a severe TBI in a younger person.[80–82] Even the outcomes of mild TBI in the elderly are much worse, with many never returning to their pre-morbid functional status.[83] However, certain 'younger elderly' people, aged 65–75 years, could have a comparable outcome to younger adults after minor to moderate brain injury, particularly if treated more aggressively in neurosurgical and rehabilitation settings.[79]

Special Populations: Penetrating Injuries

The early mortality rate after penetrating injury is much higher than that of closed brain injury.[84] Lower GCS scores and CT findings of bilaterality or transventricular injury are associated with worse outcomes. Owing to the high early mortality rate, proportionally fewer survivors are left vegetative or severely disabled compared with the closed severe brain-injured cohort.[84] The incidence of post-traumatic epilepsy is substantially higher in patients who have a penetrating brain injury, compared with those who have a severe closed brain injury. A review article published in 2012 noted that there was limited evidence available in relation to outcome following penetrating brain injuries, partly because patients with penetrating brain injuries are often excluded from studies. However, in general, patients with a severe TBI who have sustained a penetrating injury do worse than those who have had a closed injury.[85]

Special Populations: Soldiers and Civilians Exposed to Blast Injuries

Blast-related injury during war is now very common, and has been described in 88% of military personnel treated in one medical unit in Iraq.[86] Individuals exposed to explosive blast are at increased risk of TBI that is often reported as mild. Concern has been expressed that blast-related TBI represents a neuropsychiatric spectrum disorder that clinically overlaps with chronic traumatic encephalopathy (CTE). The mechanisms of injury and biological basis underpinning blast neurotrauma and its sequelae remain largely unknown, and the outcome is currently unclear.[87,88]

Conclusion

A variety of parameters can be used to measure the nature of the outcome following a brain injury. The severity of the primary injury is of paramount importance, but other factors including age and the burden of secondary insults are important. Repeated trauma and genetic factors may contribute to long-term sequelae, as may comorbidities such as alcohol and substance abuse.

References

1. Teasdale G, Jennett B. Assessment and prognosis of coma after head injury. *Acta Neurochir* 1976;34:45–55.

2. Wedekind C, Fischbach R, Pakos P, et al. Comparative use of magnetic resonance imaging and electrophysiologic investigation for prognosis of head injury. *J Trauma* 1999;47(1):44–9.

3. Firsching R, Woischneck D, Klein S, et al. Classification of severe head injury based on magnetic resonance imaging. *Acta Neurochir.* 2001;143:263–71.

4. Carpentier A, Galanaud D, Puybasset L, et al. Early morphologic and spectroscopic magnetic resonance in severe traumatic brain injuries can detect 'invisible brain stem damage' and predict 'vegetative states'. *J Neurotrauma* 2006;23(5):674–85.

5. Sidaros A, Engberg Aw, Sidaros K, et al. Diffusion tensor imaging during recovery from severe traumatic brain injury and relation to clinical outcome: a longitudinal study. *Brain* 2008;131:559–72.

6. Langares A, Ramos A, Perez-Nunez A, et al. The role of MR imaging in assessing prognosis after severe and moderate head injury. *Acta Neurochir (Wein)* 2009;151 (4):341–56.

7. Skandsen T, Kvistad KA, Solheim O, et al. Prevalence and impact of diffuse axonal injury in patients with moderate and severe head injury: a cohort study of early magnetic resonance imaging findings and 1-year outcome. *J Neurosurg* 2010;113:556–63.

8. Skandsen T, Kvistad KA, Solheim O, et al. Prognostic value of magnetic resonance imaging in moderate and severe head injury: a prospective study of early MRI and one-year outcome. *J Neurotrauma* 2011;28:691–9.

9. Haghbayan H, Boutin A, Laflamme M, et al. The prognostic value of MRI in moderate and severe traumatic brain injury: a systematic review and meta-analysis. [Review]. *Crit Care Med* 2017;45(12):e1280–8.

10. Yuh EL, Mukherjee P, Lingsma HF, et al. MRI improves 3-month outcome prediction in mild traumatic brain injury. *Ann Neurol* 2013;73(2):224–35.

11. Shendon ME, Hamoda HM, Schneiderman JS, et al. A review of magnetic resonance imaging and diffusion tensor imaging findings in mild traumatic brain injury. *Brain Imag Behav* 2012;6 (2):137–92.

12. Kothari S. Prognosis after severe TBI: a practical, evidence based approach. In: Zasler ND, Katz DI, Zalfonte RD, eds. *Brain injury medicine, principles and practice*. New York: Demos Medical Publishing; 2007.

13. Perel P, Arango M, Clayton T, MRC CRASH trial Collaborators. Predicting outcome after traumatic brain injury: practical prognostic models based on large cohort of international patients. *BMJ* 2008;336:425.

14. Jennett B, Bond M. Assessment of outcome after severe brain damage: a practical scale. *Lancet* 1975;1:480–4.

15. Jennett B, Snoek J, Bond MR, Brooks N. Disability after severe head injury: observations on the use of the Glasgow Outcome Scale. *J Neurol Neurosurg Psychiatr* 1981;44:285–93.

16. Maas AIR, Braakman R, Schouten HJA, Minderhoud JM, Van Zomeren AH. Agreement between physicians on assessment of outcome following severe head injury. *J Neurosurg* 1983;58:321–5.

17. Rappaport M, Hall KM, Hopkins K, Belleza T, Cope DN. Disability Rating Scale for severe head trauma: coma to community. *Arch Phys Med Rehabil* 1982;63:118–23.

18. Mahoney FI, Barthel DW. Functional evaluation: the Barthel Index. *Maryland State Med J* 1965;14:61–5.

19. Uniform Data Systems. *The functional independence measure*. New York: State University of Buffalo; 1987.

20. Uniform Data System for Medical Rehabilitation. *Guide for the uniform data state for medical rehabilitation (adult FIM)*, version 4.0. Buffalo: State University of New York at Buffalo; 1993.

21. Turner-Stokes L. Goal attainment scaling (GAS) in rehabilitation: a practical guide. *Clin Rehabil* 2009;23:362–70.

22. Hurn J, Kneebone I, Cropley M. Goal setting as an outcome measure: a systematic review. *Clin Rehabil* 2006;20:756–72.

23. Maas A, Marmarou A, Murray GD. Prognosis and clinical trial design in traumatic brain injury: the IMPACT study. *J Neurotrauma* 2007;24(2):232–8.

24. Lingsma HF, Roozenbeek B, Steyerberg EW, et al. Early prognosis in traumatic brain injury: from prophesies to predictions. *Lancet Neurol* 2010;9:543–54.

25. McMillan R, Strang I, Jennett B. Head injuries in primary surgical wards in Scottish hospitals: Scottish head injury management study. *Health Bull* 1979;37:75–81.

26. Field JH. *Epidemiology of head injuries in England and Wales*. London: Research Division, Department of Health and Social Security; 1975.

27. Bryden J. How many head injuries? The epidemiology of post head injury disability. In: Wood R, Eames P, eds. *Models of brain injury rehabilitation*. Baltimore: Johns Hopkins University Press; 1989.

28. Kraus JF. Epidemiology of head injury. In: Cooper PL, ed. *Head injury*. 3rd edn. London: Williams and Wilkins; 1993.

29. Thornhill S, Teasdale GM, Murray GD, et al. Disability in young people and adults one year after head injury: prospective cohort study. *Br Med J* 2000;320:1631–5.

30. Maas AIR, Stocchetti N, Bullock R. Moderate and severe traumatic brain injury in adults. *Lancet* 2008;7(8): 728–41.

31. Laureys S, Celesia GG, Cohadon F, et al. Unresponsive wakefulness syndrome: a new name for the vegetative state or apallic syndrome. *BMC Med* 2010;8:68–71.

32. Monti MM, Laureys S, Owen AM. The vegetative state. *Br Med J* 2010;341:292–6.

33. American Academy of Neurology. Practice parameter: assessment and management of patients in the persistent vegetative state. *Neurology* 1995;45:1015–18.

34. Giacino J, Ashwal S, Childs N, et al. The minimally conscious state: definition and diagnostic criteria. *Neurology* 2002;58:349–53.

35. Coleman MR, Davis MH, Rodd JM, et al. Towards the routine use of brain imaging to aid the clinical diagnosis of disorders of consciousness. *Brain* 2009;132(9):2541–52.

36. Bekinschtein TA, Shalom DE, Forcato C, et al. Classical conditioning in the vegetative and minimally conscious state. *Nat Neurosci* 2009;12:1343–9.

37. Monti MM, Vanhaudenhuyse A, Coleman MR, et al. Willful modulation of brain activity in disorders of consciousness. *N Engl Med* 2010;362:579–89.

38. Multi-Society Task Force on PVS. Medical aspects of the persistent vegetative state (part 2). *N Engl J Med* 1994;330:1572–9.

39. Luaute J, Maucort-Boulch D, Tell L, et al. Long-term outcomes of chronic minimally conscious and vegetative states. *Neurology* 2010;75(3):246–52.

40. Stender JS, Gosseries O, Bruno MA, et al. Diagnostic precision of PET imaging and functional MRI in disorders of consciousness: a clinical validation study. *Lancet* 2014;384(9942):514–22.

41. van der Naalt J. Prediction of outcome in mild to moderate head injury: a review. *J Clin Exp Neuropsychol* 2001;23:837–51.

42. Stein SC. Outcome from moderate head injury. In: Narayan RK, Wilberger JE, Povlishock JT, eds. *Neurotrauma.* New York: McGraw-Hill; 1996.

43. Sureyya SS, Corrigan J, Levin HS, et al. Cognitive outcome following traumatic brain injury. *J Head Trauma Rehabil* 2009;24:430–8.

44. Andriessen TM, Horn J, Franschman G, et al. Epidemiology, severity classification, and outcome of moderate and severe traumatic brain injury: a prospective multicenter study. *J Neurotrauma* 2011;28:2019–31.

45. Mild Traumatic Brain Injury Committee American Congress of Rehabilitation Medicine, Head Injury Interdisciplinary Special Interest Group. Definition of mild traumatic brain injury. *J Head Trauma Rehabil* 1993;8:86–7.

46. Williams DH, Levin HS, Eisenberg HM. Mild head injury classification. *Neurosurgery* 1990;27:422–8.

47. Miller H. Accident neurosis. *Br Med J* 1961;1:919.

48. Miller H. Mental after-effects of head injury. *Proc R Soc Med* 1966;59: 257–61.

49. Shulkla D, Devi BI. Mild traumatic brain injuries in adults. *J Neurosci Rural Pract* 2010;1(2):82–8.

50. Karr JE, Areshenkoff JE, Corson N, et al. The neuropsychological outcomes of concussion: a systematic review of meta-analyses on the cognitive sequelae of mild traumatic brain injury. *Neuropsychology* 2014;28(3): 321–36.

51. Gopinath SP, Robertson CS, Constant CF, et al. Jugular venous desaturation and outcome after head injury. *J Neurol Neurosurg Psychiatry* 1994;57:717–23.

52. McHugh GS, Engel DC, Butcher I, et al. Prognostic value of secondary insults in traumatic brain injury: results from the IMPACT study. *J Neurotrauma* 2007;24 (2):287–93.

53. Li W, Risacher S, McAllister T, et al. Traumatic brain injury and age at onset of cognitive impairment in older adults. *J Neurol* 2016;263:1280–5.

54. Lye TC, Shores EA. Traumatic brain injury as a risk factor for Alzheimer's disease:

a review. *Neuropsychol Rev* 2000;10:115–29.

55. Moretti L, Cristofori I, Weaver SM, Chau A, Portelli JN, Grafman J Cognitive decline in older adults with a history of traumatic brain injury Lancet Neurol 2012;11:1103–12.

56. Johnson VE, Stewart W, Smith DH. Traumatic brain injury and amyloid-β pathology: a link to Alzheimer's disease? *Nat Rev Neurosci* 2010;11:361–70.

57. Fann JR, Ribe AR, Pedersen HS, et al. Long-term risk of dementia among people with traumatic brain injury in Denmark: a population-based observational cohort study. *Lancet Psychiatr*, in press.

58. Godbolt AK, Cancelliere C, Hincapie CA, et al. Systematic review of the risk of dementia and chronic cognitive impairment after mild traumatic brain injury: results of the international collaboration on mild traumatic brain injury prognosis. *Arch Phys Med Rehabil* 2014;95(3):S245–56.

59. Deckers K, van Boxtel MP, Schiepers OJ, et al. Target risk factors for dementia prevention: a systematic review and Delphi consensus study on the evidence from observational studies. *Int J Geriatr Psychiatry* 2015;30:234–46.

60. Washington PM, Villapol S, Burns MP. Polypathology and dementia after brain trauma: does brain injury trigger distinct neurodegenerative diseases, or should they be classified together as traumatic encephalopathy? *Exp Neurol* 2016;275:381–8.

61. Walsh S, Donnan J, Fortin Y, et al. A systematic review of the risk factors associated with the onset and natural progression of epilepsy. *Neurotoxicology* 2017;61:64–77.

62. Burke JF, Stulc JL, Skolarus LE, et al. Traumatic brain injury may be an independent risk factor for stroke. *Neurology* 2013;81:33–9.

63. Liao C-C, Chou Y-C, Yeh C-C, et al. Stroke risk and outcomes in patients with traumatic brain injury: 2 nationwide studies. *Mayo Clin Proc* 2014;89:163–72.

64. Jafari S, Etminan M, Aminzadeh F, et al. Head injury and risk of Parkinson's disease: a systematic review and meta-analysis. *Mov Disord* 2013;28:1222–9.

65. Gardner RC, Burke JF, Nettiksimmons J, et al. Traumatic brain injury in later life increases risk for Parkinson's disease. *Ann Neurol* 2015;77:987–95.

66. Crane PK, Gibbons LE. Association of traumatic brain injury with late-life neurodegenerative conditions and neuropathological findings. *JAMA Neurol* 2016;73:1062–9.

67. McMillan TM, Teasdale GM, Weir CJ, et al. Death after head injury: the 13 year outcome of a case control study. *J Neurol Neurosurg Psychiatry* 2011;82:931–5.

68. Teasdale TW, Engberg AW. Suicide after traumatic brain injury: a population study. *J Neurol Neurosurg Psychiatry* 2001;71:436–40.

69. Corsellis JAN. Boxing and the brain. *Br Med J* 1989;289:105.

70. Corsellis JAN, Bruton CJ, Freeman-Browne D. The aftermath of boxing. *Psychol Med* 1973;3:270.

71. Collins MW, Iverson GL, Gaetz M, et al. Sport-related concussion. In: Zasler ND, Katz DI, Zalfonte RD, eds. *Brain injury medicine, principles and practice*. New York: Demos Medical Publishing; 2007.

72. Asken BM, Sullan MJ, Snyder AR, et al. Factors influencing clinical correlates of chronic traumatic encephalopathy (CTE): a review. *Neuropsychol Rev* 2016;26:340–63.

73. Stewart W. Five minutes with . . . Willie Stewart: neuropathologist tells Anne Gulland of his footballers' dementia risk study. *BMJ* 2018;360:88.

74. Coleman M, Handler M, Martin C. Update on apolipoprotein E state of the art. *Hosp Phys* 1995;31:22–4.

75. Teasdale GM, Nicoli JA, Murray G, et al. Association of apolipoprotein E polymorphism with outcome after head injury. *Lancet* 1997;350:1069–71.

76. Nathoo N, Chetty R, van Dellen JR, Barnett GH. Genetic vulnerability following

traumatic brain injury: the role of apolipoprotein E. *Mol Pathol* 2003;56:132–6.

77. Zhou W, Xu D, Peng X, et al. Meta-analysis of APOE4 allele and outcome after traumatic brain injury. *J Neurotrauma* 2008;25(4):279–90.

78. Kurowski B, Martin LJ, Wade SL. Genetics and outcomes after traumatic brain injury (TBI): what do we know about pediatric TBI? *J Pediatr Rehabil Med* 2012;5 (3):217–31.

79. Calvin H, Mak K, Wong H, et al. Traumatic brain injury in the elderly: is it as bad as we think? *Curr Transl Geriatr Exp Gerontol Rep* 2012;1(3):171–8.

80. Ross AM, Pitts LH, Kobayashi S. Prognosticators of outcome after major head injury in the elderly. *J Neurosci Nurs* 1992;24:88–93.

81. Pentland B, Jones PA, Roy CW, et al. Head injury in the elderly. *Age Aging* 1986;15:193–202.

82. Rothweiler B, Temkin NR, Dikmen SS. Ageing effect on psychosocial outcome in traumatic brain injury. *Arch Phys Med Rehabil* 1998;79:881–7.

83. Maurice-Williams RS. Head injuries in the elderly. *Br J Neurosurg* 1999;13:5–8.

84. Pruitt BA Jr. Part 2: prognosis in penetrating brain injury. *J Trauma* 2001;51:S44–86.

85. Santiago LA, Oh BC, Dash PK, et al. A clinical comparison of penetrating and blunt traumatic brain injuries. *Brain Injury* 2012;26(2):107–25.

86. Taber KH, Warden DL, Robin A, et al. Blast-related traumatic brain injury: what is known? *J Neuropsychiatr Clin* 2006;18:141–5.

87. Elder GA, Cristian A. Blast-related mild traumatic brain injury: mechanisms of injury and impact on clinical care. *Mount Sinai J Med* 2009;76(2):111–18.

88. Goldstein LE, Fisher AM, Tagge CA, et al. Chronic traumatic encephalopathy in blast- exposed military veterans and a blast neurotrauma mouse model. *Sci Transl Med* 2012;4(134):1–17.

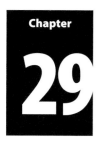

Medicolegal Aspects of Traumatic Brain and Cervical Spine Injury

Peter C. Whitfield and Peter J. Hutchinson

Introduction

Medical experts may be instructed by designated bodies such as the coroner or the court, to provide expert witness statements concerning patients treated under their care. Such reports are factual and are prepared on the basis of the medical records and personal recollection of events. Other authorities such as the Driving Vehicle and Licensing Agency can also seek information on patients with traumatic brain injury. In the civil court, experts may advise on matters relating to personal injury and medical negligence. Reports are usually based upon review of records, and often medical examination of the claimant. The expert may be instructed to provide reports on condition, prognosis and/or causation. This chapter discusses liaison with the various authorities that require medico-legal input relevant to head injury and whiplash. Although focusing on UK practice, the principles apply to other jurisdictions

Personal Injury

Authorities requesting medical reports include solicitors (personal injury claims), insurance companies, the police and the coroner. Reports need to be tailored to address the specific instructions of the requesting authority, for example an opinion on the mechanism of injury, an opinion on current condition and prognosis or an opinion on issues of causation, addressing whether the injury has caused the disability.

Personal Injury Reports

Instructions can be received from solicitors representing the claimant or the defendant. In some cases an expert may be jointly instructed by both parties: a 'single joint expert'. Medico-legal reports must be addressed to the court and need to acknowledge that it is the duty of an expert to help the Court on matters within his/her own expertise, and that this duty is paramount and overrides any obligation to the person from whom the expert has received instructions, or by whom he/she is paid. The Civil Procedure Rules Part 35 provide detailed information on the duties of the expert and the requirements that must be met in the preparation of the report (www.justice.gov.uk/courts/procedure-rules/civil/rules/part35).

The date of report and presence of accompanying persons at the time of examination should be recorded. In head injury and whiplash reports the background history is critical. Accurate recording of pre-event history and relationship with post-event symptoms is essential. Specific pre-event neurological, psychological and psychiatric symptoms should be determined. The patient's description of past medical history should be placed in the context of the medical records, from both primary and secondary care. The patient's social and employment status should also be included.

The mechanism of injury should be explained in detail and include the duration of loss of consciousness, retrograde and post-traumatic amnesia. Differentiation is required between the patient's recollection of events and what they have been subsequently told (often on many occasions). Specific points, such as whether a seat-belt was in place and whether airbags deployed, are noted. The acute symptoms experienced by the patient in the immediate aftermath of the injury should be documented in detail. Both physical symptoms such as headache, dizziness, focal deficits and psychological symptoms such as short-term memory problems should be described. The time course of the symptoms leading up to the current status of the patient should be noted. The treatment administered should be clearly described. Prognosis in terms of ongoing symptoms and future pattern, and the effect on lifestyle is crucial. The impact on activities of daily living, hobbies, family relationships and employment should be described. A statement on dependence on others and capacity both now and in the future is required. Specific factors in terms of prognosis include risk of seizures and life expectancy. Recommendations for ongoing treatment should be given and finally a summary and opinion. This is characterised as what would have happened to the patient in the absence of the index event (the 'but for' test) and what has happened to the patient as a consequence of the index event. If there is a range of medical opinion regarding the diagnosis, prognosis or significance of the injury to the constellation of symptoms and signs, this should be stipulated. The report should make it clear if any of these areas/opinions lie outside the specialist's expertise.

The risk of seizure depends on the severity of injury as defined by the Glasgow Coma Score and other specific risk factors including depressed skull fracture, intracranial haematoma and post-traumatic amnesia greater than 24 hours.[1] Population-based studies provide data on the cumulative probability of seizures. Annegers et al.[2] in a sample of 4541 patients with traumatic brain injury quote the 5 year cumulative probability of seizures as 0.7% in patients with mild injuries, 1.2% with moderate injuries and 10% with severe injuries. The equivalent figures for 30 year cumulative incidence are 2.1% (mild), 4.2 % (moderate) and 16.7% (severe). The literature, however, can only provide guidance based on population figures and the incidence for an individual can be extremely difficult to determine. The risk of seizures has major implications for driving, particularly group 2 licence holders.

The issue of life expectancy is often also very difficult to establish for an individual. It is well recognised that patients in vegetative state have reduced life expectancy. Patients with less severe degrees of disability are also at risk, for example due to the complications of aspiration and pneumonia, or sudden death following seizure. Recent evidence indicates that the overall death rate is increased for at least 7 years after head injury,[3] and that the primary causes of death after head injury are the same as those in the general population. However, on an individual basis, patients who had made a good recovery may well have a normal life expectancy.

Predicting outcome can also be notoriously difficult, particularly in the acute stages following injury. Patients who are deemed to have made a good recovery at the time of discharge are at risk of ongoing physical, psychological and psychiatric symptoms with potentially major implications for domestic life and employment. For patients with severe disability, it is usually difficult to be objective until a minimum period of 6 months has elapsed following injury and the patients may change for 2 years (often regarded as or near finality) or beyond. Serial assessment of objective outcome measures such as the Extended Glasgow Outcome Score,[4] or SF-36 quality of life questionnaire,[5] may be helpful in such situations. More detailed assessment with imaging (e.g. MRI) and neuropsychological testing may also be indicated.

Police and Coroner Reports

Reports for the coroner and police should commence with full name, medical qualifications, status and length of tenure. Reports should be detailed and factual, not assume any additional knowledge, and be written in terms that can be understood by those outside the medical profession. Police reports may require no more than a factual statement of the injuries. However, information on the mechanism of injury and prognosis may also be required. One of the commonest questions is whether the alleged mechanism of injury is consistent with the nature of the injuries sustained. Statements should begin with the sentence 'I am writing this statement in my capacity as the doctor responsible for the treatment of the said patient following his/her alleged assault on the particular date in question'. Accurate documentation particularly with regard to external signs of injury is essential in cases of alleged assault. While CT scans provide evidence of the nature of skull fractures and cerebral injury, external signs of bruising and lacerations heal with time. Photography of such injuries provides a permanent record of injuries and may be used exhibits in court cases.

Reports for the coroner need to provide a factual chronology of events, with particular regard to the mechanism of injury, description of the presenting symptoms and examination findings. In addition to recording positive examination findings, relevant negative findings should also be noted. It is also necessary to differentiate which parts of the report are based upon the medical records compared with memory of events.

Driving Licence Authorities

In terms of driving licences, requirements differ between countries. In the UK, the Driving Vehicle Licensing Authority (DVLA) is responsible for issuing and revoking licences. Reports for the UK DVLA are usually straightforward, particularly with regard to group 1 (car, motorcycle) licences. Such reports comprise the answers to specific questions on a template. The situation with regard to group 2 licences (heavy goods vehicle, bus, coach) is much more complex, particularly with regard to the risk of seizures. The DVLA produces an 'Assessing fitness to drive: a guide for medical professionals' publication', which is regularly updated and available on the internet.[6] In terms of head injury these relate to ongoing symptoms and the risk of seizures.

Current guidelines from the DVLA (group 1 licence) state that driving may resume without notification of the DVLA following a head injury on providing there is a full clinical recovery, no seizures (except at the time of impact), no post-traumatic amnesia lasting more than 24 hours and no intracranial haematoma and/or contusion on CT imaging dependent on features such as seizures, post-traumatic amnesia more than 24 hours, dural tear, haematoma and/or contusions seen on CT imaging. For more severe injuries relicensing may be considered usually after 6–12 months dependent upon features such as seizures, post-traumatic amnesia for more than 24 hours, dural tear, haematoma and/or contusions on CT imaging. Current guidelines for the DVLA (group 2 licence) are far more stringent, indicating that a group 2 licence may be returned when the risk of seizure is deemed to be less than 2% per annum and there are no debarring residual impairments.

Medical Negligence

Opinions on medical negligence, defined as a lack of proper care and attention (*Oxford Dictionary*), following the treatment of head injury and whiplash should remain in the domain

Table 29.1 Definitions

Defendant

The person against whom a legal case is filed

Plaintiff or complainant

The person, corporation or other legal entity that initiates a legal case

Duty of care

The administration of the appropriate treatment by a health care professional

Breach of duty of care

Treatment falling below the acceptable standard of a competent health care professional

Causation of injury

The demonstration that, if a breach of duty can be proved, it either directly caused the injuries or materially contributed to the injuries

Burden of proof

The burden of proof is on the claimant. It is for the claimant to prove the case to the Court

Standard of proof

The test for assessing causation of injury is 'on the balance of probabilities' (i.e. more likely than not) – a much less rigorous standard of proof than that used in the criminal courts ('beyond reasonable doubt')

of experts with extensive experience. A clear understanding of the role of the court, judge, solicitor, barrister and medical experts is required. A list of definitions is provided in Table 29.1. The role of the medical expert is to provide a detailed account of the circumstances surrounding the assessment and treatment of the patient and formulation of an opinion addressing the instructions provided by the instructing legal party. The claimant must prove that the defendant owed them a duty of care, that there was a breach in the duty of care, that the breach of duty caused damage and that the damage was not too remote from the breach of duty. Common allegations of negligence can be considered in relation to delays in diagnosis and treatment, inappropriate or incompetent management, omission of appropriate clinical care and treating without informed consent (where applicable). A report should include information on whether the alleged negligence has caused distress or impaired health. The possible consequences to the patient cover a wide spectrum from minor (of no or little consequence to the patient) to major (resulting in significant harm). When assessing outcomes it is important to consider whether the negligence has been the sole cause of harm. If a contribution to ill-health is alleged, the degree of contribution should be estimated. In some cases negligence may have caused acceleration of clinical features.

A key principle underlying the assessment of medical negligence dates back to 1957 and is known as the Bolam test[7,8] (case *Bolam v Friern Hospital Management Committee*). In this case Bolam sustained fractures during a result of electroconvulsant therapy and alleged negligent care due to the failure to administer muscle relaxant drugs. However, the use of muscle relaxants at that time during ECT was not universal. The judgement concluded that:

A medical professional is not guilty of negligence if he has acted in accordance with a practice accepted as proper by a responsible body of medical men skilled in that particular art. Putting it the other way round, a man is not negligent if he is acting in accordance with such a practice, merely because there is a body of opinion that takes a contrary view.

The medical expert should evaluate whether a reasonable standard of practice was conducted. The application of recommendations from current guidelines, for example the UK National Institute for Health and Clinical Excellence Guidelines on the initial management of adults and children with head injury NICE,[9] may provide evidence of acting in accordance with current standards of care. However, the relationship between evidence-based guidance and the determination of medical negligence is complex.[10] It is generally recognised that guidelines set standards (such that non-adherence may require explanation) but they do not constitute a *de facto* legal standard of care. They can be used, however, to provide a benchmark for the Courts to assist in the judgement of clinical conduct.

Medical negligence may apply if incorrect treatment has been administered or if appropriate treatment has not been undertaken. The case of *Bolitho v City and Hackney*[11] relates to causation where there was an omission as opposed to action. The issue to be considered was whether a doctor who delegated seeing a patient to a junior doctor, whose bleep failed to work, would have administered a particular treatment (in this case intubation of a child in respiratory distress) *if* she had attended the patient.

Many negligence claims follow from miscommunication or issues regarding consent. Accurate documentation in the medical records is essential at all stages in the assessment and treatment process.

Consent is a particularly difficult issue in the context of head injury. Patients with minor injuries may be confused and not comprehend the rationale for the treatment strategy: an assessment of mental capacity is required. Patients with major injuries will not be in a position to give consent. The doctor must undertake care in the best interest of the patient. It is good practice to inform next-of-kin of events and document the content of any discussion. When obtaining consent the extent of information to be given for neurosurgical procedures in general is the subject of strong debate, but on a background of the cases of *Sidaway v Board of Governors of the Bethlem Royal Hospital* (1985),[12] *Chester v Afshar* (2004)[13] and *Montgomery v Lanarkshire Healthboard* (2015),[14] the doctrine of fully informed consent indicates the need to inform patients and/or their next of kin of all risks to the fullest possible extent.

Many patients with neurotrauma are assessed and treated by trainee junior doctors. In terms of decision-making from the legal perspective, the courts do not make allowance for lack of experience. Junior doctors are required to apply the same standard of care as their seniors.[8]

Cervical Spine Injuries

The focus of this book has been to describe the principles of the management of head injury. Head injury is often associated with cervical spine injury. Injuries to the cervical spine carry a particularly high burden of risk from a medico-legal perspective.

Thorough assessment of the cervical spine is mandatory in any patient who has sustained a head injury. The incidence of cervical spine fracture varies with the severity of the head injury. In a series of intubated blunt trauma patients in the UK, 14% had cervical spine injuries.[15] In the NEXUS study of North American patients with head injury of any severity, the cervical fracture rate was 2.4%.[16] The Canadian study of head-injured patients with GCS of 15 reported a 2% incidence of concurrent cervical spine injury.[17] A more recent retrospective study in Finland showed that cervical fractures were more common in head injured patients with traumatic pathology on the CT brain scan.[18] Missed cervical spine injuries can lead to devastating neurological deficits that should be considered avoidable.

The identification of cervical spine injuries requires clinical evaluation, radiological imaging and careful interpretation of the findings. A systematic approach is provided by Advanced Trauma Life Support Courses.[18] The NICE guidelines provide recommendations derived mainly from a consensus view of the Canadian clinical prediction rules regarding the evaluation of the cervical spine.[19] The aim of the guidelines is to reduce the risk of missed injuries using a safe, cost-effective strategy. Even with the availability of guidelines, clinical judgement must prevail. Cervical spine immobilisation should be a treatment standard until a neck injury has been excluded in all head-injured patients with an initial GCS less than 15, and also in any patient with neck pain or symptoms and/ or signs referable to the cervical spine. Different strategies are recommended for children and adults (Table 29.2). For adults an initial decision concerning the use of a CT scan or a plain film series is required. The indications for a plain film series (AP/lateral and odontoid peg views) and for CT scanning of the cervical spine are shown in Table 29.2. The addition of oblique views to a three-view plain film series does not enhance the predictive value. A single lateral view approach is inferior, missing a significant proportion of injuries detected by a three-view series.[20] The sensitivity of plain films is inferior to that of CT scans.[21] For patients with high-risk injuries (GCS 3–12; also see Table 29.2) around 15% of fractures would be missed using plain films alone. Although many of these are not of clinical importance, CT scanning with multiplanar sagittal and coronal reformatting is recommended and should be performed concurrently with the initial CT head scan. There is no evidence to suggest that CT scans of the cervical spine must be performed in all head-injured patients regardless of severity. The role of MRI has been carefully studied in a series of 366 obtunded patients who underwent CT and MRI cervical spine imaging. MRI scanning added additional information to the CT scan in a few cases. These comprised cervical cord contusion (seven cases), single column ligament injury (four cases), disc injury (three cases) or a combination of injuries (one case). None of these injuries was considered unstable. The authors concluded that CT scanning of the entire cervical spine was an appropriate technique for the exclusion of unstable neck injuries in all obtunded trauma patients without the need for MR imaging.[22]

Once a cervical spine injury has been identified, several management options exist, including conservative management alone, application of a collar, internal fixation and external fixation using a Halo jacket.

Whiplash-Associated Disorders

The Quebec Task Force (QTF) defined 'whiplash' as 'an acceleration–deceleration mechanism of energy transfer to the neck [that] may result from rear-end or side-impact motor vehicle collisions, but can also occur during diving or other mishaps. The impact may result in bony or soft tissue injuries (whiplash injury), which may lead to a variety of clinical manifestations (whiplash associated disorders).[23] The QTF defined 6 months post-trauma as the time differentiating acute from chronic injury. A 5-point scale of injury severity for whiplash associated disorder (WAD) from grade 0 (no symptoms or

Table 29.2 Summary of NICE recommendations: the cervical spine

NICE cervical spine recommendations for children

- In general, the use of CT scans should be minimised (due to risk to thyroid of ionising radiation)

  - **three-view plain films** (lateral, AP and if child able to open mouth odontoid peg view) in children with **GCS of 13 to 15** if there is no indication for a CT scan and there was a **(1) dangerous mechanism of injury** (fall >1 m or five stairs; axial load to the head, e.g. diving, roll-over crash, high-speed MVA, ejection from vehicle, bicycle collision, motorised recreational vehicle) or **(2) unsafe to assess range of movement**. Low-risk features enabling assessment of movement include a simple rear end motor vehicle collision, comfortable sitting in emergency department, ambulatory at any time since the injury, no midline tenderness, delayed onset of neck pain.

  - **CT of the cervical spine** should only be used in children with any of the following: GCS <13 on initial assessment, intubated, focal peripheral neurological signs, paraesthesiae in the upper or lower limbs, a definitive diagnosis of cervical spine injury is required, other regions are being scanned due to polytrauma, a strong suspicion of injury despite normal plain films (e.g. neurological symptoms), inadequate plain films or a significant bony injury on plain films. This imaging should be within 1 hour of presentation.

NICE cervical spine recommendations for adults

- All patients who have sustained a head injury and present with any of the following risk factors should have full **cervical spine immobilisation** attempted:

  - GCS less than 15 on initial assessment
  - Neck pain or tenderness
  - Focal neurological deficit
  - Paraesthesia in the extremities
  - Any other clinical suspicion of cervical spine injury

- Cervical spine immobilisation should be maintained until full clinical (and radiological if deemed necessary) assessment indicates it is safe to remove the immobilisation device.
- Safe clinical assessment can be carried out if the patient:

  - Was involved in a simple rear-end motor vehicle collision
  - Is comfortable in a sitting position in the emergency department
  - Has been ambulatory at any time since injury with no midline cervical spine tenderness
  - Presents with delayed onset of neck pain

- **Indications for immediate cervical spine imaging request in adults:**
- Neck pain or midline tenderness with:

  - Age 65 or older, or
  - Dangerous mechanism of injury (fall >1 m or five stairs; axial load to the head, e.g. diving, roll-over crash, high-speed MVA, ejection from vehicle, bicycle collision, motorised recreational vehicle)
  - Considered unsafe to assess the range of movement of the cervical spine for reasons other than those above.
  - The patient cannot actively rotate 45° to the left and right.
  - A definitive diagnosis of cervical spine injury is required urgently (e.g. before surgery).

Table 29.2 (cont.)

- The radiological investigation of the cervical spine should be by CT or three-view plain films. The indications for CT are:

  - Adult patients should have CT imaging of the cervical spine performed within 1 hour if:

    - GCS below 13 on initial assessment
    - Intubated
    - Technically inadequate plain films
    - Suspicious or abnormal plain films
    - A definitive diagnosis of cervical spine injury is needed urgently (e.g. before surgery)
    - The patient is being scanned for multi-region trauma

  - The patient is alert and stable but there is clinical suspicion of cervical spine injury and:

    - age 65 and over
    - dangerous mechanism (fall > 1 m; five steps; axial load to head; high-speed motor vehicle accident; roll-over motor accident; motorised recreational vehicle; bicycle collision
    - focal neurological limb deficit
    - paraesthesia in upper or lower limbs

Radiological considerations

- Cervical spine imaging should be performed simultaneously with head imaging if this is also considered urgent.
- CT scans should cover any areas of concern or uncertainty on plain films or clinical grounds.
- The occipital condyle region of the skull should be examined on bone window settings.
- Facilities for multiplanar reformatting and interactive viewing should be available.
- MRI is indicated in the presence of neurological symptoms and signs referable to the cervical spine and if there is suspicion of a vascular lesion (e.g. fracture through the foramen transversarium; lateral masses or a posterior circulation syndrome).

Source: Adapted from National Institute for Health and Clinical Excellence[34]

---

signs) to grade IV (fracture/dislocation) was proposed (Table 29.3). Although neck pain is the key clinical feature, most patients are poly-symptomatic with any of the following: neck stiffness, headache, low back pain, shoulder pain, dizziness and non-specific visual disturbance. Risk factors for chronic WAD include older age, female sex, a high level of symptoms at onset, pre-traumatic headache, pre-existing degenerative disease and multiple symptoms.[24]

When a radiologically overt bony and/or ligamentous injury has been identified, a clear explanation for neurological symptoms and signs can be assigned. In cases of lesser severity, where imaging investigations are normal, explaining the persistence of symptoms and signs is more difficult. Biomechanical studies on volunteer cases identify predictable biophysical changes in the spine during a whiplash injury. These include straightening of the spine (loss of lordosis) followed by flexion and compressive axial forces within the upper cervical spine. Finally, extension of the head and neck occurs. During the latter phase, EMG recordings

Table 29.3 The Quebec Classification of whiplash-associated disorders

Grade	Clinical presentation
0	No symptoms or signs
I	Neck pain, stiffness or tenderness. No signs
II	Neck pain and musculoskeletal signs which may include decreased range of motion and point tenderness
III	Neck complaint and neurological signs
IV	Fracture and/or dislocation

Source: Spitzer et al.[35] Reproduced with permission from Lippincott, Williams and Wilkins.

indicate that sternocleidomastoid muscle contraction attempts to counteract extension of the spine.[25] While such mechanisms can readily explain a short-lived musculoskeletal injury pattern, chronic symptoms are more difficult to explain.

The incidence of WAD has been estimated at around 70/100 000 (Canadian provinces) to 300/100 000 in the USA and Europe and up to 325/100 000 in the Netherlands.[26,27] Recovery rates from WAD differ in different countries. In general, patients who remain symptomatic at 3 months usually continue to experience symptoms at 2 years.[28,29] It has been estimated that 40%–66% of cases are pain free by 3 months, increasing to 58%–82% by 6 months and then only around 55%–86% >6 months post-injury.[30] Studies from the litigation-free Lithuanian city of Kaunas reported initial neck and/or head pain in 35%–47% of whiplash cases. The maximum duration of symptoms was 20 days. Four percent of the 200 cases reported neck pains at least 7 days per month after 1 year, compared with 4.1% of the control population.[30] In a retrospectively studied group, 9.4% of the whiplash cases experienced neck pains compared with 5.9% of control patients; this difference was not statistically significant. Pre-accident symptoms were reported to be important.[32] The authors concluded that cultural factors are of importance in generating the clinical picture of WAD. They postulated that a large number of WAD cases are caused by an expectation of disability and attribution of pre-existing symptoms to the neck trauma.[31,32] Owing to the methodology of this study these conclusions are open to challenge. The majority of whiplash case series identify patients from Emergency Department records whereas in Lithuania patients were identified from police accident record files. This bias selection may be sufficient to explain the findings. Other research workers have found any link between symptoms and compensation to be tenuous and have suggested that psychological factors interact with symptoms to lead to different social outcomes in patients with different psychological profiles.

The persistence of post-whiplash neck symptoms has been reviewed with clarity by an experienced medico-legal expert.[30] When compiling a report, the clinician must consider the various possible explanations that can explain a chronic state. These include:

1 **Structural damage to the spine as a result of injury.** Imaging investigations need careful scrutiny to detect injuries. In the majority of patients with WAD, investigations are normal. The QTF considered imaging unnecessary for grade I WAD.[23]

2   **Acceleration of symptoms due to cervical spondylosis.** Radiological cervical spondylosis is considered normal in patients over 40 years of age. However, the conversion from an asymptomatic state to one with symptoms and signs is frequently cited as an explanation for WAD cases with pre-existing radiological degenerative disease. The link between radiological abnormality and clinical symptoms is usually based upon conjecture rather than by positive identification. These symptoms may be generated by muscular or ligamentous dysfunction or by intervertebral disc degeneration, and facet or zygapophysial joint arthrosis, although the exact cause of the pain is usually unknown. The nature of the injury and the temporal association between injury and symptoms are the key factors to consider when adopting this explanation.

3   **Unreported pre-accident symptoms.** Several studies indicate that pre-existing neck symptoms are commonly present in patients sustaining whiplash injuries.[30,31] In addition, some patients may have experienced pre-traumatic symptoms at a level that the claimant did not consider worthy of medical attention. A pitfall is to overlook such pre-existing symptoms and attribute their post-traumatic correlates to the index accident. Careful scrutiny of medical and physiotherapy records may be required to detect the presence of such symptoms.

4   **Psychological illness.** Patients with a WAD can develop a reactive depressive episode associated with emotional changes, a fear of travel, poor concentration and sleep disturbance. This may lead to a state of negativity, exaggerated symptomatology and catastrophising. Symptom amplification in which the patient attributes all clinical manifestations to the accident may then lead to perpetuation of symptoms. A psychiatric report to assess the severity and cause of such features may be useful in establishing causation. A prospective study of the psychological profiles of 117 'whiplash' patients did not identify specific pre-disposing factors that correlated with somatic features.[33]

5   **Conscious exaggeration of symptoms.** Given the financial terms of compensation settlements and the attention afforded to chronic illness patients, conscious exaggeration of symptoms may occur. This is suggested by discordance between the injury and the severity and extent of symptoms and signs, inconsistencies during examination and the universal failure of treatments to afford some degree of benefit. Such behaviour may continue after settlement, due to the patient adopting chronic illness behaviour.

The management of patients with WAD is guided by a large number of small and generally poor quality clinical trials. The Cochrane Review considered the evidence too sparse to advocate either active strategies or passive treatments as the mainstay therapeutic modality.[26]

Support Services

There are several organisations that can provide support for patients and relatives. The type and availability varies between countries. In the UK the Brain and Spine Foundation produces a number of publications relevant to head injury in terms of patient and relative information booklets. Headway, the charity for the brain-injured, also publishes a number of booklets. Specific advice and carer support is also available. Headway can also provide advice on the medico-legal process with a list of approved solicitors on the Headway panel. Other sources of support include the Citizens' Advice Bureau. Patients and/or relatives who are concerned regarding treatment that has been received can contact the patient advice and liaison service, Information Complaints' Advocacy Service or Health ombudsman.

Conclusion

Expert medical advice is increasingly being sought in relation to criminal, insurance, personal injury and negligence issues. Guidelines and the literature, both original publications, reviews and books, can assist in the preparation of such reports. However, these are based primarily on population data, and individual opinion based on the experience and synthesis of the literature by the medical expert is paramount in the compilation and interpretation of medical evidence.

References

1. Jennett B. *Epilepsy after non-missile head injuries.* London: William Heinemann Medical Books; 1975.

2. Annegers JF, Hauser WA, Coan SP, Rocca WA. A population-based study of seizures after traumatic brain injury. *N Engl J Med* 1998;338:20–4.

3. McMillan TM, Teasdale GM. Death rate is increased for at least 7 years after head injury: a prospective study. *Brain* 2007;130:2520–7.

4. Wilson JT, Pettigrew LE, Teasdale GM. Structured interviews for the Glasgow Outcome Scale and the extended Glasgow Outcome Scale: guidelines for their use. *J Neurotrauma* 1998;15:573–85.

5. Jenkinson C, Wright L, Coulter A. Criterion validity and reliability of the SF-36 in a population sample. *Qual Life Res* 1994;3:7–12.

6. Assessing Fitness to Drive. A guide for professionals. DVLA 2019. https://www.gov.uk/government/publications/assessing-fitness-to-drive-a-guide-for-medical-professionals

7. Bolam v Friern Hospital Management Committee (1957) 2 *A11 ER* 118.

8. Jones JW. The healthcare professional and the Bolam test. *Br Dent J* 2000;188 (5):237–40.

9. NICE guidance: Head Injury: assessment and early management. www.nice.org.uk/guidance/cg176

10. Hurwitz B. How does evidence based guidance influence determinations of medical negligence? *Br Med J* 2004;329:1024–8.

11. Bolitho v City and Hackney Health Authority (1997) 39 *BMLR* 1; (1998) 1 Lloyds Rep Med 26.

12. Sidaway v Bethlem Royal Hospital Governors (1985) 1 *A11 ER* 635.

13. Chester v Afshar (2004) *UKHL* 41.

14. Montgomery v Lanarkshire Healthboard (2015) UKSC 11.

15. Brohi K, Healy M, Fotheringham T, et al. Helical computed tomographic scanning for the evaluation of the cervical spine in the unconscious, intubated trauma patient. *J Trauma* 2005;58(5): 897–901.

16. Hoffman JR, Mower WR, Wolfson AB, Todd KH, Zucker MI. Validity of a set of clinical criteria to rule out injury to the cervical spine in patient with blunt trauma. National Emergency X-Radiography Utilization Study Group. *N Engl J Med* 2000;343(2): 94–9.

17. Thesleff T, Kataja A, Ohman J, Luoto TM. Head injuries and risk of concurrent cervical spine fractures. *Acta Neurochir (Wien)* 2017;159(5):907–14.

18. Stiell IG, Wells GA, Vandemheen KL, et al. The Canadian C-spine rule for radiography in alert and stable trauma patients. *J Am Med Assoc* 2001;286 (15):1841–8.

19. Spinal Injury and assessment. Nice Guideline 41. https://www.nice.org.uk/guidance/ng41. Published 2016.

20. Cohn SM, Lyle WG, Linden CH, Lancey RA. Exclusion of cervical spine injury: a prospective study. *J Trauma* 1991;31(4):570–4.

21. Holmes JF, Akkinepalli R. Computed tomography versus plain radiography to screen for cervical spine injury: a

meta-analysis. *J Trauma* 2005;58(5): 902–5.

22. Hogan GJ, Mirvis SE, Shanmuganathan K, Scalea TM. Exclusion of unstable cervical spine injury in obtunded patients with blunt trauma: is MR imaging needed when multi-detector row CT findings are normal? *Radiology* 2005;237:106–13.

23. Spitzer WO, Skovron ML, Salmi LR, et al. Scientific monograph of the Quebec Task-Force on whiplash-associated disorders – redefining whiplash and its management. *Spine* 1995;20(8): S1–73.

24. McClune T, Burton AK, Waddell G. Whiplash associated disorder: a review of the literature to guide patient information and advice. *Emerg Med J* 2002;19:499–506.

25. Brault JR, Siegmund GP, Wheeler JB. Cervical muscle response during whiplash: evidence of a lengthening muscle contraction. *Clin Biomech* 2000;15 (6):426–35.

26. Verhagen AP, Scholten-Peeters GGGM, van Wijngaarden S, de Bie RA, BiermaZeinstra SMA. Conservative treatments for whiplash. *Cochrane Database Syst Rev* 2007;2:CD003338. DOI:10.1002/14651858. CD003338.pub3.

27. Carroll L, Holm L, Hogg-Johnson S, Cote P, Cassidy D, Haldeman S, et al. Course and prognostic factors for neck pain in whiplash-associated disorders (WAD): results of the bone and joint decade 1000–2010 task force on neck pain and its associated disorders. *Spine* 2008;33:583–92.

28. Gargan MF, Bannister GC. The rate of recovery following whiplash injury. *Eur Spine J* 1994;3:162–4.

29. Maimaris C, Barnes MR, Allen MJ. Whiplash injuries of the neck: a retrospective study. *Injury* 1998;19:393–6.

30. Pearce JMS. A critical appraisal of the chronic whiplash syndrome (editorial). *J Neurol Neurosurg Psychiatry* 1999;66:272–6.

31. Obelieniene D, Schrader H, Bovim G, Miseviciene I, Sand T. Pain after whiplash: a prospective controlled inception cohort study. *J Neurol Neurosurg Psychiatr* 1999;66:279–83.

32. Schrader H, Obelieniene D, Bovim G, et al. Natural evolution of the late whiplash syndrome outside the medicolegal context. *Lancet* 1996;347:1207–11.

33. Radanov BP, Di Stefano G, Schnidrig A, Sturzenegger M. Common whiplash: psychosomatic or somatopsychic? *J Neurol Neurosurg Psychiatr* 1994;57:486–90.

34. National Institute for Health and Clinical Excellence. CG176 *Head injury: Triage, assessment, investigation and early management of head injury in infants, children and adults.* London: NICE; 2014. www.nice.org.uk/CG176

35. Spitzer WO, et al. Scientific monograph of the Quebec Task Force on Whiplash – associated disorders: redefining 'whiplash' and its management. *Spine* 1995;20(8S).

Index